Essential Endocrinology and Diabetes

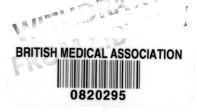
KT-430-774

Essential Endocrinology and Diabetes

Richard IG Holt

Professor in Diabetes and Endocrinology
Faculty of Medicine
University of Southampton

Neil A Hanley

Professor of Medicine
Faculty of Medical & Human Sciences
University of Manchester

Sixth edition

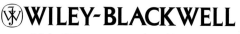

WILEY-BLACKWELL

A John Wiley & Sons, Ltd., Publication

Blackwell Publishing was acquired by John Wiley & Sons in February 2007. Blackwell's publishing program has been merged with Wiley's global Scientific, Technical and Medical business to form Wiley-Blackwell.

Registered office: John Wiley & Sons, Ltd, The Atrium, Southern Gate, Chichester, West Sussex, PO19 8SQ, UK

Editorial offices: 9600 Garsington Road, Oxford, OX4 2DQ, UK
The Atrium, Southern Gate, Chichester, West Sussex, PO19 8SQ, UK
111 River Street, Hoboken, NJ 07030-5774, USA

For details of our global editorial offices, for customer services and for information about how to apply for permission to reuse the copyright material in this book please see our website at www.wiley.com/wiley-blackwell

Library of Congress Cataloging-in-Publication Data

Holt, Richard I. G.
  Essential endocrinology and diabetes. – 6th ed. / Richard I.G. Holt, Neil A. Hanley.
      p. ; cm. – (Essentials)
  Includes bibliographical references and index.
  ISBN-13: 978-1-4443-3004-5 (pbk. : alk. paper)
  ISBN-10: 1-4443-3004-7 (pbk. : alk. paper)   1. Endocrinology–Case studies.   2. Diabetes–Case studies.   I. Hanley, Neil A.   II. Title.   III. Series: Essentials (Wiley-Blackwell)
  [DNLM: 1. Endocrine Glands–physiology.   2. Diabetes Mellitus.   3. Endocrine System Diseases.   4. Hormones–physiology.   WK 100]
  RC648.H65 2012
  616.4–dc23

                                        2011024249

A catalogue record for this book is available from the British Library.

Set in 10 on 12 pt Adobe Garamond Pro by Toppan Best-set Premedia Limited
Printed and bound in Malaysia by Vivar Printing Sdn Bhd

1 2012

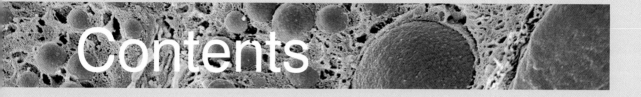

Contents

Preface   vii
List of abbreviations   x
How to get the best out of your textbook   xii

PART 1: Foundations of Endocrinology   1

1 Overview of endocrinology   3
2 Cell biology and hormone synthesis   14
3 Molecular basis of hormone action   27
4 Investigations in endocrinology and diabetes   48

PART 2: Endocrinology – Biology to Clinical Practice   63

5 The hypothalamus and pituitary gland   65
6 The adrenal gland   99
7 Reproductive endocrinology   127
8 The thyroid gland   165
9 Calcium and metabolic bone disorders   190
10 Pancreatic and gastrointestinal endocrinology and
   endocrine neoplasia   213

PART 3: Diabetes and Obesity   233

11 Overview of diabetes   235
12 Type 1 diabetes   257
13 Type 2 diabetes   285
14 Complications of diabetes   311
15 Obesity   343

Index   360

Preface

There have been significant advances and developments in the 4 years since we wrote the last edition. Consequently, many areas of the book have required substantial updating and extensive re-writing. Nevertheless, the structure of the book has remained similar to the last edition, which seemed popular around the world.

The first part strives to create a knowledgeable reader prepared for the clinical sections. Recognizing that many students now come to medicine from non-scientific backgrounds, we have tried to limit assumptions on prior knowledge. For instance, the concept of negative feedback regulation, covered in Chapter 1, is mandatory for understanding almost all endocrine physiology and is vital for the interpretation of many clinical tests. Similarly, molecular diagnostics has advanced far beyond the historical development of immunoassays. New modalities, such as molecular genetics, mass spectrometry and sophisticated imaging, are already standard practice and it is important that aspiring clinicians, as well as scientists, appreciate their methodology, application and limitations. The second part retains a largely organ-based approach. The introductory basic science in these chapters aims to be concise yet sufficient to understand, diagnose and manage the associated clinical disorders. The chapter on endocrine neoplasia, including hormone-secreting tumours of the gut, has been expanded in recognition of the increasing array of hormones discovered from the pancreas and gastrointestinal tract. In previous editions these hormones have lacked attention. However, many of them are now emerging as key regulators that are exploited in new therapies. For instance, augmentation of glucagon-like peptide 1 signalling is an effective treatment for diabetes. The third part on diabetes and obesity was entirely new in the last edition and these chapters have undergone the greatest change here. Over the last 4 years we have seen significant advances in the treatment of type 2 diabetes such as the new incretin-based therapies and the withdrawal of other treatments due to safety concerns. Clinical algorithms have also changed and these have been updated.

The textbook aims to bridge the gap from basic science training, through clinical training, to the knowledge required for the early postgraduate years and specialist training. The text goes beyond core undergraduate medical education. Learning objectives, boxes, and concluding 'key points' aim to emphasize the major topics. There is hopefully useful detail for more advanced clinicians who, like the authors, enjoy trying to interpret clinical medicine scientifically, but for whom memory occasionally fails. Although the structure of the book is largely unchanged from the previous edition, readers of the old edition will recognize welcome developments. For the first time, the book is in full colour, which has allowed us to include colour photographs in the relevant chapter. We have introduced recap and cross-reference guides at the beginning of each of the clinical chapters to help the reader find important information in other parts of the book more easily. The case histories that were introduced in the last edition proved to be a success and these have been expanded to provide greater opportunity to put theory into practice.

We have brought our clinical and research experiences together to create this book. While it has been a truly collaborative venture and the book is designed to read as a whole, inevitably one of us has taken a lead with each chapter depending on our own interests. As such, NAH was responsible for writing Part 1 and Part 2, while RIGH was responsible for Part 3.

Finally, we must thank a number of people without whom this book would not have come to fruition. We are grateful for the skilled help of Wiley-Blackwell Publishing and remain indebted to our predecessors up to and including the 4th edition, Charles Brook and Nicholas Marshall, for their excellent starting point. We are also grateful to our families without whose support this book would not have been possible and to whom we dedicate this edition.

R.I.G. Holt
University of Southampton
N.A. Hanley
University of Manchester

The authors

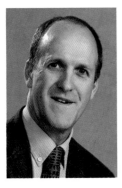

Richard Holt is Professor in Diabetes and Endocrinology at the University of Southampton School of Medicine and Honorary Consultant in Endocrinology at Southampton University Hospitals NHS Trust. His research interests are broadly focused around clinical diabetes with particular interests in diabetes in pregnancy and young adults, and the relation between diabetes and mental illness. He also has a long-standing interest in growth hormone.

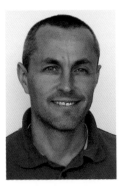

Neil Hanley is Professor of Medicine and Wellcome Trust Senior Fellow in Clinical Science at the University of Manchester. He is Honorary Consultant in Endocrinology at the Central Manchester University Hospitals NHS Foundation Trust where he provides tertiary referral endocrine care. His main research interests are human developmental endocrinology and stem cell biology.

Both authors play a keen role in the teaching of undergraduate medical students and doctors. RIGH is a Fellow of the Higher Education Academy. NAH is Director of the Academy for Training & Education at the Manchester Biomedical Research Centre.

Further reading

The following major international textbooks make an excellent source of secondary reading:

Melmed S, Polonsky KS, Reed Larsen P, Kronenberg HM, eds. *Williams Textbook of Endocrinology*, 12th edn. Saunders, 2011.

Holt RIG, Cockram C, Flyvbjerg A, Goldstein BJ. *Textbook of Diabetes*, 4th edn. Wiley-Blackwell, 2010.

In addition, the following textbooks cover topics, relevant to some chapters, in greater detail:

Delves PJ, Martin SJ, Burton DR, Roitt IM. *Roitt's Essential Immunology*, 12th edn. Wiley-Blackwell, 2011.

Johnson M. *Essential Reproduction*, 6th edn. Wiley-Blackwell, 2007.

Nelson DL, Cox MM. *Lehninger Principles of Biochemistry*, 5th edn. W.H. Freeman, 2008.

List of abbreviations

5-HIAA	5-hydroxyindoleacetic acid	GC	gas chromatography
5-HT	5-hydroxytryptophan	GDM	gestational diabetes
αMSH	α-melanocyte stimulating hormone	GFR	glomerular filtration rate
ACTH	adrenocorticotrophic hormone	GH	growth hormone (somatotrophin)
ADH	vasopressin/antidiuretic hormone	GHR	GH receptor
AFP	α-fetoprotein	GHRH	growth hormone-releasing hormone
AGE	advanced glycation end-product	GI	glycaemic index
AGRP	Agouti-related protein	GIP	glucose-dependent insulinotrophic peptide (gastric inhibitory peptide)
AI	angiotensin I		
AII	angiotensin II	GLUT	glucose transporter
ALS	acid labile subunit	GnRH	gonadotrophin-releasing hormone
AMH	anti-Müllerian hormone	GPCR	guanine-protein coupled receptor
AR	androgen receptor	GR	glucocorticoid receptor
APS-1	type 1 autoimmune polyglandular syndrome	Grb2	type 2 growth factor receptor-bound protein
APS-2	type 2 autoimmune polyglandular syndrome	hCG	human chorionic gonadotrophin
		hMG	human menopausal gonadotrophin
CAH	congenital adrenal hyperplasia	HMGCoA	hydroxymethylglutaryl coenzyme A
cAMP	cyclic adenosine monophosphate	HNF	hepatocyte nuclear factor
CBG	cortisol binding globulin	HPLC	high performance liquid chromatography
cGMP	guanosine monophosphate		
CRE	cAMP response element	HRE	hormone response element
CREB	cAMP response element-binding protein	HRT	hormone replacement therapy
		ICSI	intracytoplasmic sperm injection
CNS	central nervous system	IDDM	insulin-dependent diabetes mellitus
CRH	corticotrophin-releasing hormone	IFG	impaired fasting glycaemia
CSF	cerebrospinal fluid	IFMA	immunofluorometric assay
CT	computed tomography	IGF	insulin-like growth factor
CVD	cardiovascular disease	IGFBP	IGF-binding protein
DAG	diacylglycerol	IGT	impaired glucose tolerance
DEXA	dual energy X-ray absorptiometry	IP	inositol phosphate
DHEA	dehydroepiandrosterone	IPF	insulin promoter factor
DHT	5α-dihydrotestosterone	IR	insulin receptor
DI	diabetes insipidus	IRMA	intraretinal microvascular abnormalities (Chapter 14)
EGF	epidermal growth factor		
EPO	erythropoietin	IRMA	immunoradiometric assay (Chapter 4)
ER	oestrogen receptor		
FFA	free fatty acid	IRS	insulin receptor substrate
FGF	fibroblast growth factor	IVF	*in vitro* fertilization
FIA	fluoroimmunoassay	JAK	Janus-associated kinase
FISH	fluorescence *in situ* hybridization	LDL	low-density lipoprotein
FSH	follicle-stimulating hormone	LH	luteinizing hormone
fT_3	free tri-iodothyronine	MAO	monoamine oxidase
fT_4	free thyroxine	MAPK	mitogen-activated protein kinase

MEN	multiple endocrine neoplasia	RANK	receptor activator of nuclear factor-kappa B
MIS	Müllerian inhibiting substance		
MODY	maturity-onset diabetes of the young	RER	rough endoplasmic reticulum
MR	mineralocorticoid receptor	RIA	radioimmunoassay
MRI	magnetic resonance imaging	rT_3	reverse tri-iodothyronine
MS	mass spectrometry	RXR	retinoid X receptor
MSH	melanocyte-stimulating hormone	SERM	selective ER modulator
NEFA	non-esterified fatty acid	SHBG	sex hormone-binding globulin
NICTH	non-islet cell tumour hypoglycaemia	SIADH	syndrome of inappropriate antidiuretic hormone
NIDDM	non–insulin-dependent diabetes mellitus		
		SoS	son of sevenless protein
NPY	neuropeptide Y	SRE	serum response element
NVD	new vessels at the disc	SS	somatostatin
NVE	new vessels elsewhere	StAR	steroid acute regulatory protein
OGTT	oral glucose tolerance test	STAT	signal transduction and activation of transcription protein
PCOS	polycystic ovarian syndrome		
PCR	polymerase chain reaction	T1DM	type 1 diabetes
PDE	phosphodiesterase	T2DM	type 2 diabetes
PGE2	prostaglandin E_2	$t_{1/2}$	half-life
PI	phosphatidylinositol	T_3	tri-iodothyronine
PIT1	pituitary-specific transcription factor 1	T_4	thyroxine
		TGFβ	transforming growth factor β
PKA	protein kinase A	TK	tyrosine kinase
PKC	protein kinase C	TPO	thyroid peroxidase
PLC	phospholipase C	TR	thyroid hormone receptor
PNMT	phenylethanolamine *N*-methyl transferase	TRE	thyroid hormone response element
		TRH	thyrotrophin-releasing hormone
POMC	pro-opiomelanocortin	TSH	thyroid-stimulating hormone
PPAR	peroxisome proliferator-activated receptor	UFC	urinary free cortisol
		V	vasopressin/antidiuretic hormone (previously also known as arginine vasopressin)
PRL	prolactin		
PTH	parathyroid hormone		
PTHrP	parathyroid hormone-related peptide	VEGF	vascular endothelial growth factor
PTU	propylthiouracil	VIP	vasoactive intestinal peptide

How to get the best out of your textbook

Welcome to the new edition of *Essential Endocrinology and Diabetes*. Over the next few pages you will be shown how to make the most of the learning features included in the textbook.

The anytime, anywhere textbook ▶

For the first time, your textbook comes with free access to a Wiley Desktop Edition – a digital, interactive version of this textbook which you own as soon as you download it. Your Wiley Desktop Edition allows you to:

Search: Save time by finding terms and topics instantly in your book, your notes, even your whole library (once you've downloaded more textbooks)

Note and Highlight: Colour code highlights and make digital notes right in the text so you can find them quickly and easily

Organize: Keep books, notes and class materials organized in folders inside the application

Share: Exchange notes and highlights with friends, classmates and study groups

Upgrade: Your textbook can be transferred when you need to change or upgrade computers

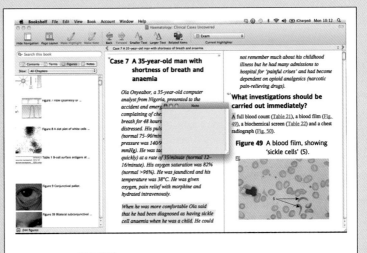

To access your Wiley Desktop Edition:

- Find the redemption code on the inside front cover of this book and carefully scratch away the top coating of the label.
- Visit **www.vitalsource.com/software/bookshelf/downloads** to download the Bookshelf application to your computer, laptop or mobile device
- Open the Bookshelf application on your computer and register for an account.
- Follow the registration process and enter your redemption code to download your digital book.

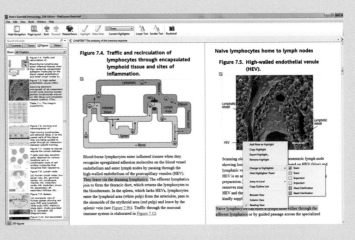

CourseSmart gives you instant access (via computer or mobile device) to this Wiley-Blackwell eTextbook and its extra electronic functionality, at 40% off the recommended retail print price. See all the benefits at: **www.coursesmart.com/students**.

Instructors . . . receive your own digital desk copies! ▶

It also offers you an immediate, efficient, and environmentally-friendly way to review this textbook for your course. For more information visit: **www.coursesmart.com/instructors.**
With CourseSmart, you can create lecture notes quickly with copy and paste, and share pages and notes with your students. Access your Wiley CourseSmart digital textbook from your computer or mobile device instantly for evaluation, class preparation, and as a teaching tool in the classroom.

Simply sign in at:
http://instructors.coursesmart.com/bookshelf to download your Bookshelf and get started. To request your desk copy, hit 'Request Online Copy' on your search results or book product page.

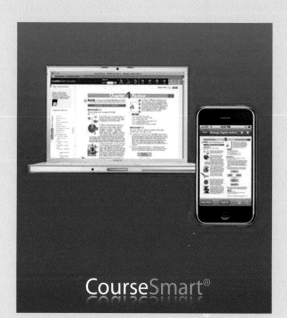

Features contained within your textbook

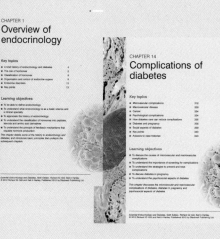

◀ Every chapter has its own chapter-opening page that offers a list of key topics and learning objectives pertaining to the chapter

Throughout your textbook you will find this icon which points you to cases with self-test questions. You will find the answers at the end of each chapter.

You will also find a helpful list of key points at the end of each chapter which give a quick summary of important principles.

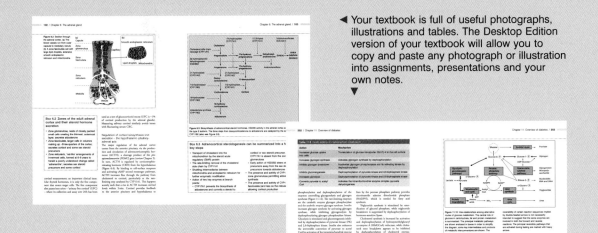

◀ Your textbook is full of useful photographs, illustrations and tables. The Desktop Edition version of your textbook will allow you to copy and paste any photograph or illustration into assignments, presentations and your own notes.

▼

Cross-reference

■ The development of the parathyroid and parafollicular C-cells is described alongside the thyroid in Chapter 8

■ Tumours of the parathyroid glands are an important component of multiple endocrine neoplasia, covered in Chapter 10

■ Other hormones such as cortisol (see Chapter 6) and sex hormones (see Chapter 7) affect mineralization of the bones

◀ At the beginning of some chapters you will also find cross-references which make it easy to locate related information quickly and efficiently.

We hope you enjoy using your new textbook. Good luck with your studies!

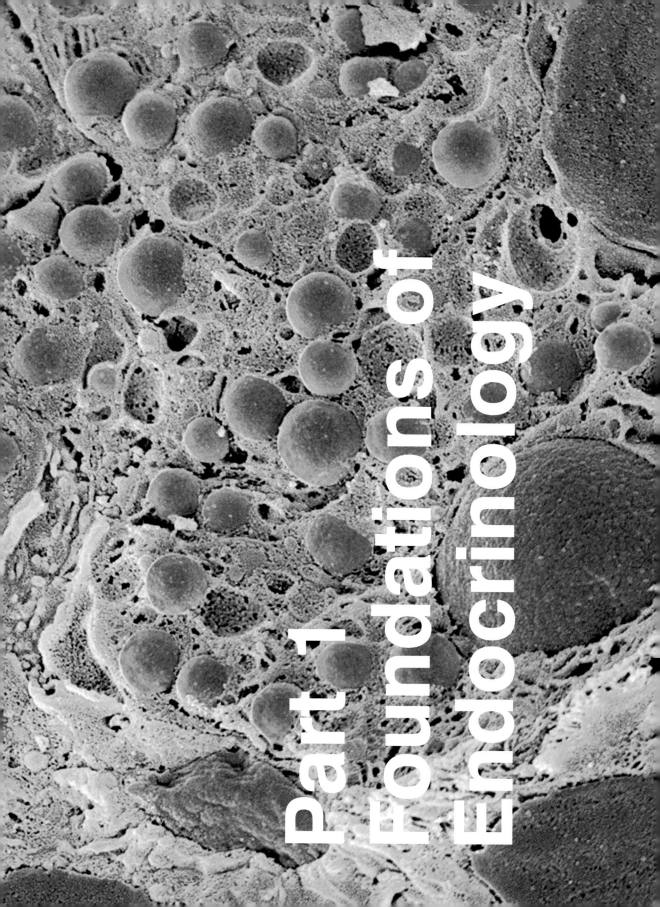

Part 1
Foundations of
Endocrinology

CHAPTER 1

Overview of endocrinology

Key topics

- A brief history of endocrinology and diabetes   4
- The role of hormones   5
- Classification of hormones   8
- Organization and control of endocrine organs   9
- Endocrine disorders   13
- Key points   13

Learning objectives

- To be able to define endocrinology
- To understand what endocrinology is as a basic science and a clinical specialty
- To appreciate the history of endocrinology
- To understand the classification of hormones into peptides, steroids and amino acid derivatives
- To understand the principle of feedback mechanisms that regulate hormone production

This chapter details some of the history to endocrinology and diabetes, and introduces basic principles that underpin the subsequent chapters

Essential Endocrinology and Diabetes, Sixth Edition. Richard IG Holt, Neil A Hanley.
© 2012 Richard IG Holt and Neil A Hanley. Publlished 2012 by Blackwell Publishing Ltd.

An organism comprised of a single or a few cells analyzes and responds to its external environment with relative ease. No cell is more than a short diffusion distance from the outside world or its neighbours, allowing a constancy of internal environment ('homeostasis'). This simplicity has been lost with the evolution of more complex, larger, multicellular organisms. Simple diffusion has become inadequate in larger animal species where functions localize to specific organs. In humans, there are $\sim 10^{14}$ cells of 200 or more different types. With this compartmentalized division of purpose comes the need for effective communication to disseminate information throughout the whole organism – only a few cells face the outside world, yet all respond to it. Two communication systems facilitate this: the endocrine and nervous systems (Box 1.1).

The specialized ductless glands and tissues of the endocrine system release chemical messengers – hormones – into the extracellular space, from where they enter the bloodstream. It is this blood-borne transit that defines endocrinology; however, the principles are similar for hormone action on a neighbouring cell ('*para*crinology') or, indeed, itself ('*auto-* or *intra-*crinology') (Figure 1.1).

The nervous and endocrine systems interact. Endocrine glands are under both nervous and hormonal control, while the central nervous system is affected by multiple hormonal stimuli – features reflected by the composite science of neuroendocrinology (Figure 1.1).

A brief history of endocrinology and diabetes

The term 'hormone', derived from the Greek word 'hormaein' meaning 'to arouse' or 'to excite', was first used in 1905 by Sir Ernest Starling in his Croonian Lecture to the Royal College of Physicians;

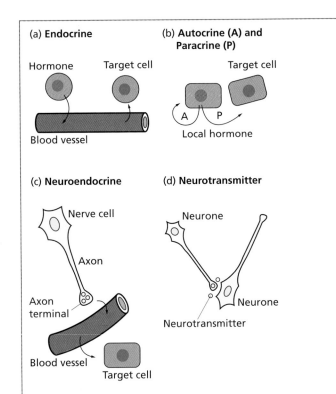

Figure 1.1 Cells that secrete regulatory substances to communicate with their target cells and organs. (a) Endocrine. Cells secrete hormone into the blood vessel, where it is carried, potentially over large distances, to its target cell. (b) Autocrine (A): hormones such as insulin-like growth factors can act on the cell that produces them, representing autocrine control. Paracrine (P): cells secrete hormone that acts on nearby cells (e.g. glucagon and somatostatin act on adjacent β-cells within the pancreatic islet to influence insulin secretion). (c) Stimulated neuroendocrine cells secrete hormone (e.g. the hypothalamic hormones that regulate the anterior pituitary) from axonic terminals into the bloodstream. (d) Neurotransmitter cells secrete substances from axonic terminals to activate adjacent neurones.

Box 1.1 Functions of the endocrine and nervous systems, the two main communication systems

- To monitor internal and external environments
- To allow appropriate adaptive changes

  } maintain homeostasis

- To communicate via chemical messengers

however, the specialty is built on foundations that are far older. Aristotle described the pituitary, while the associated condition, gigantism, due to excess growth hormone (GH), was referred to in the Old Testament, two millennia or so before the 19th century recognition of the gland's anterior and posterior components by Rathke, and Pierre Marie's connection of GH-secreting pituitary tumours to acromegaly.

Diabetes was recognized by the ancient Egyptians. Areteus later described the disorder in the second century AD as 'a melting down of flesh and limbs into urine' – diabetes comes from the Greek word meaning siphon. The pancreas was only implicated relatively recently when Minkowski realized in 1889 that the organ's removal in dogs mimicked diabetes in humans.

The roots of reproductive endocrinology are equally long. The Bible refers to eunuchs and Hippocrates recognized that mumps could result in sterility. Oophorectomy in sows and camels was used to increase strength and growth in ancient Egypt. The association with technology is also longstanding. For instance, it took the microscope in the 17th century for Leeuwenhoek to visualize spermatozoa and later, in the 19th century, for the mammalian ovum to be discovered in the Graafian follicle.

During the last 500 years, other endocrine organs and axes have been identified and characterized. In 1564, Bartolommeo Eustacio noted the presence of the adrenal glands. Almost 300 years later (1855), Thomas Addison, one of the forefathers of clinical endocrinology, described the consequences of their inadequacy. Catecholamines were identified at the turn of the 19th century, in parallel with Oliver and Schaffer's discovery that these adrenomedullary substances raise blood pressure. This followed shortly after the clinical features of myxoedema were linked to the thyroid gland, when, in 1891, physicians in Newcastle treated hypothyroidism with sheep thyroid extract. This was an important landmark, but long after the ancient Chinese recognized that seaweed, as a source of iodine, held valuable properties in treating 'goitre', swelling of the thyroid gland.

Early clinical endocrinology and diabetes tended to recognize and describe the features of the endocrine syndromes. Since then, our understanding has advanced through:

- Successful quantification of circulating hormones
- Pathophysiological identification of endocrine dysfunction
- Molecular genetic diagnoses
- Molecular unravelling of complex hormone action.

Some of the landmarks from the last 100 years are shown in Box 1.2, and those researchers who have been awarded the Nobel Prize for Medicine, Physiology or Chemistry for discoveries that have advanced endocrinology and diabetes are listed in Table 1.1.

Traditionally, endocrinology has centred on specialized hormone-secreting organs (Figure 1.2), largely built on the 'endocrine postulates' of Edward Doisy (Box 1.3). While the focus of this textbook remains with these organs, many tissues display appreciable degrees of hormone biosynthesis, and, equally relevant, modulate hormone action. All aspects are important for a complete appreciation of endocrinology and its significance.

The role of hormones

Hormones are synthesized by specialized cells (Table 1.2), which may exist as distinct endocrine glands or be located as single cells within other organs, such as the gastrointestinal tract. The chapters in Part 2 are largely organized on this anatomical basis.

Endocrinology is defined by the secretion of hormones into the bloodstream; however, autocrine or paracrine actions are also important, often modulating the hormone-secreting cell type. Hormones act by binding to specific receptors, either on the surface of or inside the target cell, to initiate a cascade of intracellular reactions, which frequently amplifies the original stimulus and generates a final response. These responses are altered in hormone deficiency and excess: for instance, GH deficiency leads to short stature in children, while excess causes over-growth (either gigantism or acromegaly; Chapter 5).

Box 1.2 Some landmarks in endocrinology over the last 100 years or so

1905	First use of the term 'hormone' by Starling in the Croonian Lecture at the Royal College of Physicians
1909	Cushing removed part of the pituitary and saw improvement in acromegaly
1914	Kendall isolated an iodine-containing substance from the thyroid
1921	Banting and Best extracted insulin from islet cells of dog pancreas and used it to lower blood sugar
Early 1930s	Pitt-Rivers and Harrington determined the structure of the thyroid hormone, thyroxine
1935–40	Crystallization of testosterone
1935–40	Identification of oestrogen and progesterone
1940s	Harris recognized the relationship between the hypothalamus and anterior pituitary in the 'portal-vessel chemotransmitter hypothesis'
1952	Gross and Pitt-Rivers identified tri-iodothyronine in human serum
1955	The Schally and Guillemin laboratories showed that extracts of hypothalamus stimulated adrenocorticotrophic hormone (ACTH) release
1956	Doniach, Roitt and Campbell associated antithyroid antibodies with some forms of hypothyroidism – the first description of an autoimmune phenomenon
1950s	Adams and Purves identified thyroid stimulatory auto-antibodies
	Gonadectomy and transplantation experiments by Jost led to the discovery of the role for testosterone in rabbit sexual development
1955	Sanger reported the primary structure of insulin
1957	Growth hormone was used to treat short stature in patients
1966	First transplant of human pancreas to treat type 1 diabetes by Kelly, Lillehei, Goetz and Merkel at the University of Minnesota
1969	Hodgkin reported the three-dimensional crystallographic structure of insulin
1969–71	Discovery of thyrotrophin-releasing hormone (TRH) and gonadotrophin-releasing hormone (GnRH) by Schally's and Guillemin's groups
1973	Discovery of somatostatin by the group of Guillemin
1981–2	Discovery of corticotrophin-releasing hormone (CRH) and growth hormone-releasing hormone (GHRH) by Vale
1994	Identification of leptin by Friedman and colleagues
1994	First transplantation of pancreatic islets to treat type 1 diabetes by Pipeleers and colleagues in Belgium
1999	Discovery of ghrelin by Kangawa and colleagues
1999	Sequencing of the human genome – publication of the DNA code for chromosome 22
2000	Advanced islet transplantation using modified immunosuppression by Shapiro and colleagues to treat type 1 diabetes

Thyroid hormone acts on many, if not all, of the 200 plus cell types in the body. The basal metabolic rate increases if it is present in excess and declines if there is a deficiency (see Chapter 8). Similarly, insulin acts on most tissues, implying its receptors are widespread. Its importance is also underlined by its role in the survival and growth of many cell types in laboratory culture. In contrast, other hormones may act only on one tissue. Thyroid-stimulating hormone (TSH), adrenocorticotrophic hormone (ACTH) and the gonadotrophins are secreted by the anterior pituitary and have specific target tissues

Table 1.1 Nobel prize winners for discoveries relevant to endocrinology and diabetes

Year	Prize winner(s)	For work on . . .
1909	Emil Theodor Kocher	Physiology, pathology and surgery of the thyroid gland
1923	Frederick Grant Banting and John James Richard Macleod	Discovery of insulin
1928	Adolf Otto Reinhold Windhaus	Constitution of the sterols and their connection with the vitamins
1939	Adolf Friedrich and Johann Butenandt	Sex hormones
1943	George de Hevesy	Use of isotopes as tracers in the study of chemical processes
1946	James Batcheller Summer, John Howard Northrop and Wendell Meredith Stanley	Discovery that enzymes can be crystallized and prepared in a pure form
1947	Carl Ferdinand Cori, Getty Theresa Cori (neé Radnitz) and Bernardo Alberto Houssay	Discovery of the course of the catalytic conversion of glycogen
1950	Edwin Calvin Kendall, Tadeus Reichstein and Philip Showalter Hench	Discoveries relating to the hormones of the adrenal cortex, their structure and biological effects
1955	Vincent du Vigneaud	Biochemically important sulphur compounds, especially for the first synthesis of a polypeptide hormone
1958	Frederick Sanger	Structures of proteins, especially that of insulin
1964	Konrad Bloch and Feodor Lynen	Discoveries concerning the mechanism and regulation of cholesterol and fatty acid metabolism
1966	Charles Brenton Huggins	Discoveries concerning hormonal treatment of prostatic cancer
1969	Derek HR Barton and Odd Hassel	Development of the concept of conformation and its application in chemistry
1970	Bernard Katz, Ulf von Euler and Julius Axelrod	Discoveries concerning the humoral transmitters in the nerve terminals and the mechanism for their storage, release and inactivation
1971	Earl W Sutherland Jr	Discoveries concerning the mechanisms of the action of hormones
1977	Roger Guillemin, Andrew V Schally and Rosalyn Yalow	Discoveries concerning peptide hormones in the production in the brain and the development of radioimmunoassay from peptide hormones
1979	Allan M Cormack and Godfrey N Hounsfield	Development of computer-assisted tomography

(Continued)

Table 1.1 *(Continued)*

Year	Prize winner(s)	For work on . . .
1982	Sune K Bergström, Bengt I Samuelson and John R Vane	Discoveries concerning prostaglandins and related biologically active substances
1985	Michael S Brown and Joseph L Goldstein	Discoveries concerning the regulation of cholesterol metabolism
1986	Stanley Cohen and Rita Levi-Montalcini	Discoveries of growth factors
1992	Edmond H Fischer and Edwin G Krebs	Discoveries concerning reversible protein phosphorylation as a biological regulatory mechanism
1994	Alfred G Gilman and Martin Rodbell	Discovery of G-proteins and the role of these proteins in signal transduction in cells
2003	Peter Agre and Roderick MacKinnon	Discovery of water channels, and the structural and mechanistic studies of ion channels
2003	Paul Lauterbur and Sir Peter Mansfield	Discoveries concerning magnetic resonance imaging
2010	Robert G Edwards	Development of *in vitro* fertilization

– the thyroid gland, the adrenal cortex and the gonads, respectively (Table 1.2).

Classification of hormones

There are three major groups of hormones according to their biochemistry (Box 1.4). Peptide or protein hormones are synthesized like any other cellular protein. Amino acid-derived and steroid hormones originate from a cascade of biochemical reactions catalyzed by a series of intracellular enzymes.

Peptide hormones

The majority of hormones are peptides and range in size from very small, only three amino acids [thyrotrophin-releasing hormone (TRH)], to small proteins of over 200 amino acids, such as TSH or luteinizing hormone (LH). Some peptide hormones are secreted directly, but most are stored in granules, the release from which is commonly controlled by another hormone, as part of a cascade, or by innervation.

Some peptide hormones have complex tertiary structures or are comprised of more than one peptide chain. Oxytocin and vasopressin, the two posterior pituitary hormones, have ring structures linked by disulphide bridges. Despite being remarkably similar in structure, they have very different physiological roles (Figure 1.3). Insulin consists of α- and β-chains linked by disulphide bonds. Like several hormones, it is synthesized as an inactive precursor that requires modification prior to release and activity. To some extent this regulation protects the synthesizing cell from being overwhelmed by its own hormone action. The gonadotrophins, follicle-stimulating hormone (FSH) and LH, TSH and human chorionic gonadotrophin (hCG) also have two chains. However, these α- and β-subunits are synthesized quite separately, from separate genes. The α-subunit is common; the distinctive β-subunit of each confers biological specificity.

Amino acid derivatives

These hormones are small water-soluble compounds. Melatonin is derived from tryptophan, whereas tyrosine derivatives include thyroid hor-

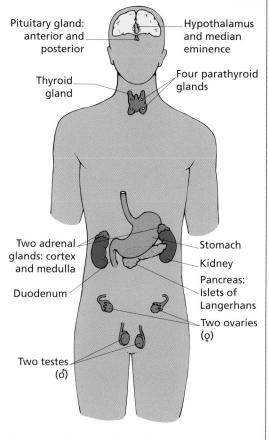

Pituitary gland: anterior and posterior

Hypothalamus and median eminence

Thyroid gland

Four parathyroid glands

Two adrenal glands: cortex and medulla

Stomach

Kidney

Duodenum

Pancreas: Islets of Langerhans

Two ovaries (♀)

Two testes (♂)

Figure 1.2 The sites of the principal endocrine glands. The stomach, kidneys and duodenum are also shown. Not shown, scattered cells within the gastrointestinal tract secrete hormones.

Box 1.3 The 'Endocrine Postulates': Edward Doisy, St Louis University School of Medicine, USA, 1936

- The gland must secrete something (an 'internal secretion')
- Methods of detecting the secretion must be available
- Purified hormone must be obtained from gland extracts
- The pure hormone must be isolated, its structure determined and synthesized

To this could be added:
- The hormone must act on specific target cells via a receptor such that excess or deficiency results in a specific phenotype

stituent of the cell membrane. Produced by the adrenal cortex, gonad and placenta, steroid hormones are insoluble in water and largely circulate bound to plasma proteins.

Organization and control of endocrine organs

The synthesis and release of hormones is regulated by control systems, similar to those used in engineering. These mechanisms ensure that hormone signals can be limited in amplitude and duration. Central to the regulation of many endocrine organs is the anterior pituitary gland, which, in turn, is controlled by a number of hormones and factors released from specialized hypothalamic neurones (see Chapter 5). Thus, major endocrine axes comprise the hypothalamus, anterior pituitary and end organ, such as the adrenal cortex, thyroid, testis or ovary. An understanding of these control mechanisms is crucial for appreciating both regulation of many endocrine systems and their clinical investigation.

mones, catecholamines, and dopamine, which regulates prolactin secretion in the anterior pituitary. The catecholamines from the adrenal medulla, epinephrine (adrenaline) and norepinephrine (noradrenaline), are also sympathetic neurotransmitters, emphasizing the close relationship between the nervous and endocrine systems (see Figure 1.2). Like peptide hormones, they are stored in granules prior to release.

Steroid hormones

Steroid hormones are lipid-soluble molecules derived from cholesterol, which is itself a basic con-

Simple control

An elementary control system is one in which the signal itself is limited, either in magnitude or

Table 1.2 The endocrine organs and their hormones*

Gland	Hormone	Molecular characteristics
Hypothalamus/ median eminence	Releasing and inhibiting hormones:	
	Thyrotrophin-releasing hormone (TRH)	Peptide
	Somatostatin (SS; inhibits GH))	Peptide
	Gonadotrophin-releasing hormone (GnRH)	Peptide
	Corticotrophin-releasing hormone (CRH)	Peptide
	Growth hormone-releasing hormone (GHRH)	Peptide
	Dopamine (inhibits prolactin)	Tyrosine derivative
Anterior pituitary	Thyrotrophin or thyroid-stimulating hormone (TSH)	Glycoprotein
	Luteinizing hormone (LH)	Glycoprotein
	Follicle-stimulating hormone (FSH)	Glycoprotein
	Growth hormone (GH) (also called somatotrophin)	Protein
	Prolactin (PRL)	Protein
	Adrenocorticotrophic hormone (ACTH)	Peptide
Posterior pituitary	Vasopressin [also called antidiuretic hormone (ADH)]	Peptide
	Oxytocin	Peptide
Thyroid	Thyroxine (T4) and tri-iodothyronine (T3)	Tyrosine derivatives
	Calcitonin	Peptide
Parathyroid	Parathyroid hormone (PTH)	Peptide
Adrenal cortex	Aldosterone	Steroid
	Cortisol	Steroid
	Androstenedione	Steroid
	Dehydroepiandrosterone (DHEA)	Steroid
Adrenal medulla	Epinephrine (also called adrenaline)	Tyrosine derivative
	Norepinephrine (also called noradrenaline)	Tyrosine derivative
Stomach[†]	Gastrin	Peptide
Pancreas (islets of Langerhans)[†]	Insulin	Protein
	Glucagon	Protein
	Somatostatin (SS)	Protein
Duodenum and jejunum[†]	Secretin	Protein
	Cholecystokinin	Protein

Gland	Hormone	Molecular characteristics
Liver	Insulin-like growth factor I (IGF-I)	Protein
Ovary	Oestrogens	Steroid
	Progesterone	Steroid
Testis	Testosterone	Steroid

Table 1.2 (*Continued*)

* The distinction between peptide and protein is somewhat arbitrary. Shorter than 50 amino acids is termed a peptide in this table.
[†] The list is not exhaustive for the gastrointestinal tract and the pancreas (see Chapter 11).

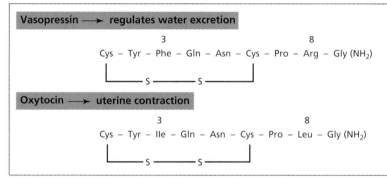

Figure 1.3 The structures of vasopressin and oxytocin are remarkably similar, yet the physiological effects of the two hormones differ profoundly.

Box 1.4 Major hormone groups

- Peptides and proteins
- Amino acid derivatives
- Steroids

duration, so as to induce only a transient response. Certain neural impulses are of this type. Refinement allows discrimination of a positive signal from background 'noise' to ensure that the target cell cannot or does not respond below a certain threshold level. An example is the pulsatile release of gonadotrophin-releasing hormone (GnRH) from the hypothalamus.

Negative feedback

Negative feedback is the commonest form of regulation used by many biological systems. For example,

in enzymology, the product frequently inhibits further progress of the catalyzed reaction. In endocrinology, a hormone may act on its target cell to stimulate a response (often secretion of another hormone) that then inhibits production of the first hormone (Figure 1.4a). Hormone secretion may also be regulated by metabolic processes. For instance, the pancreatic β-cell makes insulin in response to high ambient glucose. The effect is to lower glucose, which, in turn, inhibits further insulin production. The hypothalamic–anterior pituitary–end organ axes are a more complex extension of this model. The hypothalamic hormone [e.g. corticotrophin-releasing hormone (CRH)] stimulates release of anterior pituitary hormone (e.g. ACTH) to increase peripheral hormone production (e.g. cortisol), which then feeds back on the anterior pituitary and hypothalamus to reduce the original secretions. Figure 1.4b illustrates the anterior pituitary and end-organ components of this model.

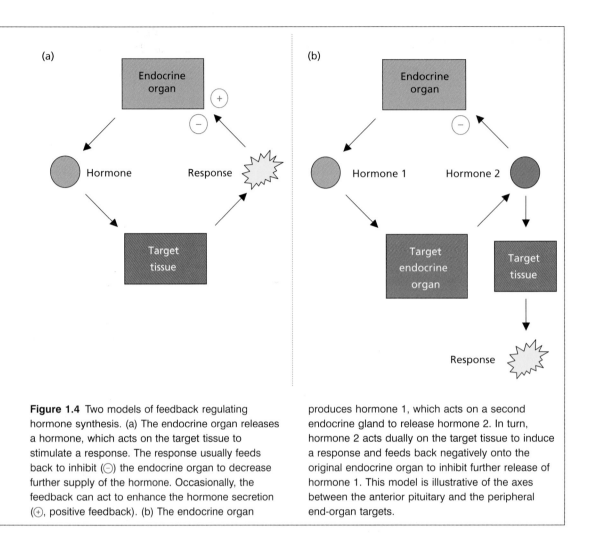

Figure 1.4 Two models of feedback regulating hormone synthesis. (a) The endocrine organ releases a hormone, which acts on the target tissue to stimulate a response. The response usually feeds back to inhibit (⊝) the endocrine organ to decrease further supply of the hormone. Occasionally, the feedback can act to enhance the hormone secretion (⊕, positive feedback). (b) The endocrine organ produces hormone 1, which acts on a second endocrine gland to release hormone 2. In turn, hormone 2 acts dually on the target tissue to induce a response and feeds back negatively onto the original endocrine organ to inhibit further release of hormone 1. This model is illustrative of the axes between the anterior pituitary and the peripheral end-organ targets.

Positive feedback

Under certain, more unusual, circumstances, hormone feedback enhances, rather than inhibits, the initial response. This is called positive feedback (an example is shown alongside the more usual negative feedback in Figure 1.4a). This is intrinsically unstable. However, in some biological systems it can be transiently beneficial: for instance, the action of oestrogen on the pituitary gland to induce the ovulatory surge of LH and FSH (see Chapter 7); or during childbirth, stretch receptors in the distended vagina and nerves to the brain stimulate oxytocin release. This hormone causes the uterus to contract, further activating the stretch receptors to establish positive feedback that is only terminated by delivery of the baby. The role of oxytocin in the suckling–milk ejection reflex is similar – a positive feedback loop that is only broken by cessation of the baby's suckling.

Inhibitory control

The secretion of some hormones is under inhibitory as well as stimulatory control. Somatostatin, a hypothalamic hormone, prevents the secretion of GH, such that when somatostatin secretion is diminished, GH secretion is enhanced. Prolactin is similarly controlled, under tonic inhibition from dopamine.

Box 1.5 Endocrine cycles

Circadian = 24-h cycle
• Circa = about, dies = day

Ultradian < 24-h cycle
• E.g. GnRH release

Infradian > 24-h cycle
• E.g. menstrual cycle

Endocrine rhythms

Many of the body's activities show periodic or cyclical changes (Box 1.5). Control of these rhythms commonly arises from the nervous system, e.g. the hypothalamus. Some appear independent of the environment, whereas others are coordinated and 'entrained' by external cues (e.g. the 24-h light/dark cycle that becomes temporarily disrupted in jetlag). Cortisol secretion is maximal between 0400h and 0800h as we awaken and minimal as we retire to bed. In contrast, GH and prolactin are secreted maximally ~1 h after falling asleep. Clinically, this knowledge of endocrine rhythms is important as investigation must be referenced according to hour-by-hour and day-to-day variability. Otherwise, such laboratory tests may be invalid or, indeed, misleading.

Endocrine disorders

The chapters in Part 2 largely focus on organ-specific endocrinology and associated endocrine disorders. Diabetes in Part 3, incorporating obesity, has now become its own specialized branch of endocrinology. Nevertheless, it is possible to regard all endocrine abnormalities as *disordered, too much* or *too little* production of hormone. Some clinical features can occur because of compensatory overproduction of hormones. For example, Addison disease is a deficiency of cortisol from the adrenal cortex (see Chapter 6), which reduces negative feedback on ACTH production at the anterior pituitary. ACTH rises and stimulates melanocytes in the skin to increase pigmentation – a cardinal sign of Addison disease.

Imbalanced hormone production may occur when a particular enzyme is missing because of a genetic defect. For example, in congenital adrenal hyperplasia, the lack of 21-hydroxylase causes failure to synthesize cortisol (see Chapter 6). Other pathways remain intact, leading to excess production of sex steroids that can masculinize aspects of the female body. Endocrine disorders may also arise from abnormalities in hormone receptors or downstream signalling pathways. The commonest example is type 2 diabetes, which arises in part from resistance to insulin action in target tissues (see Chapter 13).

For those endocrine glands under regulation by the hypothalamus and anterior pituitary, disorders can also be categorized according to site. Disease in the end organ is termed 'primary'. When the end organ is affected downstream of a problem in the anterior pituitary (either underactivity or overactivity), it is secondary, while in tertiary disease, the pathology resides in the hypothalamus.

Like in other specialties, tumourigenesis impacts on clinical endocrinology. Most commonly, these tumours are sporadic and benign, but they may oversecrete hormones, and are described in the appropriate organ-specific chapters in Part 2. However, endocrine tumourigenesis may also form part of recognized multiorgan clinical syndromes. These are described in Chapter 10.

⚷ Key points

• Endocrinology is the study of hormones and forms one of the body's major communication systems
• A hormone is a chemical messenger, commonly distributed via the circulation, that elicits specific effects by binding to a receptor on or inside target cells
• The three major types of hormones are peptides, and the derivatives of amino acids and cholesterol
• Negative and, occasionally, positive feedback, and cyclical mechanisms operate to regulate hormone production, commonly as part of complex multiorgan systems or axes
• Clinical endocrine disorders usually arise through too much, too little or disordered hormone production

CHAPTER 2
Cell biology and hormone synthesis

Key topics

- Chromosomes, mitosis and meiosis   15
- Making a protein or peptide hormone   16
- Making a hormone derived from amino acids or cholesterol   20
- Hormone transport   24
- Key points   26

Learning objectives

- To appreciate the organization, structure and function of DNA
- To understand mitosis and meiosis
- To understand protein synthesis and peptide hormone production
- To understand the function of enzymes and how enzyme cascades generate steroid and amino acid-derived hormones

This chapter aims to introduce some of the basic principles that are needed to understand later chapters

Essential Endocrinology and Diabetes, Sixth Edition. Richard IG Holt, Neil A Hanley.
© 2012 Richard IG Holt and Neil A Hanley. Publlished 2012 by Blackwell Publishing Ltd.

This chapter introduces five major themes: chromosomes and DNA; protein (and peptide) hormone synthesis; hormones derived from amino acids; steroid hormones and vitamin D; and hormone transport in the circulation. How hormones exert their actions is covered in Chapter 3.

The human genome is made up of deoxyribonucleic acid (DNA), assembled into 46 chromosomes, and resides in the nucleus (Box 2.1). The DNA contains the 'blueprints', called genes, for synthesizing proteins. There are approximately 30,000 human genes. Each gene serves as the template for generating many copies of messenger ribonucleic acid (mRNA) by a process called gene expression that amplifies the information contained in a single gene into the building blocks for many replica proteins. Specific proteins define the phenotype of a particular cell type (e.g. a thyroid cell that synthesizes thyroid hormone); more commonplace proteins carry out basic functions, e.g. the metabolic processes common to all cells. Proteins on the cell surface act as receptors that initiate intracellular signalling, which in turn is reliant on proteins that function as enzymes. Eventually, signalling information reaches the nucleus and the proteins within it, called transcription factors. These latter proteins bind or release themselves from areas of DNA around genes to determine whether a gene is switched on ('expressed', when mRNA is transcribed) or silenced.

Chromosomes, mitosis and meiosis

Genomic DNA in most human cells is packaged into chromosomes by being wrapped around proteins called histones – the DNA–histone complex is referred to as chromatin. There are 22 pairs of 'autosomes' and two sex chromosomes – two Xs in females, one X and a Y in males. This composition makes females 46,XX and males 46,XY. Distinct chromosomes are only apparent when they are lined up in preparation for cell division, either 'mitosis' or 'meiosis' (Figure 2.1). Mitosis generates two daughter cells, each with a full complement of 46 chromosomes, and occurs ~10^{17} times during human life. Meiosis creates the gametes (i.e. spermatozoan or ovum), each with 23 chromosomes so that full diploid status is reconstituted at fertilization.

Several chromosomal abnormalities can result in endocrinopathy. During meiosis, if a chromosome fails to separate properly from its partner or if migration is delayed, a gamete might result that lacks a chromosome or has too many. Thus, it is easy to appreciate Turner syndrome (45,XO), where one sex chromosome is missing; or Klinefelter syndrome (47,XXY), where there is an extra X. Similarly, breaks and rejoining across or within chromosomes produce unusual 'derivative' chromosomes or ones with duplicated or deleted regions (see Figure 4.4). If such events occur close to genes, function can be disrupted, e.g. congenital loss of a hormone. Duplication can be equally significant; on the X chromosome, a double dose of a region that includes the *dosage-sensitive sex reversal, adrenal hypoplasia critical region gene 1* (DAX1) causes female development in a 46,XY fetus.

Box 2.1 The structure of DNA

- A molecule of deoxyribose (a 5-carbon sugar) is linked covalently to one of two types of nitrogenous bases:
  - Purine – adenine (A) or guanine (G)
  - Pyrimidine – thymine (T) or cytosine (C)
  - The base plus the sugar is termed a 'nucleoside', e.g. adenosine
- The addition of a phosphate group to a nucleoside creates a nucleotide, e.g. adenosine mono-, di- or tri-phosphate (according to how many phosphate groups have been added)
- Phosphodiester bonds polymerize the nucleotides into a single strand of DNA
- Two strands, running in opposite directions, 5 prime (5′; upstream) to 3′ (downstream) assemble as a double helix:
  - Hydrogen bonds form between the strands, between the base pairs A–T and G–C
- ~3 billion base pairs comprise the human genome

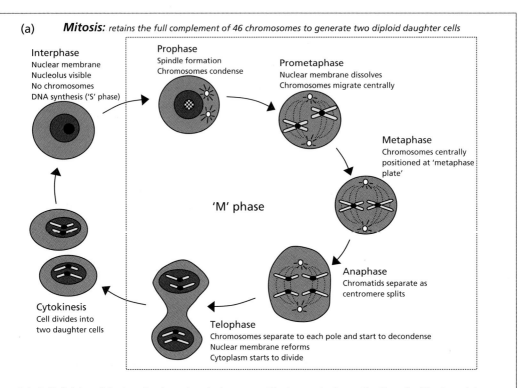

(a) **Mitosis:** *retains the full complement of 46 chromosomes to generate two diploid daughter cells*

Interphase
Nuclear membrane
Nucleolus visible
No chromosomes
DNA synthesis ('S' phase)

Prophase
Spindle formation
Chromosomes condense

Prometaphase
Nuclear membrane dissolves
Chromosomes migrate centrally

Metaphase
Chromosomes centrally
positioned at 'metaphase
plate'

'M' phase

Anaphase
Chromatids separate as
centromere splits

Cytokinesis
Cell divides into
two daughter cells

Telophase
Chromosomes separate to each pole and start to decondense
Nuclear membrane reforms
Cytoplasm starts to divide

Figure 2.1 Cell division. Prior to mitosis and meiosis the cell undergoes a period of DNA synthesis ('S' phase) so that the normal diploid status of DNA (2n) temporarily becomes 4n. (a) The stages of mitosis result in each daughter cell containing diploid 2n quantities of DNA. (b, opposite) Meiosis is split into two stages, each of which comprises prophase, prometaphase, metaphase, anaphase and telophase. During prophase of meiosis I, the maternally and paternally derived chromosomes align to allow crossing over ('recombination'), a critical aspect of genetic diversity. The two sister chromatids do not separate, so that the secondary oocyte and spermatocytes each contains 2n quantities of DNA. During the second stage of meiosis, separation of the chromatids results in haploid cells (n). In males, meiosis is an equal process resulting in four spermatids. In contrast, in females, only one ovum is produced from a primary oocyte, smaller polar bodies being extruded at both stages of meiosis.

Making a protein or peptide hormone

Gene transcription and its regulation

The production of mRNA from a gene is called transcription. Within most genes, the stretches of DNA that encode protein, called exons, are separated by variable lengths of non-coding DNA called introns (Figure 2.2). Upstream of the first exon is the 5′ flanking region of the gene, which contains multiple promoter elements, usually within a few hundred base pairs. Transcription factors bind to these elements either to promote (i.e. turn on) or to repress (i.e. turn off) the production of mRNA by RNA polymerase, the enzyme that 'reads' the DNA code. Commonly, the signal that recruits RNA polymerase to the DNA occurs at a 'TATA' box, a short run of adenosines and thymidines, ~30 base pairs upstream of exon 1 (Figure 2.2) or an area rich in G and C residues.

Superimposed on this, gene expression can be further increased or diminished by more cell- or tissue-specific transcription factors potentially

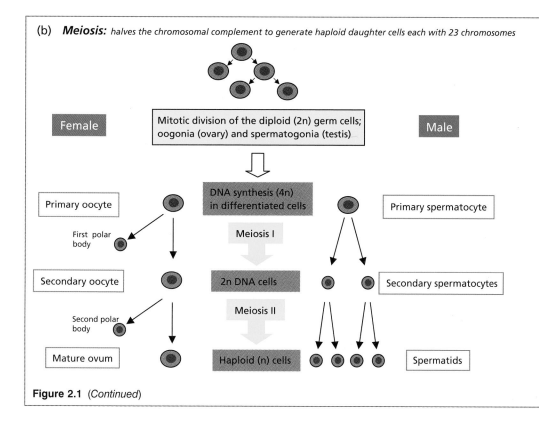

(b) *Meiosis:* halves the chromosomal complement to generate haploid daughter cells each with 23 chromosomes

Figure 2.1 *(Continued)*

binding to more distant stretches of DNA (either 'enhancer' or 'repressor' elements). For instance, the transcription factor, steroidogenic factor-1 (SF-1), turns on many genes specific to the adrenal cortex and gonad; when SF-1 is absent, both organs fail to form. These alterations to expression are dependent on the exact DNA sequence recognized by specific proteins. There is another layer of complexity governing how genes are expressed. Epigenetics is the study of how gene expression is regulated by mechanisms beyond the precise DNA sequence, e.g. by methylation of the DNA around genes, which tends to silence expression; or by modifications to histones, such as acetylation or methylation, which alter the chromatin structure and make stretches of DNA containing genes accessible or inaccessible to transcription factors. Acetylation tends to open up the structure, facilitating gene expression, whereas methylation tends to close it down, silencing transcription. Genomic imprinting is an epigenetic phenomenon involving DNA methylation and modifications to histones such that gene expression varies according to which parent the particular chromosome came from.

RNA contains ribose sugar moieties rather than deoxyribose. RNA polymerase 'sticks' ribonucleotides together to generate a single strand of mRNA that correlates to the DNA code of the gene, except that in place of thymidine, a very similar nucleoside, uridine, is incorporated. The initial mRNA strand (pre-mRNA) is processed so that intronic gene regions are excluded and only the exonic sequences are 'spliced' together. Not all exonic regions encode protein; stretches at either end constitute the 5′ and 3′ untranslated regions (UTRs) (Figure 2.2). Within the 3′ UTR, mRNA transcription is terminated by a specific purine-rich motif, the polyadenylation signal, ~20 base pairs upstream of where the mRNA gains a stretch of adenosine residues. This poly-A tail provides stability as the mRNA is moved from the nucleus to the cytoplasm for translation into protein.

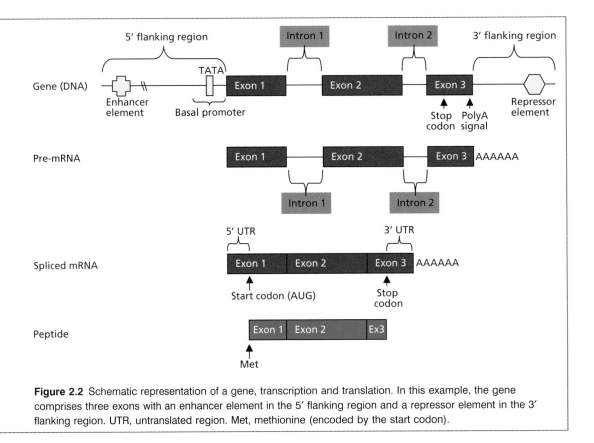

Figure 2.2 Schematic representation of a gene, transcription and translation. In this example, the gene comprises three exons with an enhancer element in the 5′ flanking region and a repressor element in the 3′ flanking region. UTR, untranslated region. Met, methionine (encoded by the start codon).

Translation into protein

mRNA is transported to the ribosomes, where protein synthesis occurs by translation (Figure 2.3a). The ribosomes are attached to the outside of the endoplasmic reticulum (ER), leading to the description of rough ER.

The ribosome is an RNA–protein complex that 'reads' the mRNA sequence. On the first occasion that sequential A–U–G nucleotides are encountered (corresponding to ATG in the genomic DNA), translation starts (see Figure 2.2). From this point, every three nucleotides represent an amino acid. This nucleotide triplet is called a codon, AUG being a start codon that specifies the amino acid methionine. Similarly, translation continues until a 'stop' codon is encountered (UAA, UGA or UAG).

By understanding these normal events of gene transcription and protein translation, it becomes possible to appreciate how mutations (sequence errors) in the genomic DNA lead to a miscoded, and consequently malfunctional, protein (Box 2.2). An entire gene may be missing ('deleted') or duplicated. An erroneous base pair in the promoter region may impair a critical transcription factor from binding. A similar error in an exonic coding sequence might translate a different amino acid or even create a premature stop codon. Small deletions or insertions of one or two base pairs throw the whole triplet code out of frame. A mutation at the boundary between an intron and an exon can prevent splicing so that the intron becomes included in the mature mRNA. All of these events affect endocrinology either as congenital defects (i.e. during early development so that the fault is present in the genome of many cells) or as acquired abnormalities later in life, potentially predisposing to the formation of an endocrine tumour (see Chapter 10).

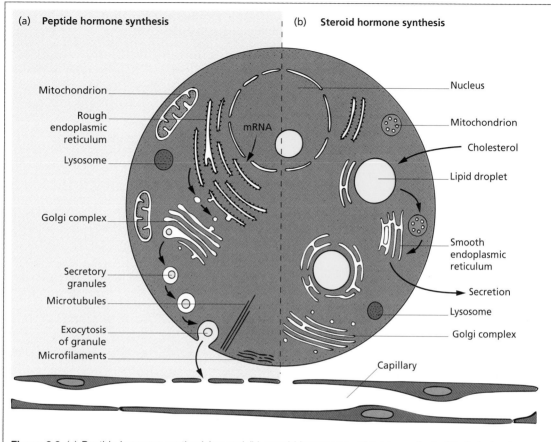

Figure 2.3 (a) Peptide hormone-synthesizing and (b) steroid hormone-synthesizing cells. In (b) cholesterol enters the cell via the low-density lipoprotein receptor which is internalized.

Post-translational modification of peptides

Some polypeptides can function as hormones after little more than removal of the starting methionine, e.g. thyrotrophin-releasing hormone (TRH), which consists of only three amino acids. Others undergo further modification or potentially fold together as different subunits of a hormone, e.g. luteinizing hormone (LH). Peptides with any degree of complexity fold into three-dimensional structures, which may contain helical or pleated domains. These shapes provide stability and affect how one protein interacts with another (e.g. how a hormone might bind to its receptor).

For hormones that require secretion out of the cell, additional modifications are common and important (Figure 2.4). The precursor peptide, called a pre-prohormone, carries a lipophilic signal peptide at the amino terminus. This sequence is recognized by channel proteins so that the immature peptide can cross the ER membrane. Once inside the ER, the signal peptide is excised in preparation for other post-translational changes (Figure 2.4a–d).

Disulphide bridges are formed in certain proteins (e.g. growth hormone or insulin; Figure 2.4a and c). Certain carbohydrates may be added to form glycoproteins (Figure 2.4d). Some prohormones (e.g. pro-opiomelanocortin and proglucagon) need processing to give rise to several final products, whereas others are assembled as a combination of distinct peptide chains, each synthesized from different genes, e.g. thyroid-stimulating hormone (TSH).

Box 2.2 Genetic, genomic and epigenetic abnormalities that can result in endocrinopathy

Abnormalities in DNA (genetic)
- Base substitution – swapping different nucleotides
- Insertion or deletion – alters frame if exonic and not a multiple of three

Chromosomal abnormalities (genomic)
- Numerical – three copies as in Down syndrome (trisomy 21)
- Structural:
  - Inversions – region of a chromosome is turned upside down
  - Translocations – regions swapped between chromosomes
  - Duplications – region of a chromosome is present twice
  - Deletions – region of a chromosome is excised and lost

Imprinting abnormalities (epigenetic)
- Methylation – altered methylation changing local gene expression, such as Beckwith–Wiedemann syndrome with neonatal hypoglycaemia or transient neonatal diabetes associated with overexpression of the gene called *ZAC*
- Structural chromosomal abnormalities (as above) can also cause imprinting errors

---

Box 2.3 Role of post-translational modifications

Post-translational modifications are important so that:
- Great diversity of hormone action is generated from a more limited range of encoding genes
- Active hormone is saved for its intended site of action
- The synthesizing cell is protected from a barrage of its own hormone action

---

ules. Movement of these vesicles to a position near the cell membrane is influenced by two types of filamentous structure: microtubules and microfilaments (see Figure 2.3a). Secretion of the stored hormone tends to be rapid but only occurs after appropriate stimulation of the cell. Whether this is hormonal, neuronal or nutritional, it usually involves a change in cell permeability to calcium ions. These divalent metal ions are required for interaction between the vesicle and plasma membrane, and for the activation of enzymes, microfilaments and microtubules. The secretory process is called exocytosis (see Figure 2.3a). The membrane of the storage granule fuses with the cell membrane at the same time as vesicular endopeptidases are activated so that active hormone is expelled into the extracellular space from where it enters the blood vessels. The vesicle membrane is then recycled within the cell.

The completed protein is then packaged into membrane-bound vesicles, which may contain specific 'endopeptidases'. These enzymes are responsible for final hormone activation – cleaving the 'pro-'portion of the protein chain, as occurs with the release of C-peptide and insulin (Figure 2.4c). Such post-translational modifications are essential stages in hormone synthesis (Box 2.3).

Storage and secretion of peptide hormones

Endocrine cells usually store newly synthesized peptide hormone in small vesicles or secretory gran-

Making a hormone derived from amino acids or cholesterol

In addition to peptides or proteins, hormones can also be synthesized by sequential enzymatic modification of the amino acids tyrosine and tryptophan, or of cholesterol.

Enzyme action and cascades

Enzymes can be divided into classes according to the reactions that they catalyze (Table 2.1). In endocrinology, they frequently operate in cascades where the

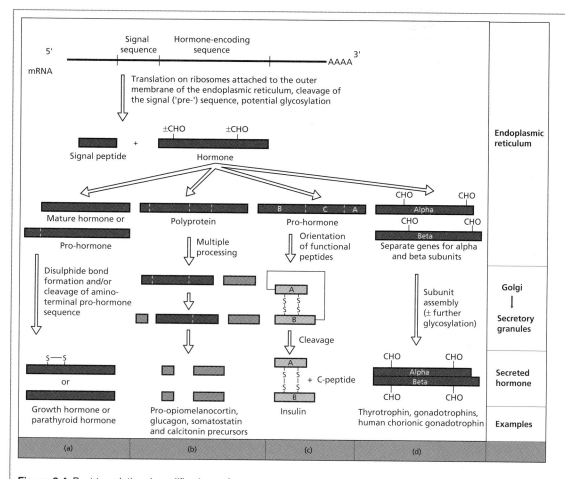

Figure 2.4 Post-translational modifications of peptide hormones. Four types are shown. (a) Simple changes such as removal of the amino terminal 'pro-'extension prior to secretion (e.g. parathyroid hormone) or the addition of intra-chain disulphide bonds (e.g. growth hormone). (b) Multiple processing of a 'polyprotein' into a number of different peptide hormones (e.g. pro-opiomelanocortin can give rise to adrenocorticotrophic hormone plus melanocyte-stimulating hormone and β-endorphin). (c) Synthesis of insulin requires folding of the peptide and the formation of disulphide bonds. The active molecule is created by hydrolytic removal of a connecting (C)-peptide, i.e. proinsulin gives rise to insulin plus C-peptide in equimolar proportion. (d) Synthesis of larger protein hormones (e.g. thyroid-stimulating hormone, luteinizing hormone, follicle-stimulating hormone and human chorionic gonadotrophin) from two separate peptides that complex together. The four hormones share the same α-subunit with a hormone-specific β-subunit.

product of one reaction serves as the substrate for the next. Most simplistically, enzyme action is achieved by protein–protein interaction between the substrate and the enzyme at the latter's 'active site'. This causes a modification to the substrate to form a product which no longer binds to the active site and is thus released. Other macromolecules bind else-where to the enzyme and function as co-factors, adding more complex regulation to the biochemical reaction.

Patients can present with many endocrine syndromes because of loss of enzyme function. For instance, gene mutation might lead to substitution of an amino acid at a key position of an enzyme's

Table 2.1 Definition and classification of enzymes

Definition

An enzyme is a biological macromolecule – most frequently a protein – that catalyzes a biochemical reaction

Catalysis increases the rate of reaction, e.g. the disappearance of substrate and generation of product

Enzyme action is critical for the synthesis of hormones derived from amino acids and cholesterol

Classification

Enzyme	Catalytic function	Example (and relevance)
Hydrolases	Cleavage of a bond by the addition of water	Cytochrome P450 11A1/cholesterol side-chain cleavage (CYP11A1; early step in steroid hormone biosynthesis)
Lyases	Removal of a group to form a double bond or addition of a group to a double bond	Cytochrome P450 17α-hydroxylase/17–20 lyase (CYP17A1; step in synthesis of steroid hormones other than aldosterone)
Isomerases	Intramolecular rearrangments	3β-hydroxysteroid dehydrogenase/delta 4,5 isomerase isoforms (HSD3B; step in synthesis of all major steroid hormones)
Oxidoreductase	Oxidation and reduction	11β-hydroxysteroid dehydrogenase isoforms (HSD11B; inter-conversion of cortisol and cortisone)
Ligases or synthases	Joins two molecules together	Thyroid peroxidase (TPO; step in synthesis of thyroid hormone)
Transferases	Transfer of a molecular group from substrate to product	Phenol ethanolamine *N*-methyl transferase (PNMT; conversion of norepinephrine to epinephrine)

active site. The three-dimensional structure might be affected so significantly that the substrate may no longer convert to product. In the enzyme cascade that synthesizes cortisol, this causes various forms of congenital adrenal hyperplasia (CAH) (see Chapter 6). Understanding the biochemical cascade allows accurate diagnosis as the substrate builds up in the circulation and its excess can be measured, e.g. by immunoassay or mass spectrometry (see Chapter 4).

Synthesizing hormones derived from amino acids

The amino acid tyrosine can be modified by sequential enzyme action to give rise to several hormones (Box 2.4). The precise synthetic pathways for dopamine and catecholamines are described in

---

Box 2.4 Hormones derived from tyrosine

- Thyroid hormones: sequential addition of iodine and coupling of two tyrosines together (see Chapter 8)
- Adrenomedullary hormones: hydroxylation steps and decarboxylation to form dopamine and catecholamines (see Chapter 6)
- Hypothalamic dopamine formed by hydroxylation and decarboxylation (see Chapter 5)

Chapter 6 (Figure 6.11) and for thyroid hormones in Chapter 8 (Figures 8.3 and 8.4). Melatonin, important in endocrine circadian rhythms with a new link to type 2 diabetes (see Chapter 5), is generated from the amino acid tryptophan via synthesis of the neurotransmitter serotonin.

Synthesizing hormones derived from cholesterol

Steroid hormones are generated by enzyme cascades that modify the four-carbon ring structure of cholesterol (see Figure 2.6). The precise sequence of enzymes determines which steroids are generated as the final product (Box 2.4). In addition to making steroid hormones, cholesterol is a critical building block of all mammalian cell membranes and the starting point for synthesizing vitamin D, which functions, and can be classified, as a hormone (see Chapter 9). Cholesterol is acquired in approximately equal measure from the diet and *de novo* synthesis (mostly in the liver; Box 2.5). From the diet, cholesterol is delivered to cells as a complex with low-density lipoprotein (LDL–cholesterol). Intracellular uptake is via the cell-surface LDL receptor and endocytosis (see Figure 2.3b). *De novo* biosynthesis commences with co-enzyme A (CoA), itself synthesized from pantothenate, cysteine and adenosine, and proceeds via hydroxymethylglutaryl co-enzyme A (HMGCoA) and mevalonic acid (Figure 2.5). The rate-limiting step is the reduction of HMGCoA by the enzyme HMGCoA reductase. Pharmacological inhibition of this enzyme to treat hypercholesterolaemia and lessen cardiovascular disease has led to the most widely prescribed drug family in the world (the 'statins') and the award of the Nobel Prize to Michael Brown and Joseph Goldstein (see Table 1.2).

Box 2.5 Hormones derived from cholesterol

Cholesterol derived from the diet and *de novo* synthesis used to synthesize:
- Vitamin D (see Chapter 10)
- Steroid hormones:
  - Adrenal cortex: aldosterone, cortisol and sex steroid precursors (see Chapter 6)
  - Testis: testosterone (see Chapter 7)
  - Ovary and placenta: oestrogens and progesterone (see Chapter 7)

In steroidogenic cells, cholesterol is largely deposited as esters in large lipid-filled vesicles (see Figure 2.3b). Upon stimulation, cholesterol is released from its stores and transported into the mitochondria, a process that is facilitated by the steroid acute regulatory (StAR) protein in the adrenal and gonad and by the related protein, start domain containing 3 (STARD3), in the placenta. The first step in the synthesis of a steroid hormone is the rate-limiting conversion of cholesterol to pregnenolone. Pregnenolone then undergoes a range of further enzymatic modifications in the mitochondria or the ER to make active steroid hormones.

Nomenclature of steroidogenic pathways

Figure 2.6 shows a generic representation of human steroid hormone biosynthesis. Many of the enzymes that catalyze steps in these pathways are encoded by the cytochrome P450 (*CYP*) family of related genes that is also critical for hepatic detoxification of drugs. Some of the enzymes are important in both the adrenal cortex and gonad (e.g. CYP11A1), whereas others are restricted and thus create the distinct steroid profiles of each tissue (e.g. CYP21A2, needed for cortisol and aldosterone biosynthesis, is very largely limited to the adrenal cortex).

Historically, the enzymes have been named according to function (e.g. hydroxylation) at a specific carbon atom, with a Greek letter indicating orientation above or below the four-carbon ring structure (e.g. 17α-hydroxylase attaches a hydroxyl group in the alpha position to carbon 17; Figure 2.6).

The common names used for steroids also adhere to a loose convention. The suffix -ol indicates an important hydroxyl group, as in cholester*ol* or cortis*ol*, whereas the suffix -one indicates an important ketone group (testoster*one*). The extra presence of -di, as in -diol (oestra*diol*) or -dione (androstene*dione*), reflects two of these groups, respectively; '-ene' (andros*tene*dione) within the name indicates a significant double bond in the steroid nucleus.

Storage of steroid hormones

Unlike cells making peptide hormones, most steroid-secreting cells do not store hormones but

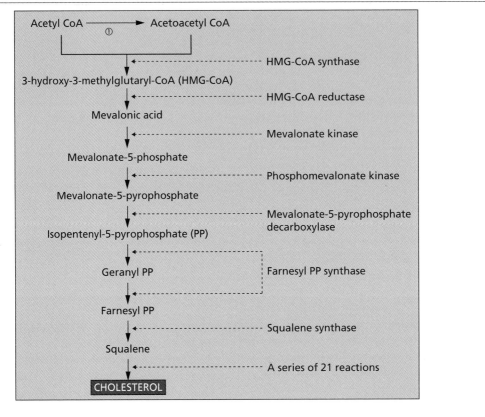

Figure 2.5 Synthesis of cholesterol. Step ① is catalyzed by the enzyme thiolase; otherwise the enzymes are shown to the right of the cascade. The individual steps between squalene and cholesterol have been omitted.

synthesize them as required. As a consequence, there is a slower onset of action for steroid hormones following the initial stimulation of the steroidogenic organ.

Hormone transport

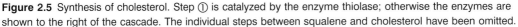

Most peptide hormones are hydrophilic, so they generally circulate free in the bloodstream with little or no association with serum proteins. In contrast, steroid hormones and thyroid hormones circulate bound to proteins because, like cholesterol, they are hydrophobic. There are relatively specific transport proteins for many of the steroid hormones, e.g. cortisol-binding globulin (CBG) and sex hormone-binding globulin (SHBG), as well as for thyroid hormones [thyroxine-binding globulin (TBG)]. Many hormones also loosely associate with other circulating proteins, especially albumin.

The equilibrium between protein-bound and unbound ('free') hormone determines activity, as only free hormone readily diffuses into tissues. This is relevant to many hormone assays where total hormone is measured. Results may be markedly altered by changes in the concentration of binding protein, but the change in free hormone concentration may be very small and biological activity remains unaltered. For instance, women on the combined oral contraceptive pill have raised serum CBG and increased total cortisol; however, free cortisol is unaltered.

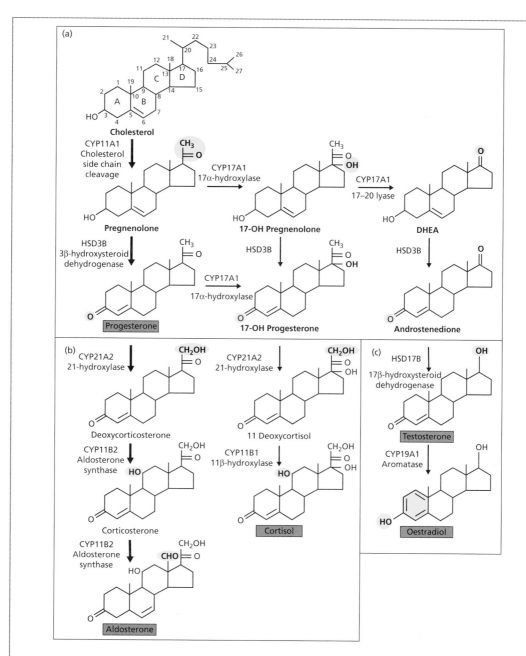

Figure 2.6 Overview of the major steroidogenic pathways. Yellow shading indicates the enzymatic change since the last step. The enzymes are shown by proper name and common name according to their action. Note some enzymes perform multiple reactions (e.g. CYP17A1 acts as both a hydroxylase and lyase) and some reactions are performed by multiple enzyme isoforms (e.g. HSD3B exists as HSD3B1 and HSD3B2). For 17-OH progesterone, the enzymatic change illustrated is that catalyzed by HSD3B activity rather than CYP17A1. The simplified pathways are grouped into three blocks: (a) common to both the adrenal cortex and the gonad; (b) adrenocortical steroidogenesis; and (c) pathways characteristic of the testis (testosterone) or ovary and placenta (oestradiol). OH, hydroxy; DHEA, dehydroepiandrosterone.

Key points

- Mutations in DNA and chromosomal abnormalities cause congenital and sporadic endocrine disease
- Meiosis is central to reproductive endocrinology
- Genes are stretches of DNA responsible for encoding protein
- Many protein hormones are synthesized as prohormones requiring post-translational modification and processing before they become active
- Enzyme cascades synthesize hormones derived from amino acids and cholesterol
- Unlike peptide hormones, steroid hormones are not stored in cells but made 'on demand'
- Many peptide hormones are free in the circulation, unlike steroid or thyroid hormones, which associate with binding proteins

CHAPTER 3
Molecular basis of hormone action

Key topics

- Cell-surface receptors   28
- Tyrosine kinase receptors   31
- G-protein–coupled receptors   34
- Nuclear receptors   40
- Key points   47

Learning objectives

- To understand the principles of hormone–receptor interaction
- To understand the biology of the different families of hormone receptors
  - ☐ Tyrosine kinase receptors and associated signalling pathways
  - ☐ G-protein–coupled receptors and associated signalling pathways
  - ☐ Nuclear receptors and their influence on gene expression
- To appreciate the role of transcription factors that are important in endocrine development and function
- To appreciate how abnormalities in hormone receptors or their downstream signalling can cause endocrinopathy

This chapter describes the key events that occur within the cell following stimulation by hormone

Essential Endocrinology and Diabetes, Sixth Edition. Richard IG Holt, Neil A Hanley.
© 2012 Richard IG Holt and Neil A Hanley. Publlished 2012 by Blackwell Publishing Ltd.

Hormones act by binding to receptors. There are two superfamilies of hormone receptor: the cell-surface receptors and nuclear receptors, named according to their site of action, and which display characteristic features (Figure 3.1 and Box 3.1).

Cell-surface receptors

Cell-surface receptors comprise three components, each with characteristic structural features that reflect their location and function (Figure 3.2).

Stage 1: Binding of hormone to receptor

Historically, hormone–receptor interactions (Box 3.2) have been characterized using radiolabelled hormones and isolated preparations of receptors to define two properties:

• The hormone–receptor interaction is saturable (Figure 3.3)
• The hormone–receptor interaction is reversible (Figure 3.4).

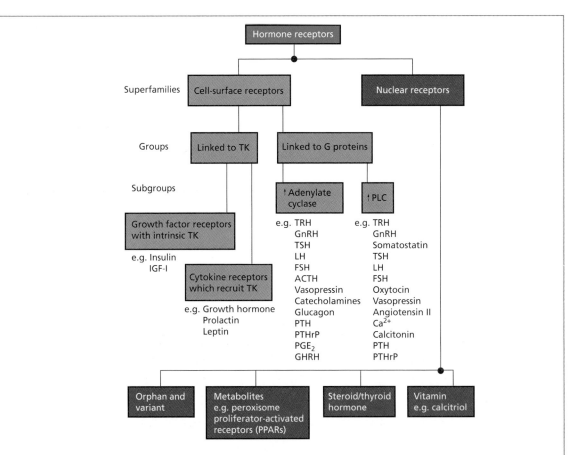

Figure 3.1 The different classes of hormone receptor. Some cell-surface receptors, e.g. the parathyroid hormone (PTH) receptor, can link to different G-proteins, which couple to either adenylate cyclase or phospholipase C (PLC). TK, tyrosine kinase; TRH, thyrotrophin-releasing hormone; GnRH, gonadotrophin-releasing hormone; TSH, thyroid-stimulating hormone; LH, luteinizing hormone; FSH, follicle-stimulating hormone; ACTH, adrenocorticotrophic hormone; PTHrP, parathyroid hormone-related peptide; PGE_2, prostaglandin E_2; GHRH, growth hormone releasing hormone; IGF-I, insulin-like growth factor I.

Box 3.1 Some basic facts about hormone receptors

- Tissue distribution of receptor determines the scope of hormone action:
  - Thyroid-stimulating hormone (TSH) receptor largely limited to thyroid, therefore TSH action restricted to the thyroid
  - Thyroid hormone receptor is widespread, therefore thyroid hormone action is diverse
- Binding of hormone induces a conformational change in the receptor that initiates downstream signalling
- Downstream signalling differs across cell types to produce potentially diverse hormonal effects
- Control is exerted through the constant synthesis, degradation and localization of hormone receptors – most target cells have 2000–100,000 receptors for a particular hormone

Hormone receptor superfamilies
- Water-soluble hormones (e.g. peptide hormones):
  - Plasma membrane is impenetrable
  - Cell-surface receptors transduce signal through membrane
  - Activate intracellular signalling pathways
  - Fast responses (seconds) as well as slow ones
- Lipid-soluble hormones (e.g. steroid and thyroid hormones):
  - Pass through plasma membrane
  - Receptors function as transcription factors in the nucleus
  - Activate or repress gene expression
  - Tend to be relatively slow responses (hours–days)

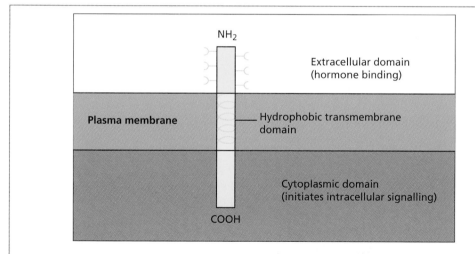

Figure 3.2 A membrane-spanning cell-surface receptor. The hormone acts as ligand. The ligand-binding pocket in the extracellular domain is comparatively rich in cysteine residues that form internal disulphide bonds and repeated loops to ensure correct folding. For some hormones, e.g. growth hormone, this extracellular domain can circulate as a potential binding protein. Circulating fragments of the thyroid-stimulating hormone receptor may be immunogenic for antibody formation in autoimmune thyroid disease. The α-helical membrane-spanning domain is rich in hydrophobic and uncharged amino acids. The C-terminal cytoplasmic domain either contains, or links to, separate catalytic systems, which initiate the intracellular signals after hormone binding.

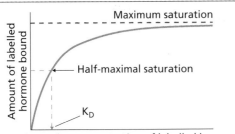

Figure 3.3 Hormone–receptor systems are saturable. Increasing amounts of labelled hormone are incubated with a constant amount of receptor. The amount of bound labelled hormone increases as more is added until the system is saturated. At this point, further addition fails to increase the amount bound to receptors. The concentration of hormone that is required for half-maximal saturation of the receptors is equal to the dissociation constant (K_D) of the hormone–receptor interaction.

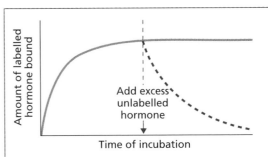

Figure 3.4 Hormone–receptor interactions are reversible. Constant amounts of labelled hormone and receptors are incubated together for different times. The bound label increases with time until it reaches a plateau, when the bound and free hormone have reached a dynamic equilibrium. In a dynamic equilibrium, hormone continually associates and dissociates from its receptor. By adding excess unlabelled hormone, competition with the labelled hormone is established for access to the receptors. Consequently, the amount of bound labelled hormone decreases with extended incubation (dashed line).

Box 3.2 Binding characteristics of hormone receptors

- *High affinity*: hormones circulate at low concentrations – receptors are like 'capture systems'
- *Reversible binding*: one reason for the transient nature of endocrine responses
- *Specificity*: receptors distinguish between closely related molecular structures

Using methodology similar to that for immunoassays (see Chapter 4), constant amounts of labelled hormone and receptor preparations can be incubated with increasing, known amounts of unlabelled hormone for a specified time. Separating and measuring the receptor-bound labelled fraction allows curves to be plotted and mathematical modelling of the hormone (H)–receptor (R) interaction; e.g. whether it is conforms to the equation $H + R \leftrightarrows HR$. Ultimately, these types of experi-

ment can allow estimation of the number of hormone receptors present on each target cell.

Stage 2: Signal transduction

When a hormone binds to a cell-surface receptor, the cascade of cytoplasmic responses is mediated through protein phosphorylation by kinase enzymes or the generation of 'second messengers' via coupling to guanine ('G') proteins. Signalling through either process amplifies the hormone response as many protein phosphorylation events or second messenger molecules are produced for each hormone–receptor interaction. They also distinguish the two major groups of cell-surface receptor: tyrosine kinase receptors and G-protein–coupled receptors (Figure 3.1 and Box 3.3).

Protein phosphorylation is a key molecular switch. Approximately 10% of proteins are phosphorylated at any given time in a mammalian cell. The phosphate group is donated from ATP during catalysis by the 'kinase' enzyme. It is accepted by the polar hydroxyl group of serine, threonine or

Box 3.3 Categories of cell-surface receptors

Tyrosine kinase receptors
- Signal via phosphorylation of the amino acid, tyrosine

G-protein–coupled receptors
- Activate or inhibit adenylate cyclase and/or phospholipase C (PLC)
- Signal via second messengers: cyclic adenosine monophosphate (cAMP), inositol triphosphate (IP_3), diacylglycerol (DAG) and intracellular calcium
- Signal via phosphorylation of serine and threonine amino acids

tyrosine (Figure 3.5a) and causes a conformational change in the three-dimensional shape of the protein (Figure 3.5b). In many signalling pathways, the phosphorylated protein can also act as a kinase and phosphorylate the next protein in the sequence. In this way, a phosphorylation cascade is generated, which relays and amplifies the intracellular signal generated by the hormone binding to its receptor (Figure 3.5c).

Tyrosine kinase receptors

Phosphorylation of tyrosine kinase (TK) receptors can occur through:

- Intrinsic TK activity located in the cytosolic domain of the receptor; or
- Separate TKs recruited after receptor activation (see Figure 3.1).

By either mechanism, conformational change induced by phosphorylation creates 'docking' sites for other proteins. Frequently, this occurs via conserved motifs within the target protein, known as 'SH2' or 'SH3' domains. These domains may be involved in the activation of downstream kinases or they may stabilize other signalling proteins within a phosphorylation cascade.

Receptors with intrinsic tyrosine kinase activity

Intrinsic TK receptors autophosphorylate upon binding of the appropriate hormone. This group includes the receptor for insulin and those for epidermal growth factor (EGF), fibroblast growth factor (FGF) and insulin-like growth factor I (IGF-I). The EGF and FGF receptors exist as monomers that dimerize upon hormone binding to activate tyrosine phosphorylation. Those for insulin and IGF-I exist in their unoccupied state as preformed dimers. The signalling pathways for all these receptors are heavily involved in cell growth and proliferation.

Insulin signalling pathways

The dimerized insulin receptor (IR) is composed of two α- and two β-subunits linked by a series of disulphide bridges (Figure 3.6; see Chapter 11). The earliest response to insulin binding is autophosphorylation of the cytosolic domains of the β-subunit. The activated receptor then phosphorylates two key intermediaries, insulin receptor substrate (IRS) 1 or 2, which are thought to be essential for almost all biological actions of insulin. IRS1 has many potential tyrosine phosphorylation sites, at least eight of which are phosphorylated by the activated IR.

Multiple phosphorylation of IRS1 or 2 leads to the docking of several proteins with SH2 domains, and the activation of divergent intracellular signalling. For example, docking of phosphatidylinositol-3-kinase (PI3-kinase) leads to deployment of the glucose transporter (GLUT) family members. For instance, in adipose tissue and muscle, GLUT-4 translocates from intracellular vesicles to the cell membrane, allowing glucose uptake into the cell. The mitogenic effects of insulin are mediated via a different intracellular pathway. Activated IRS1 docks with the SH2/SH3 domains of the type 2 growth factor receptor-bound (Grb2) protein. This adaptor protein links IRS1 to the son of sevenless (SoS) protein and, ultimately, to activation of the mitogen-activated protein kinase (MAPK) pathway, leading to gene expression that promotes mitosis and growth.

(a) Amino acids that can be phosphorylated.

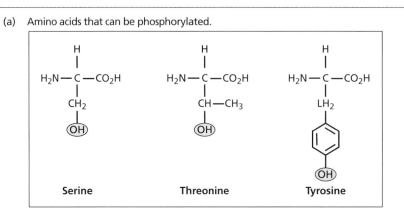

(b) Phosphorylation of protein 1 induces an activating conformational change due to the energetically favourable phosphorylation (P) of a hydroxyl group (OH).

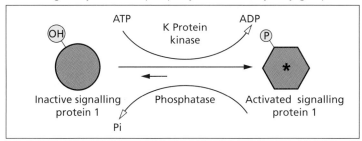

(c) The initiation of a phosphorylation cascade. Phosphorylated protein 1 acts as a kinase and phosphorylates protein 2.

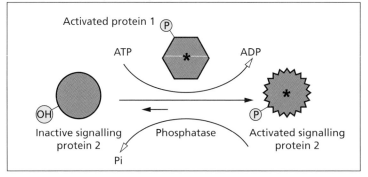

Figure 3.5 Intracellular signalling via phosphorylation. (a) Amino acids serine, threonine and tyrosine carry polar hydroxyl (OH) groups that can be phosphorylated. Over 99% of all protein phosphorylation occurs on serine and threonine residues; however, phosphorylation of tyrosine, the only amino acid with a phenolic ring, generates particularly distinctive intracellular signalling pathways. (b) Protein 1 is inactive until its hydroxyl group is phosphorylated by the action of a kinase enzyme. This induces a conformational change, resulting in an activated phosphorylated protein. Energy for the transfer of the phosphate group comes from the hydrolysis of ATP to ADP. The reverse reaction, from active to inactive states, is catalyzed by a phosphatase and releases inorganic phosphate (Pi) for reincorporation back into ATP. (c) The initiation of a signalling cascade. Activated phosphorylated protein 1 itself acts as a kinase and catalyzes the phosphorylation of protein 2. Amino acid specificity means that serine/threonine kinases usually show no activity with tyrosine residues and tyrosine kinases normally do not phosphorylate serine or threonine residues.

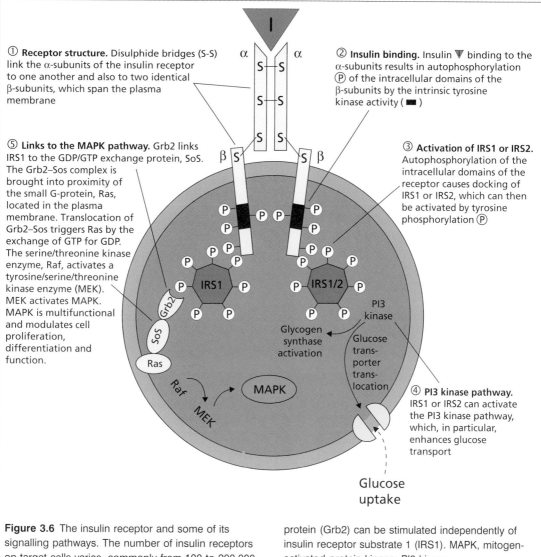

① **Receptor structure.** Disulphide bridges (S-S) link the α-subunits of the insulin receptor to one another and also to two identical β-subunits, which span the plasma membrane

② **Insulin binding.** Insulin ▼ binding to the α-subunits results in autophosphorylation ⓟ of the intracellular domains of the β-subunits by the intrinsic tyrosine kinase activity (■)

⑤ **Links to the MAPK pathway.** Grb2 links IRS1 to the GDP/GTP exchange protein, SoS. The Grb2–Sos complex is brought into proximity of the small G-protein, Ras, located in the plasma membrane. Translocation of Grb2–Sos triggers Ras by the exchange of GTP for GDP. The serine/threonine kinase enzyme, Raf, activates a tyrosine/serine/threonine kinase enzyme (MEK). MEK activates MAPK. MAPK is multifunctional and modulates cell proliferation, differentiation and function.

③ **Activation of IRS1 or IRS2.** Autophosphorylation of the intracellular domains of the receptor causes docking of IRS1 or IRS2, which can then be activated by tyrosine phosphorylation ⓟ

④ **PI3 kinase pathway.** IRS1 or IRS2 can activate the PI3 kinase pathway, which, in particular, enhances glucose transport

Glucose uptake

Figure 3.6 The insulin receptor and some of its signalling pathways. The number of insulin receptors on target cells varies, commonly from 100 to 200,000, with adipocytes and hepatocytes expressing the highest numbers. Not all insulin-signalling pathways are shown, e.g. type 2 growth factor receptor-bound protein (Grb2) can be stimulated independently of insulin receptor substrate 1 (IRS1). MAPK, mitogen-activated protein kinase; PI3 kinase, phosphatidylinositol-3-kinase; SoS, son of sevenless protein; I, insulin.

These molecular events lie at the heart of insulin's clinical action (see Part 3). Defects in the signalling pathway can result in resistance to insulin action either as rare monogenic syndromes (Box 3.4) or as a considerable part of the type 2 diabetes phenotype (see Chapters 11 and 13).

Receptors that recruit tyrosine kinase activity

The sub-family of receptors that bind growth hormone (GH) and prolactin (PRL) includes those for numerous cytokines and the hormones leptin

---

Box 3.4 Defects in the insulin signalling pathways and 'insulin resistance' syndromes

Over 50 mutations have been reported in the insulin receptor (IR) that impair glucose metabolism and raise serum insulin ('insulin resistance'). Historically, these have been discovered as different congenital syndromes; however, the advance of molecular genetics has unified these diagnoses as a phenotypic spectrum according to the severity of IR inactivation. Patients with milder insulin resistance and less affected IR signalling are usually only diagnosed at puberty, whereas what was known as 'Leprachaunism', with an effective absence of functional IR, manifests as severe intrauterine growth retardation. These latter patients rarely survive beyond the first year of life. Interestingly, the *IR* gene is seemingly normal in most patients with milder congenital insulin resistance, suggestive of abnormalities in other components of insulin signalling pathways. Indeed, some of these monogenic causes of insulin resistance have now been discovered. Impaired insulin signalling is also a very significant component of type 2 diabetes (see Chapters 11 and 13).

---

and erythropoietin (EPO). The basic receptor composition, shown in Figure 3.2, contains major homology between family members in the extracellular domain.

Growth hormone and prolactin signalling pathways – the Janus family of tyrosine kinases

Similar mechanisms govern GH and PRL receptor binding and signal transduction. Two different sites on the hormone are capable of binding receptors that dimerize. The hormone–dimerized receptor interaction leads to conformational change in the cytoplasmic regions and signal transduction. Discovery of this phenomenon has been utilized in drug design to combat excessive GH action in acromegaly (Figure 3.7). The EPO receptor also forms homodimers, i.e. two identical receptors bind together. The cytokine receptors tend to form heterodimers with diverse partner proteins.

Activation of the hormone receptor rapidly recruits one of four members of the 'Janus-associated kinase' (JAK) family of TKs (Figure 3.8), so named after the two-faced Roman deity, Janus, because of distinctive, tandem kinase domains at their carboxy-terminals. GH, PRL and EPO receptor dimerization brings together JAK2 molecules that become phosphorylated. The major downstream substrates of JAK are the STAT family of proteins (hence the term 'JAK-STAT' signalling; Figure 3.8). The name STAT comes from dual function: *s*ignal *t*ransduction, located in the cytoplasm, and nuclear *a*ctivation of *t*ranscription. Both activities rely on phosphorylation by JAK (Figure 3.8). Phosphorylated STAT proteins dissociate from the occupied receptor–kinase complex and, themselves, dimerize to gain access to the nucleus. There, they activate target genes, commonly those that regulate proliferation or the differentiation status of the target cell. One of the major targets of GH is the *IGF-I* gene (Box 3.5). JAK signalling does not focus exclusively on STAT. The GH receptor (GHR) also signals through MAPK and PI3-kinase pathways. This overlap may account for some of the rapid metabolic effects of GH (Figure 3.8).

Defects in the GH signalling pathway can result in rare syndromes of resistance to GH action (Box 3.6 and Figure 3.9).

G-protein–coupled receptors

The commonest subset of cell-surface receptors (>140 members) couple to G-proteins at the inner surface of the cell membrane, leading to the generation of intracellular second messengers such as adenosine-3′, 5′-cyclic monophosphate (cyclic AMP or cAMP), diacylglycerol (DAG) and inositol triphosphate (IP$_3$). In addition to hormones, G-protein–coupled receptors (GPCRs) also exist for glutamate, thrombin, odourants and the visual transduction of light.

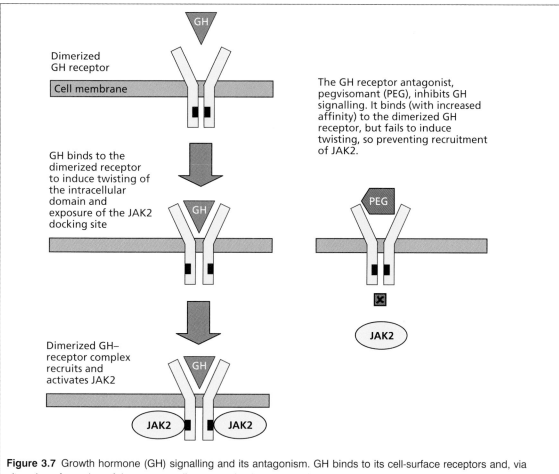

Figure 3.7 Growth hormone (GH) signalling and its antagonism. GH binds to its cell-surface receptors and, via altered conformation of the receptor dimer, recruits Janus-associated kinase 2 (JAK2). This model led to the design of the GH receptor antagonist, pegvisomant.

Box 3.5 One of the major targets of GH signalling is the *IGF-I* gene

- Measuring serum IGF-I is a useful measure of GH activity in the body

The most striking structural feature of all these receptors lies in the transmembrane domain, comprising hydrophobic helices, which cross the lipid bilayer of the plasma membrane seven times (Figure 3.10). GPCR signalling involves the hydrolysis of GTP to GDP. In their resting state, the G-proteins exist in the cell membrane as heterotrimeric complexes with α, β and γ subunits. In practice, the β and γ subunits associate with such affinity that the functional units are Gα and Gβ/γ. Hormone occupancy results in conformational change of receptor structure. In turn, this causes a conformational change in the α-subunit, leading to an exchange of GDP for GTP. The acquisition of GTP causes the α-subunit to dissociate from the Gβ/γ subunits and bind to a downstream catalytic unit, either adenylate cyclase in the generation of cAMP or phospholipase C (PLC) to produce DAG/IP₃ from phosphatidylinositol (Figures 3.10 and 3.11). The energy to activate these target enzymes comes

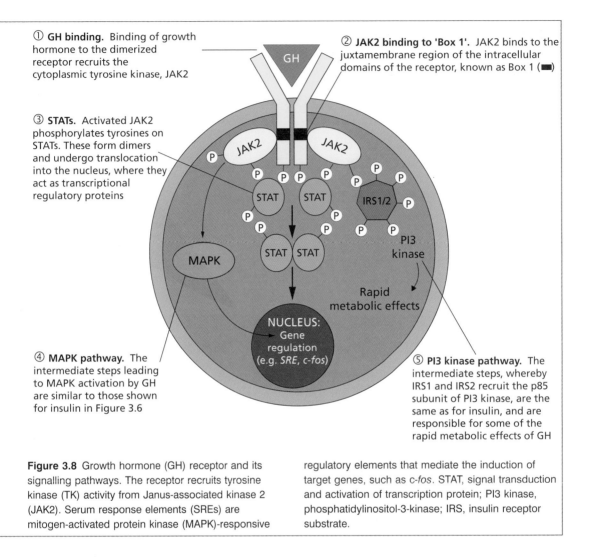

① **GH binding.** Binding of growth hormone to the dimerized receptor recruits the cytoplasmic tyrosine kinase, JAK2

② **JAK2 binding to 'Box 1'.** JAK2 binds to the juxtamembrane region of the intracellular domains of the receptor, known as Box 1 (■)

③ **STATs.** Activated JAK2 phosphorylates tyrosines on STATs. These form dimers and undergo translocation into the nucleus, where they act as transcriptional regulatory proteins

④ **MAPK pathway.** The intermediate steps leading to MAPK activation by GH are similar to those shown for insulin in Figure 3.6

⑤ **PI3 kinase pathway.** The intermediate steps, whereby IRS1 and IRS2 recruit the p85 subunit of PI3 kinase, are the same as for insulin, and are responsible for some of the rapid metabolic effects of GH

Figure 3.8 Growth hormone (GH) receptor and its signalling pathways. The receptor recruits tyrosine kinase (TK) activity from Janus-associated kinase 2 (JAK2). Serum response elements (SREs) are mitogen-activated protein kinase (MAPK)-responsive regulatory elements that mediate the induction of target genes, such as *c-fos*. STAT, signal transduction and activation of transcription protein; PI3 kinase, phosphatidylinositol-3-kinase; IRS, insulin receptor substrate.

from the cleavage of phosphate from GTP. This regenerates Gα-GDP, which no longer associates with adenylate cyclase or PLC, thus switching off the cascade and recycling the Gα-GDP back to the start.

There are over 20 isoforms of the Gα subunit that may be grouped into four major sub-families (Box 3.7). These are involved differentially with the various hormone receptor signalling pathways (Table 3.1). More than half of GPCRs can interact with different Gα subunits and thus signal through contrasting, and sometimes opposing, intracellular

second messenger systems (Figure 3.12). In part, this promiscuity can be attributed to the degree of hormonal stimulation or activation of different receptor sub-types. For instance, at low concentrations, TSH, calcitonin and LH receptors associate with $G_s\alpha$ to activate adenylate cyclase, whereas higher concentrations recruit $G_q\alpha$ to activate PLC. Calcitonin receptor sub-types are differentially expressed according to the stage of the cell cycle. Defects in the G-protein signalling pathways can result in many endocrine disorders (Box 3.8; Figures 3.13 and 3.14).

Box 3.6 Defects in growth hormone signalling pathways and growth hormone resistance syndromes

Severe resistance to GH, mainly secondary to mutations in the GH receptor that commonly affect the hormone-binding domain, is characterized by grossly impaired growth and is termed Laron syndrome, eponymously named after it was first reported by Laron in 1966 (Figure 3.9). It is an autosomal recessive disorder with a variable phenotype typified by normal or raised circulating GH and low levels of serum IGF-I.

For other patients, no *GHR* mutations have been identified, implicating genes that encode downstream components or related aspects of GH signalling. For instance, defects in the *IGF-I* gene have been associated with severe intrauterine growth retardation, mild mental retardation, sensorineural deafness and postnatal growth failure.

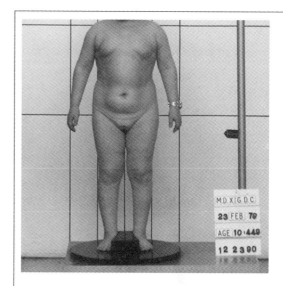

Figure 3.9 Laron syndrome showing truncal obesity. This boy presented aged 10.4 years but with a height of 95 cm – equivalent to that of a 3-year-old. In addition to truncal obesity, there is a very small penis. These features could represent severe growth hormone (GH) deficiency. However, serum GH levels were elevated with undetectable insulin-like growth factor I (IGF-I) indicative of GH resistance. Laron syndrome was diagnosed due to an inactivating mutation of the gene encoding the GH receptor. Other clinical features include a prominent forehead, depressed nasal bridge and under-development of the mandible.

Second messenger pathways

Cyclic adenosine monophosphate

Activation of membrane-bound adenylate cyclase catalyzes the conversion of ATP to the potent second messenger cAMP (see Figure 3.11). cAMP interacts with protein kinase A (PKA) to unmask its catalytic site, which phosphorylates serine and threonine residues on a transcription factor called cAMP response element binding protein (CREB) (Figure 3.15). CREB then translocates to the nucleus where it binds to a short palindromic sequence in the regulatory regions of cAMP-regulated genes. This signalling pathway controls major metabolic pathways, including those for lipolysis, glycogenolysis and steroidogenesis.

The cAMP response is terminated by a large family of phosphodiesterases (PDEs), which can be activated by a variety of systems, including phos-

phorylation by PKA in a negative feedback loop. PDEs rapidly hydrolyze cAMP to the inactive 5′-AMP. In addition, activated PKA can phosphorylate serine and threonine residues of the GPCR to cause receptor desensitization.

Diacylglycerol and Ca²⁺

Signalling from hormones, such as TRH, GnRH and oxytocin, recruits G-protein complexes containing the Gqα subunit. This activates membrane-associated PLC, which catalyzes the conversion of PI 4,5-bisphosphate (PIP_2) to DAG and IP_3 (Figures 3.11 and 3.16). IP_3 stimulates the transient release of calcium from the endoplasmic reticulum to activate several calcium-sensitive enzymes, including

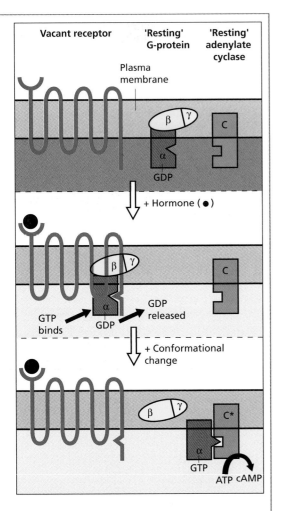

Figure 3.10 G-protein–coupled receptors. The extracellular domain is ligand specific and, hence, less conserved across family members (e.g. only 35–45% for the TSH, LH and FSH receptors). The transmembrane domain has a characteristic heptahelical structure, most of which is embedded in the cell membrane and provides a hydrophobic core. Conserved cysteine residues can form a disulphide bridge between the second and third extracellular loops. The cytoplasmic domain links the receptor to the signal-transducing G-proteins and, in this example, is linked to membrane-bound adenylate cyclase. The activation of adenylate cyclase is depicted by the conversion of C to C*.

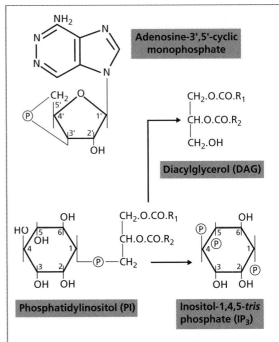

Figure 3.11 Second messengers that mediate G-protein–coupled receptor signalling. The symbol P is the abbreviation for a phosphate group. Carbon atoms are numbered in their ring position. R_1 and R_2 represent fatty acid chains.

Box 3.7 Sub-families of Gα protein subunits

- $G_s\alpha$: activates adenylate cyclase
- $G_i\alpha$: inhibits adenylate cyclase
- $G_q\alpha$: activates PLC
- $G_o\alpha$: activates ion channels

isoforms of protein kinase C (PKC), and proteins like calmodulin (Figure 3.16). Calcium ions also activate cytosolic guanylate cyclase, an enzyme that catalyzes the formation of cyclic guanosine monophosphate (cGMP). The effects of atrial natriuretic peptide are mediated by receptors linked to guanylate cyclase.

The major target of DAG signalling is PKC, which activates phospholipase A_2 to liberate arachidonic acid from phospholipids and generate potent eicosanoids, including thromboxanes, leucotrienes,

Table 3.1 Use of different G-protein α-subunits by various hormone signalling pathways	
Hormone	**Dominant G-protein α-subunit(s)**
Thyrotrophin-releasing hormone (TRH)	Gqα
Corticotrophin-releasing hormone (CRH)	Gsα
Gonadotrophin-releasing hormone (GnRH)	Gqα
Somatostatin (SS)	Giα/Gqα
Thyroid-stimulating hormone (TSH)	Gsα/Gqα
Luteinizing hormone (LH)/human chorionic gonadotrophin (hCG)	Gsα/Gqα
Follicle-stimulating hormone (FSH)	Gsα/Gqα
Adrenocorticotrophic hormone (ACTH)	Gsα
Oxytocin	Gqα
Vasopressin	Gsα/Gqα
Catecholamines (β-adrenergic)	Gsα
Angiotensin II (AII)	Giα/Gqα
Glucagon	Gsα
Calcium	Gqα/Giα
Calcitonin	Gsα/Giα/Gqα
Parathyroid hormone (PTH)/PTH-related peptide (PTHrP)	Gsα/Gqα
Prostaglandin E$_2$	Gsα

For signalling by SS, vasopressin, AII, calcitonin and PTH/PTHrP, different receptor sub-types, potentially in different tissues, determine α-subunit specificity. This provides opportunities for selective antagonist therapies.

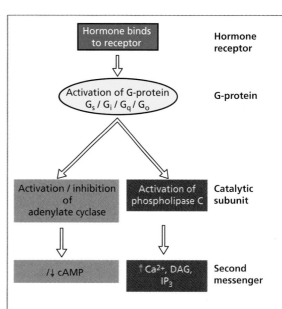

Figure 3.12 Hormonal activation of G-protein–coupled receptors can link to different second messenger pathways. The two alternative pathways are not mutually exclusive and may, in fact, interact.

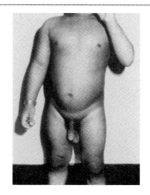

Figure 3.13 Familial male precocious puberty ('testotoxicosis'). This 2-year-old presented with signs of precocious puberty. Note the musculature, pubic hair and size of the testes and penis. He was the size of a 4-year-old. His overnight gonadotrophins [luteinizing hormone (LH) and follicle stimulating hormone] were undetectable as the testosterone was arising autonomously from Leydig cells due to a gain-of-function mutation in the gene encoding the LH receptor (see Box 3.8).

Box 3.8 Defects in the G-protein–coupled receptor/G-protein signalling pathways

Several endocrinopathies occur because of activating or inactivating mutations in genes encoding GPCRs or G-proteins coupled to them. Activating mutations cause constitutive overactivity; inactivating mutations cause hormone resistance syndromes characterized by high circulating hormone levels but diminished hormone action.

Gain of function
- LH receptor: male precocious puberty (Figure 3.13)
- TSH receptor: 'toxic' thyroid adenomas
- $G_s\alpha$: McCune–Albright syndrome (Figure 3.14), some cases of acromegaly and some autonomous thyroid nodules

Loss of function
- V2 receptor: nephrogenic diabetes insipidus (high vasopressin)
- TSH receptor: resistance to TSH (high TSH)
- $G_s\alpha$: pseudohypoparathyroidism (see Figure 9.9) and Albright hereditary osteodystrophy

lipoxins and prostaglandins (Figure 3.17). The latter are well-recognized paracrine and autocrine mediators capable of amplifying or prolonging a response to a hormonal stimulus.

Nuclear receptors

The second superfamily of hormone receptor is the nuclear receptors, which are classified by their ligands, small lipophilic molecules that diffuse across the plasma membrane of target cells. Once ligand bound, the receptors typically bind DNA and function as transcription factors (Figure 3.18). This need for transcription and translation to elicit an effect means that biological responses of nuclear receptors are relatively slow compared to cell-surface receptor signalling.

Distinct regions of nuclear receptors can be identified, for which evolutionary conservation can be as high as 60–90%, i.e. the receptors are structurally related (Figure 3.19). For one sub-group of the superfamily, no endogenous ligand has been identified and they are termed 'orphan' nuclear receptors. In addition, some variant receptors have atypical DNA-binding domains and potentially function via indirect interaction with the genome. All the different types are associated with endocrinopathies, usually due to loss of function.

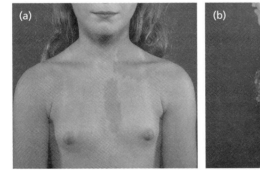
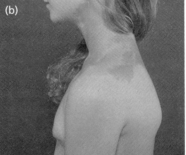

Figure 3.14 McCune–Albright syndrome. At 6 years of age, this girl presented with breast development and vaginal bleeding in the absence of gonadotrophins. An activating mutation in $G_s\alpha$ had created independence from melanocyte-stimulating hormone (MSH) causing skin pigmentation ('café-au-lait' spots) and similar constitutive activation in the ovary (i.e. independence from gonadotrophins), giving rise to premature breast development. In some cases, constitutive overactivity can manifest in bones (causing 'fibrous dysplasia'), the adrenal cortex (Cushing syndrome) and the thyroid (thyrotoxicosis). From Brook's Clinical Pediatric Endocrinology, Sixth Edition, Charles G. D. Brook, Peter E. Clayton, Rosalind S. Brown, Eds. Blackwell Publishing Limited. 2009.

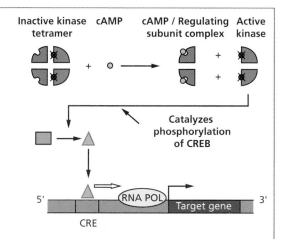

Figure 3.15 The activation of protein kinase A, a cAMP-dependent protein kinase. The four-subunit complex is inactive. When cAMP binds to the regulatory subunits (red), dissociation occurs so that the active kinase subunits (blue) are released to catalyze the phosphorylation of the cAMP response element-binding protein (CREB). This activates CREB (■ → ▲) so that it can bind to its DNA target, the cAMP response element (CRE), to switch on transcription of cAMP-inducible genes. RNA POL, RNA polymerase.

The receptors predominantly reside in the nucleus, although increasingly nuclear import and export appears to be an important regulatory mechanism, controlling access of the nuclear receptor to target gene DNA. This shuttling has been long recognized for the glucocorticoid receptor (Figure 3.18).

Target cell conversion of hormones destined for nuclear receptors

In many instances, the ligand for the nuclear receptor undergoes enzymatic modification within the target cell. This converts the circulating hormone into a more or less potent metabolite prior to receptor binding (Table 3.2). For instance, cortisol is metabolized to cortisone by type 2 11β-hydroxysteroid dehydrogenase (HSD11B2). In kidney tubular cells, this inactivation preserves aldosterone action at the mineralocorticoid receptor (MR). Without this, cortisol, present in the circulation

at much higher concentrations than aldosterone, might saturate the MR, causing inappropriate overactivity. Accordingly, impaired function of HSD11B2 leads to hypertension and hypokalaemia in the syndrome of 'apparent mineralocorticoid excess'.

Nuclear localization, DNA binding and transcriptional activation

In their resting state, unbound steroid hormone receptors associate with heat-shock proteins, which obscure the DNA-binding domain, so that they are considered incapable of binding the genome. Steroid binding causes conformational change and dissociation of the heat-shock proteins. This reveals two polypeptide loops stabilized by zinc ions, known as zinc fingers. Once two steroid receptors have dimerized, these motifs bind to target DNA at the specific hormone response element (HRE) (Figure 3.20).

The unliganded thyroid hormone receptor (TR) is located in the nucleus bound to DNA at the thyroid hormone response element (TRE). In the absence of hormone, the TR dimerizes with the retinoid X receptor and tends to recruit nuclear proteins that inhibit transcription (co-repressors). The binding of thyroid hormone leads to dissociation of these factors, the recruitment of transcriptional co-activators, and a sequence of events recruiting DNA-dependent RNA polymerase leading to transcription (Figure 3.20 and review Figure 2.2).

Resistance syndromes for nuclear receptors are similar to those for cell-surface receptors. Inactivating mutations lead to loss of receptor function, such as reduced hormone binding or impaired receptor dimerization, loss of hormone action, for instance decreased binding to the HRE, and, characteristically, raised circulating hormone levels (Table 3.3).

Orphan nuclear receptors and variant nuclear receptors

Some orphan and variant receptors play very important roles in endocrinology. For instance,

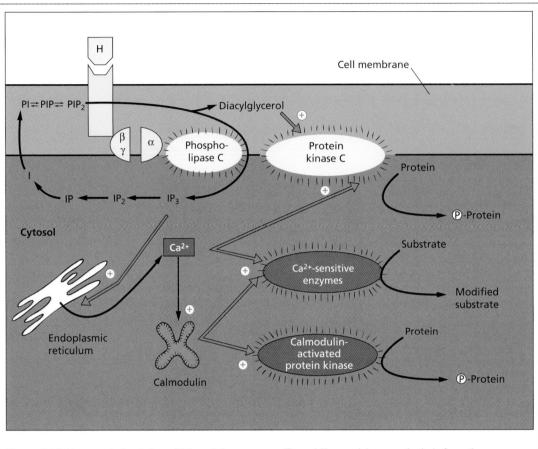

Figure 3.16 Hormonal stimulation of intracellular phospholipid turnover and calcium metabolism. Phosphatidylinositol (PI) metabolism includes the membrane intermediaries, PI monophosphate (PIP) and PI bisphosphate (PIP$_2$). Hormone action stimulates phospholipase C, which hydrolyzes PIP$_2$ to diacylglycerol (DAG) and inositol triphosphate (IP$_3$). IP$_3$ mobilizes calcium, particularly from the endoplasmic reticulum. DAG activates protein kinase C and increases its affinity for calcium ions, which further enhances activation. Collectively, these events stimulate phosphorylation cascades of proteins and enzymes that alter intracellular metabolism.

steroidogenic factor 1 (SF1, also called NR5A1) is a critical mediator of endocrine organ formation. Without it, the anterior pituitary gonadotrophs, adrenal gland and gonad fail to develop. It is also critical for the ongoing expression of many important genes within these cell types (e.g. the enzymes that orchestrate steroidogenesis; see Figure 2.6). A variant receptor with a similar expression profile is DAX1 (also called NROB1), mutation of which causes congenital adrenal hypoplasia (i.e. under-development). Duplication of the region that includes the gene encoding DAX1 causes male-to-female sex reversal (see Chapters 6 and 7). Increasingly, endogenous compounds are being identified that occupy the three-dimensional structure created by the ligand-binding domain. Whether these substances are the true hormone ligands remains debatable.

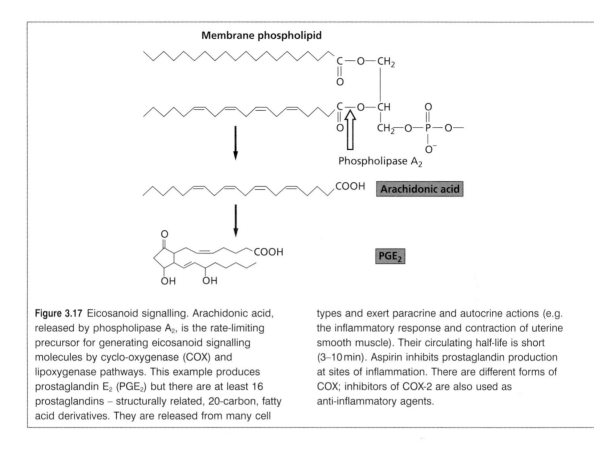

Membrane phospholipid

Phospholipase A$_2$

COOH Arachidonic acid

COOH PGE$_2$

Figure 3.17 Eicosanoid signalling. Arachidonic acid, released by phospholipase A$_2$, is the rate-limiting precursor for generating eicosanoid signalling molecules by cyclo-oxygenase (COX) and lipoxygenase pathways. This example produces prostaglandin E$_2$ (PGE$_2$) but there are at least 16 prostaglandins – structurally related, 20-carbon, fatty acid derivatives. They are released from many cell types and exert paracrine and autocrine actions (e.g. the inflammatory response and contraction of uterine smooth muscle). Their circulating half-life is short (3–10 min). Aspirin inhibits prostaglandin production at sites of inflammation. There are different forms of COX; inhibitors of COX-2 are also used as anti-inflammatory agents.

Endocrine transcription factors

Although distinct from the nuclear receptor super-family, other transcription factors play critical roles in the endocrine system, both during its development and in regulating its differentiated function (Table 3.4). This is important to the endocrinologist because inactivating mutations in the transcription factors can be a cause of endocrine pathology, particularly in the paediatric clinic, where molecular genetics can increasingly provide precise diagnostic answers (see Chapter 4). For instance, in the pituitary, pituitary-specific transcription factor 1 (PIT1) regulates the expression of genes encoding GH, PRL and the β-subunit of TSH. Patients with inactivating *PIT1* mutations show reduced, or absent, levels of these hormones, causing short stature, and are at risk of congenital secondary hypothyroidism with severe learning disability.

The development of the pancreas and, in particular, the specification and function of β-cells relies on several transcription factors. Pancreas duodenal homeobox factor 1 [PDX1, also called insulin promoter factor 1 (IPF1)] and several members of the hepatocyte nuclear factor (HNF) family are critical in this regard; inactivating mutations have been identified, which cause monogenic diabetes mellitus at an early age, called maturity-onset diabetes of the young (MODY) (see Table 11.3). Potentially, these patients never accrue a normal number of β-cells, which also fail to function properly.

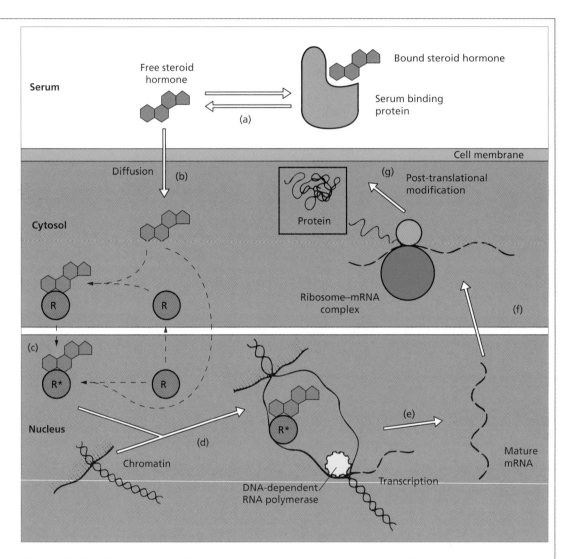

Figure 3.18 Simplified schematic of nuclear hormone action. (a) Free hormone (a steroid is shown), in equilibrium with that bound to protein, diffuses across the target cell membrane. (b) Inside the cell, free hormone binds to its receptor (Ⓡ). This may occur in the cell cytoplasm (e.g. glucocorticoid receptor) or in the cell nucleus (e.g. thyroid hormone receptor). (c) The activated hormone–receptor complex (Ⓡ*), now present in the nucleus, binds to the hormone-response element of its target genes. (d) This interaction promotes DNA-dependent RNA polymerase (Pol II) to start transcription of mRNA. (e) Post-transcriptional modification and splicing sees the mRNA exit the nucleus for translation into protein on ribosomes. Post-translational modification provides the final protein.

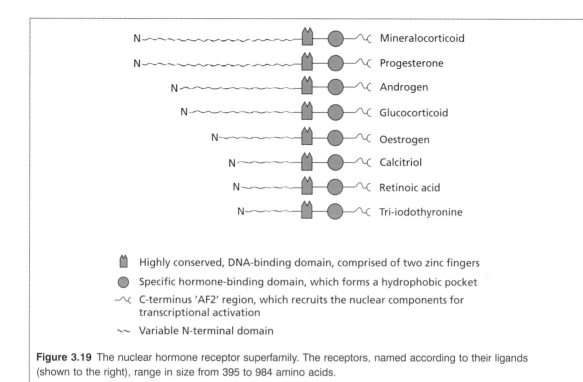

N ~~~~~~~~~~~~⌂⬤~C Mineralocorticoid

N ~~~~~~~~~~~⌂⬤~C Progesterone

N ~~~~~~~~⌂⬤~C Androgen

N ~~~~~~⌂⬤~C Glucocorticoid

N ~~~~~⌂⬤~C Oestrogen

N ~~~~⌂⬤~C Calcitriol

N ~~~⌂⬤~C Retinoic acid

N ~~~⌂⬤~C Tri-iodothyronine

⌂ Highly conserved, DNA-binding domain, comprised of two zinc fingers

⬤ Specific hormone-binding domain, which forms a hydrophobic pocket

~C C-terminus 'AF2' region, which recruits the nuclear components for transcriptional activation

~~ Variable N-terminal domain

Figure 3.19 The nuclear hormone receptor superfamily. The receptors, named according to their ligands (shown to the right), range in size from 395 to 984 amino acids.

Table 3.2 Potential modifications of hormones, their precursors and metabolites within the cell prior to nuclear receptor action

Modification that increases activity	Modification that decreases activity
Deiodination of thyroxine (T_4) to tri-iodothyronine (T_3) by type 1 and type 2 selenodeiodinase (see Figure 8.6)	Inactivation of T_4 and T_3 by the formation of reverse T_3 and di-iodothyronine (T_2) by type 3 selenodeiodinase (see Figure 8.6)
Reduction of testosterone to dihydrotestosterone (DHT) by 5α-reductase (see Figure 7.7); gain of oestrogenic activity by conversion of testosterone to oestradiol by the action of aromatase (CYP19; see Figure 2.6)	Loss of androgenic activity by conversion of testosterone to oestradiol by the action of aromatase (CYP19; see Figure 2.6)
Conversion of 25-hydroxyvitamin D to 1,25-dihydroxyvitamin D (calcitriol) by 1α-hydroxylase (see Figure 9.2)	Conversion of 25-hydroxyvitamin D to 24,25-dihydroxyvitamin D or the inactivation of 1,25-dihydroxyvitamin D to 1,24,25-trihydroxyvitamin D by 24α-hydroxylase (see Figure 9.2)
Generation of cortisol from cortisone by type 1 11β-hydroxysteroid dehydrogenase (HSD11B1; see Figure 6.4)	Inactivation of cortisol to cortisone by Type 2 11β-hydroxysteroid dehydrogenase (HSD11B2; see Figure 6.4)

The biological importance of these modifying enzymes is exemplified by rare mutations in the genes that encode them, presenting with endocrine overactivity or underactivity.

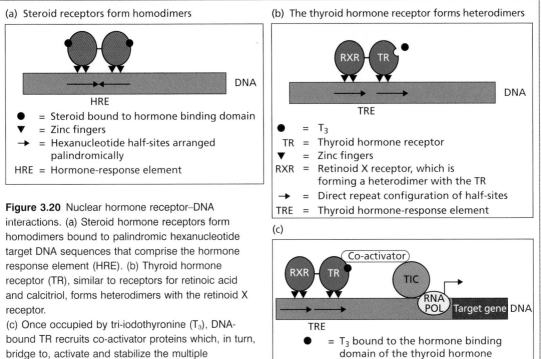

(a) Steroid receptors form homodimers

DNA

HRE

● = Steroid bound to hormone binding domain
▼ = Zinc fingers
→ = Hexanucleotide half-sites arranged palindromically
HRE = Hormone-response element

Figure 3.20 Nuclear hormone receptor–DNA interactions. (a) Steroid hormone receptors form homodimers bound to palindromic hexanucleotide target DNA sequences that comprise the hormone response element (HRE). (b) Thyroid hormone receptor (TR), similar to receptors for retinoic acid and calcitriol, forms heterodimers with the retinoid X receptor.
(c) Once occupied by tri-iodothyronine (T_3), DNA-bound TR recruits co-activator proteins which, in turn, bridge to, activate and stabilize the multiple components of the transcription initiation complex at the basal promoter of the target gene.

(b) The thyroid hormone receptor forms heterodimers

RXR TR

DNA

TRE

● = T_3
TR = Thyroid hormone receptor
▼ = Zinc fingers
RXR = Retinoid X receptor, which is forming a heterodimer with the TR
→ = Direct repeat configuration of half-sites
TRE = Thyroid hormone-response element

(c)

Co-activator

RXR TR TIC

RNA POL Target gene DNA

TRE

● = T_3 bound to the hormone binding domain of the thyroid hormone receptor (TR)
▼ = Zinc fingers
RXR = Retinoid X receptor
TIC = Transcription initiation complex
RNA POL = RNA polymerase
TRE = Thyroid hormone-response element

Table 3.3 Defects in nuclear hormone signalling

Mutations in receptor for	Clinical effects
Androgen (AR)	Partial or complete androgen insensitivity syndromes
Glucocorticoid (GR)	Generalized inherited glucocorticoid resistance
Oestrogen (ER)	Oestrogen resistance
Thyroid hormone (TR)	Thyroid hormone resistance
Vitamin D (VDR)	Vitamin D (calcitriol)-resistant rickets

Table 3.4 Some important transcription factors required for development and function of endocrine cell types and organs

Organ or cell type	Transcription factor
Adrenal gland	SF-1, DAX1, CITED2
Enteroendocrine cells	NGN3
Gonad	WT1, SRY, SOX9, SF-1, DAX1
Pancreas/islets of Langerhans	PDX1, SOX9, HLXB9, NGN3, PAX6, PAX4, RFX6, NKX2.2, NKX6.1, NeuroD1 (also see Table 13.3)
Parathyroid gland	TBX1 (part of Di George syndrome; see Figure 4.4), GATA3
Pituitary	PIT1, PROP1, HESX1, PITX2, SF-1, DAX1, LHX3, LHX4
Thyroid gland	PAX8, FOXE1, NKX2.1

Key points

- Hormones act by binding to receptors and triggering intracellular responses
- Tissue distribution of the receptor determines where a hormone will exert its effect
- The two major subdivisions of hormone receptors are classified by site of action: cell surface and nuclear
- Peptide hormones and catecholamines act via cell-surface receptors and generate fast responses in seconds or minutes
- Steroid and thyroid hormones act via nuclear receptors to alter expression of target genes; a slow response occurs because of the need to produce protein from the expression of target genes
- Mutations in genes encoding any part of the cascade from hormone receptor to action can result in underactive or overactive endocrinopathy, or potentially tumour formation

CHAPTER 4
Investigations in endocrinology and diabetes

Key topics

- Laboratory assay platforms   49
- Cell and molecular biology as diagnostic tools   56
- Imaging in endocrinology   57
- Key points   61

Learning objectives

- To understand how circulating hormones are measured by a range of different immunoassays
- To understand other laboratory investigations as applied to clinical endocrinology and diabetes
- To understand the molecular biology that underpins genetic diagnoses
- To understand the options available for imaging the endocrine system

This chapter details how clinical endocrinology and diabetes is investigated

All specialties have been advanced by methods to aid diagnosis, and monitor and assess treatment. Investigation in endocrinology and diabetes remains centred on laboratory assays that determine the concentration of hormones and metabolites usually in blood. The first challenge is correct collection; for some investigations, prior fasting is important. Appropriate conditions or preservatives are mandatory (Box 4.1). In addition to clinical biochemistry (also called chemical pathology), molecular genetics and cytogenetics are routine investigations to provide personalized genetic diagnoses that predict the course of some endocrine disorders (e.g. multiple endocrine neoplasia; see Chapter 10).

Outside of the laboratory, clinical investigation draws heavily upon expertise in radiology and nuclear medicine. Some investigations are highly specific (e.g. visual fields for pituitary tumours or retinal screening for diabetes) and these are covered in later topic-specific chapters.

Laboratory assay platforms

Immunoassays

Hormones (and other metabolites) are most commonly measured by immunoassay, although increasingly mass spectrometry is used (see below). Immunoassays, introduced in the 1960s, are sufficiently sensitive, precise and hormone specific for routine application in clinical biochemistry. Bioassays, which measure physiological responses induced by a stimulus, are near obsolete in clinical practice.

Immunoassay is a broad term for one of two different techniques: true immunoassay and immunometric assay. Both forms are based on the hormone to be measured being antigenic and bound by specific antibodies to form an antibody–antigen complex. Both forms of immunoassay also employ a label, historically a radioactive isotope [e.g. iodine-125 (I^{125})], but commonly now a fluorescent tracer, to generate a quantitative signal. Both assays also rely on comparison of the patient sample with known concentrations of a reference compound.

Box 4.1 The specifics of sample collection are mandatory

Containers for investigation of blood
- Lithium heparin: most hormones
- Fluoride oxalate: glucose
- Di-potassium EDTA: tests requiring DNA isolation

Peptide hormones and catecholamines tend to be less stable than other hormones and need prompt delivery to the laboratory on ice

Samples for which prior fasting may be required
- Glucose
- Lipids
- Calcium

Hormones that may require 9 AM collection
- Cortisol
- Testosterone

Containers for investigation of urine
- Acid: calcium, 5-hydroxyindoleacetic acid (5-HIAA), catecholamines
- No acid/simple preservative: urinary free cortisol

To set up a calibration or standard curve for the immunoassay, a constant amount of antibody is added to a series of tubes with increasing, known amounts of a reference preparation, in this example GH (Figure 4.1). This reaction is reversible with the antigen and antibody continuously associating and dissociating; however, after incubation, equilibrium is reached when tubes with more GH generate more bound complex. Measurement of the amount of bound complex (e.g. in terms of fluorescence or radioactivity) can thus be related to the quantity of GH that was originally added. This allows a calibration curve to be plotted, against which the same process can now deduce the GH concentration in a patient sample.

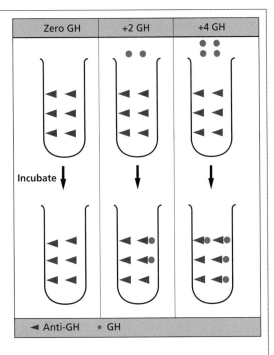

Figure 4.1 The basics of immunoassay are shown for growth hormone (GH; see text for details). For clarity, in Figures 4.1–4.3 only small numbers of hormone molecules and antibodies are shown; in practice, numbers are in the order of 10^8–10^{13}.

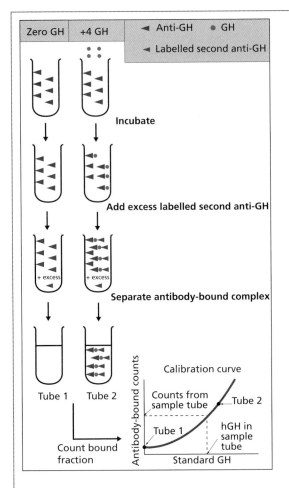

Figure 4.2 The basics of an immunometric assay for growth hormone (GH; also see text). As in Figure 4.1, in practice large numbers of molecules are present for each reagent and the incubation of the first and second antibodies is usually simultaneous. Because the hormone is bound between the two antibodies in the triple complex (◄•◄), this assay is sometimes referred to as a sandwich assay. Separation of the complex from the excess labelled second antibody is usually achieved physically, e.g. by precipitation and centrifugation (the supernatant contains the unbound antibody and is discarded). This leaves the bound labelled second antibody to be quantified by counting radioactivity or measuring fluorescence. The low measurement from the 'zero' tube, Tube 1, and the higher value from Tube 2 are plotted on the calibration curve. Tube 1 is not zero because of minor non-specific antibody binding. The calibration line is also curved, rather than straight, because of the reversible nature of the interaction between antibodies and their antigens. In practice, five to eight calibration points are used to construct the curve.

Immunometric assays – the sandwich assays

In the immunometric assay (shown for GH in Figure 4.2), a constant amount of antibody is added to each tube with increasing, known amounts of reference preparation. After incubation, the amount of GH bound to the antibody is detected by adding an excess of a second labelled antibody to all tubes. The second antibody is directed against a different antigenic site on GH from the first antibody to form a triple complex sandwiching GH between the two antibodies. Any unbound antibody is removed, leaving the amount of triple complex to be determined by quantifying the bound label (e.g. fluorescence or radioactivity). This emission is plotted for increasing, known amounts of reference compound to generate a calibration curve (Figure 4.2). In practice, five to eight concentrations of hormone standard are used to generate a precise calibration curve, against which patient samples can be interpolated. The immunometric assay is suitable only when the hormone to be measured permits discrete binding of two antibodies. This would not work for small hormones such as thyroxine (T_4) or tri-iodothyronine (T_3), for which the competitive-binding immunoassay system must be used.

Immunoassays – the competitive-binding assays

In the competitive-binding immunoassay (shown for T_4 in Figure 4.3), constant amounts of antibody and labelled antigen are added to each tube. A 'zero' tube is set up that contains labelled T_4, as well as a tube that also includes a known amount of unlabelled standard T_4. Incubation allows the antigen–antibody complex to form. Since the zero tube contains twice as much labelled T_4 as antibody, half of the labelled hormone will be bound and the other half will remain free (i.e. in excess). In the other tube, unlabelled and labelled T_4 compete for the limited opportunity to bind antibody. The total antibody-bound T_4 is separated (e.g. by precipitation) and the label measured (e.g. by fluorescence or radioactivity). There will be less signal from the second tube because of competition from the unlabelled T_4; the decrease will be a function of the amount of unlabelled T_4 added, i.e. the signal decreases as the amount of unlabelled T_4 increases, allowing the construction of a calibration curve (Figure 4.3). For clinical use, standard T_4 is replaced by the patient sample, with all other assay conditions kept the same. As for immunometric assays, a five to eight point calibration curve offers sufficient precision for patient samples to be interpolated.

Analytical methods linked to mass spectrometry

In some situations, immunoassays are unreliable or unavailable, commonly because antibodies lack sufficient specificity, or there are difficulties with measurements at low concentrations (e.g. serum testosterone in women). This leads to differences in measurements across different assay platforms that inhibit the development of internationally agreed standards for diagnosis and care. For some steroid or peptide hormones, or metabolic intermediaries, mass spectrometry (MS) is becoming increasing

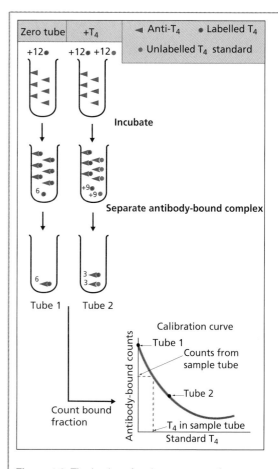

Figure 4.3 The basics of an immunoassay for thyroxine (T4; also see text). As in Figure 4.1, in practice large numbers of molecules are present for each reagent. Under the conditions shown, the competition between equal amounts of labelled and unlabelled T_4 in Tube 2 will be such that, on average, 50% of the antibody binding sites will be occupied by labelled T_4. Because of competition between labelled and unlabelled hormone for a limited amount of antibody, this type of immunoassay is sometimes called a 'competitive-binding' assay. After removing unbound label (as in Figure 4.2 legend), the fluorescent or radioactive bound fraction is quantified and a calibration curve constructed. In practice, five to eight calibration points are used to construct the curve.

helpful. It is applied either by itself or, for increased ability to resolve and measure substances, in tandem (MS/MS) or downstream of liquid chromatography (LC/MS) or gas chromatography (GC/MS). These approaches provide definitive identification of the relevant hormone or compound according to its chemical and physical characteristics, e.g. particularly useful for the unequivocal detection of performance-enhancing agents in sport.

GC allows separation of vaporized molecules according to their chemical structure. For a sample loaded on a GC column, different components exit the column and pass to the mass spectrometer at different times. MS ionizes compounds to charge them, after which the spectrometer measures mass and charge during passage through an electromagnetic field. This gives a characteristic mass-to-charge ratio for any one substance. As with immunoassays, patient samples can be judged against the performance of precisely known standards. LC/MS is similar to GC/MS; however, the initial separation is performed in the liquid rather than the gaseous phase.

Enzymatic assays

Some metabolites are assayed enzymatically, frequently using dye substrates that are catalyzed to products that are coloured or fluoresce. By incorporating known standards, the amount of colour or fluorescence can be used for precise quantification. For example, glycated haemoglobin (HbA$_{1c}$), a measure of long-term diabetes control (see Chapter 11) can be measured in an enzymatic assay as well as by immunoassay and chromatography/MS approaches. Serum glucose can be measured by oxidation to generate a product that interacts with a dye to generate colour or fluorescence in an enzymatic assay.

Reference ranges

Typical adult reference ranges are listed for a number of hormones in Table 4.1. Whenever possible, hormones are measured in molar units (e.g. pmol/L) or mass units (e.g. ng/L). However, this is not possible for complex hormones such as the glycoproteins thyroid-stimulating hormone (TSH), luteinizing hormone (LH) and follicle-stimulating hormone (FSH),

because they circulate in a variety of slightly different forms ('microheterogeneity'). In this scenario, international reference preparations are agreed, with potency expressed in 'units' (U) and their subdivisions [e.g. milliunits (mU)]. Potency is assigned after large collaborative trials involving many laboratories worldwide using a range of assay platforms and physical analytical techniques. Patient results are then expressed relative to the reference data.

Static and dynamic testing

Most of endocrinology testing is 'static'; the measurement of hormones and metabolites as they circulate at any one time. However, rhythmical, pulsatile or variable hormone secretion makes interpretation of single random samples meaningless or misleading (see Chapter 1). For some hormones, such as GH, a clinical impression can be gained from a series of six to eight measurements during the course of a day. Alternatively, dynamic testing can be necessary where, based on understanding normal physiology, responses are measured following a stimulus. This might be metabolic, such as insulin-induced hypoglycaemia to study the expected rise in serum GH and cortisol (see Chapter 5), or the administration of glucose during a glucose tolerance test to diagnose diabetes (see Chapter 11). Alternatively, the stimulus might be hormonal, such as injecting adrenocorticotrophic hormone (ACTH; the anterior pituitary hormone) to measure secretion of cortisol (the adrenocortical hormone). In this sense, fasting measurements, as required for serum lipids or commonly for glucose, could be viewed as dynamic, where fasting is the stimulus.

Dynamic tests can be split into two categories: provocative ones to interrogate suspected inadequate function; or suppression tests, taking advantage of negative feedback to investigate potential overactivity (Box 4.2). For instance, ACTH is injected to see if cortisol secretion rises in suspected adrenocortical inadequacy (Addison disease; see Chapter 6); whereas dexamethasone, a potent synthetic glucocorticoid, is given to see if pituitary ACTH and consequently cortisol secretion is appropriately diminished. If it is not, it implies that the adrenal cortex is overactive (Cushing syndrome; see Chapter 6).

Table 4.1 Endocrine reference ranges

Adult reference hormone	Range	Units	Range	Unit
17-hydroxyprogesterone (male)	0.18–9.1	nmol/L	5.9–300	ng/dL
17-hydroxyprogesterone (female)	0.6–3.0	nmol/L	20–99	ng/dL
Adrenocorticotrophic hormone (ACTH, 9 AM)	0–8.8	pmol/L	0–40	ng/L
Aldosterone (AM; out of bed for 2 h; seated 5–15 min)[a]	100–500	pmol/L	3.6–18.1	ng/dL
Androstenedione (adult male and female)	2.1–9.4	nmol/L	60–270	ng/dL
Anti-Müllerian hormone (to indicate poor ovarian reserve)[b]	>7	pmol/L	>1	ng/mL
Chromogranin A (fasting)	0–5.2	nmol/L	0–250	ng/ml
Cortisol (9 AM)[c]	140–700	nmol/L	5–25	µg/dL
Cortisol (midnight)	80–350	nmol/L	2.9–12.5	µg/dL
Cortisol (post low dose dexamethsaone)	<50	nmol/L	1.8	µg/dL
Cortisol (urinary free)	0–280	nmol/24 h	0–10	µg/24 h
Epinephrine (adrenaline)	0–546	pmol/L	0–100	pg/mL
Epinephrine (adrenaline; urine)	0–1.0	µmol/24 h	0.5–20	µg/24 h
Follicle-stimulating hormone (FSH)				
Males (adult)	1.0–8.0	U/L	–	–
Females				
Early follicular phase	1.0–11.0	U/L	–	–
Post-menopausal	>30	U/L	–	–
Gastrin (fasting)	0–40	pmol/L	0–154	pg/mL
Glucagon (fasting)	0–50	pmol/L	0–139	pg/mL
Glucose				
Fasting (normal)	<6.1	mmol/L	<110	mg/dL
Fasting (impaired fasting glycaemia; 'pre-diabetes')	6.1–6.9	mmol/L	110–125	mg/dL
Fasting (diabetes)	≥7.0	mmol/L	≥126	mg/dL
Post-glucose tolerance test (normal)	<7.8	mmol/L	<140	mg/dL

(*Continued*)

Table 4.1 (*Continued*)

Adult reference hormone	Range	Units	Range	Unit
Post-glucose tolerance test (impaired glucose tolerance; 'pre-diabetes')	7.8–11.0	mmol/L	140–200	mg/dL
Post-glucose tolerance test (diabetes)	≥11.1	mmol/L	≥200	mg/dL
Growth hormone				
After a glucose load	<0.3[d]	ng/mL	<0.8	mU/L
Stress-induced [e.g. glucose <2.2 mmol/L (<40 mg/dL)]	>6.7	ng/mL	>17	mU/L
HbA$_{1c}$ (to diagnose diabetes)[e]	≥47	mmol/mol	≥6.5	%
Insulin				
Fasting	<69.5	pmol/L	<10	mU/L
When glucose <2.5 mmol/L (<45 mg/dL)	<34.7	pmol/L	<5	mU/L
When glucose <1.5 mmol/L (<27 mg/dL)	<13.9	pmol/L	<2	mU/L
Insulin-like growth factor I[f]				
25–39 years	114–492	ng/mL	–	–
40–54 years	90–360	ng/mL	–	–
>54 years	71–290	ng/mL	–	–
Luteinizing hormone (LH)				
Males	0.5–9.0	U/L	–	–
Females				
Early follicular phase	0.5–14.5	U/L	–	–
Postmenopausal	>20	U/L	–	–
Metanephrine	0–0.5	nmol/L	0–99	pg/mL
Metanephrine (urine)	0–2.0	µmol/24 h	24–96	µg/24 h
Norepinephrine (noradrenaline)	0–3.5	nmol/L	0–600	pg/mL
Norepinephrine (urine)	0–0.2	µmol/24 h	15–80	µg/24 h
Normetanephrine	0–1.0	nmol/L	0–180	pg/mL
Normetanephrine (urine)	0–3.0	µmol/24 h	75–375	µg/24 h
Oestradiol				
Males	37–130	pmol/L	10–35	pg/mL
Females				

Table 4.1 (*Continued*)

Adult reference hormone	Range	Units	Range	Unit
Early follicular phase	70–600	pmol/L	19–160	pg/mL
Mid-cycle	700–1900	pmol/L	188–371	pg/mL
Luteal phase	300–1250	pmol/L	81–337	pg/mL
Pancreatic polypetide (fasting)	0–100	pmol/L	0–418.5	pg/mL
Parathyroid hormone (PTH)	0–4.4	pmol/L	0–41.5	pg/mL
Prolactin	80–500	mU/L	3.8–23.6	ng/mL
Progesterone (day 21, luteal phase)	>30	nmol/L	>9.4	ng/mL
Renin (AM; out of bed for 2h; seated 5–15 min)[ag]	2–30	mU/L	0.9–13.6	pg/mL
Sex hormone-binding globulin				
Females	40–120	nmol/L	–	–
Males	20–60	nmol/L	–	–
Somatostatin (fasting)	0–150	pmol/L	0–245	pg/mL
Testosterone				
Males	8–35	nmol/L	230–1000	ng/mL
Females	0.7–3.0	nmol/L	20–85	ng/mL
Thyroglobulin	1.5–30	pmol/L	1–20	μg/L
Thyroid-stimulating hormone (TSH)	0.3–5.0	mU/L	–	–
Thyroxine, free (fT_4)	9–23	pmol/L	0.7–1.8	ng/dL
Tri-iodothyronine, free (fT_3)	3.1–7.7	pmol/L	0.2–0.5	ng/dL
Vasoactive intestinal polypeptide (fasting)	0–30	pmol/L	102	pg/mL
Vitamin D (25-OH-cholecalciferol)	4–40	nmol/L	1.6–16	ng/mL
Vitamin D (1,25-OH-cholecalciferol)	48–110	pmol/L	20–45.8	pg/mL

Ranges shown are for serum unless otherwise stated. Ranges vary slightly between laboratories due to differences in the methods employed. These examples are only intended to be illustrative and readers should check with their local laboratories.

[a]Most informative as part of the aldosterone:renin ratio (see Chapter 6).

[b]Age-dependent. Low values indicate poor ovarian reserve.

[c]Salivary assays are variable and require establishment of local normal ranges.

[d]Greater suppression from glucose load can be demonstrated using newer more sensitive immunoradiometric or chemiluminescent assays.

[e]The World Health Organization and the American Diabetes Association have endorsed HbA_{1c} for the diagnosis of diabetes above or equal to these values.

[f]IGF-I values are approximate as age- and sex-adjusted ranges are required.

[g]Renin is also measured as 'plasma renin activity' when 1 mU/L equates to 1.56 pmol/L/min (0.12 ng/mL/h).

Cell and molecular biology as diagnostic tools

Karyotype

Karyotype refers to the number and microscopic appearance of chromosomes arrested at metaphase (see Chapter 2). The word also describes the complement of chromosomes within an individual's cells, i.e. the normal karyotype for females is 46,XX and for males is 46,XY. A karyogram is the reorganized depiction of metaphase chromosomes as pairs in ascending number order. An abnormal total number of chromosomes is called aneuploidy (common in malignant tumours). More detail comes from Giemsa (G) staining of metaphase chromosomes, where each chromosome can be identified by its particular staining pattern, called 'G-banding'.

Ascertaining the karyotype can be useful in congenital endocrinopathy, such as genital ambiguity (i.e. is it 46,XX or 46,XY?), or if there is concern over Turner syndrome (45,XO) or Klinefelter syndrome (47,XXY) (see Chapter 7). G-banding allows experienced cytogeneticists to resolve chromosomal deletions, duplications or translocations (when fragments are swapped between two chromosomes) to within a few megabases. Sometimes, there is evidence of mosaicism when cells from the same person show more than one karyotype. This implies that something went wrong downstream of the first cell division such that some cell lineages have a normal karyotype while others are abnormal.

Fluorescence *in situ* hybridization

When a syndrome is suspected, for which the causative gene or locus (genomic position) is known,

fluorescence *in situ* hybridization (FISH) allows assessment of duplications, deletions or translocations on a smaller scale. For instance, a locus for congenital hypoparathyroidism, as part of DiGeorge syndrome, exists on the long arm of chromosome 22 (22q). FISH utilizes the principle that complementary DNA sequences will hybridize together by hydrogen bonding. Stretches of DNA from the region of interest are fluorescently labelled and hybridized to the patient's DNA. The fluorescence is visible as a dot on each sister chromatid of each relevant chromosome (Figure 4.4). Therefore, normal autosomal copy number is viewed as two pairs of two dots; one pair indicates a deletion; and three pairs indicate either duplication or potentially a translocation breakpoint (where the probe detects

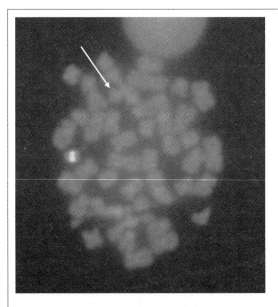

Figure 4.4 Fluorescent *in situ* hybridization in a patient with congenital hypoparathyroidism due to DiGeorge syndrome causing hypocalcaemia and congenital heart disease. Metaphase chromosomes were hybridized with a fluorescent probe from chromosome 22q11. The two bright dots indicate hybridization on the sister chromatids of the normal chromosome 22. The arrow points to the other chromosome 22 that lacks signal, indicating a deletion. Images kindly provided by Professor David Wilson, University of Southampton.

sequence either side of the breakpoint on different chromosomes).

Genome-wide microarray-based technology

Applying the principles of FISH on a genome-wide scale in a microarray format is called 'array comparative genomic hybridization' (array CGH). Short stretches of the genome are printed as thousands of microscopic spots on a glass slide (the 'microarray'). The patient's genomic DNA is fluorescently labelled and hybridized to the spots on the slide. According to the strength of the fluorescent signal, microdeletions or duplications anywhere in the whole genome can be detected in one experiment with a resolution of several kilobases.

Single nucleotide polymorphism (SNP) arrays are being used similarly. Spread across the entire genome, there are millions of very subtle variations (polymorphisms) at specific nucleotides between different individuals. On SNP arrays, the spots on the glass slide represent the different sequences at each SNP. As an individual's paired chromosomes come one from each parent, this means that at any one SNP, there are often two different sequences (one from the mother, one from the father; this is called heterozygosity). Across stretches of DNA, SNP arrays can identify regions showing 'loss of heterozygosity' (i.e. there is no variation in the signal), which is indicative of deletion of either the maternal or paternal copy, or altered ratio of signals indicative of duplication.

Diagnosing mutations in single genes by polymerase chain reaction and sequencing

With the discovery of disease-causing genes in monogenic disorders (i.e. a single gene is at fault), genetic testing is expanding rapidly into clinical endocrinology and diabetes. Increasingly precise prediction is becoming possible from correlating genotype (i.e. the gene and the position in a gene that a specific mutation lies) and phenotype (i.e. the clinical course of a patient). For instance, certain mutations in the *RET* proto-oncogene in type 2

multiple endocrine neoplasia (MEN2; see Chapter 10) have never been associated with phaeochromocytoma, normally one of the commonest features of MEN2. However, other *RET* mutations predict medullary carcinoma of the thyroid at a very young age, thus instructing when total thyroidectomy is needed. Genetically defining certain forms of monogenic diabetes is now dictating choice of therapy (see Case history 11.3).

Polymerase chain reaction (PCR) and sequencing is used to identify a mutation in a specific gene (Figure 4.5). Using DNA isolated from the patient's white blood cells, PCR amplifies the exons of the gene of interest in a reaction catalyzed by bacterial DNA polymerases that withstand high temperature (>90°C). These enzymes originate from microorganisms that replicate in hot springs. A second modified PCR reaction provides the base pair sequence of the DNA, demonstrating whether or not the gene is mutated.

Since sequencing the human genome in the last decade, technology has advanced enormously, greatly bringing down cost. What was once achieved by cutting-edge multi-million pound international consortia is now possible within an individual laboratory in a matter days or weeks for a few thousand pounds. In addition to ethical implications of holding these whole genome datasets, the bioinformatics required for their analysis is massive. Nevertheless, by 'next generation sequencing' on 'exome' arrays (i.e. all exons of nearly all genes), defining a patient's genome is fast becoming a diagnostic reality.

Imaging in endocrinology

Ultrasound

Ultrasound travels as sound waves beyond the range of human hearing and, according to the surface encountered, is reflected back towards the emitting source (the ultrasound probe). Different tissues have different reflective properties. By knowing the speed of the waves and the time between emission and detection, the distance between the reflective surfaces and the source can be calculated. These data allow a two-dimensional image to be generated

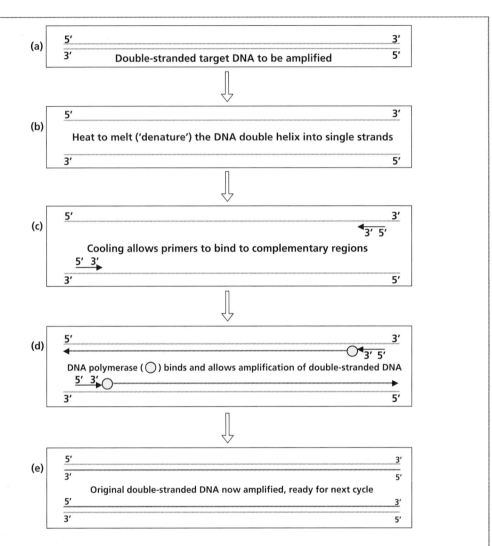

Figure 4.5 The basic principles of the polymerase chain reaction (PCR). PCR allows the amplification of a user-defined stretch of genomic DNA. In diagnostic genetics, this is commonly an exonic sequence where a mutation is suspected to underlie the patient phenotype. (a) Starting DNA. (b) The double helix is separated into two single strands by heating to ~94°C. (c) Cooling from this high temperature allows binding of user-designed short stretches of DNA (primers) that are complementary to the opposite strands at each end of the region to be amplified. (d) DNA polymerase catalyzes the addition of deoxynucleotide residues according to the complementary base pairs of the template strand. (e) Once complete, two double-stranded sequences arise from the original target DNA. Another cycle then recommences at (a) with double the amount of template, making the increase in DNA exponential. Having amplified large amounts of the desired DNA sequence, a modified PCR reaction and analysis sequences the DNA to discover the presence or absence of a mutation.

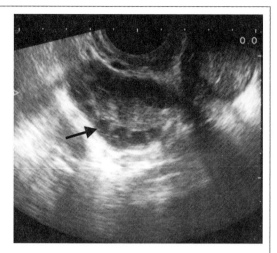

Figure 4.6 Ultrasound of a polycystic ovary. The presence of multiple small cysts (one shown by the arrow) is consistent with, but not required for, the diagnosis of polycystic ovarian syndrome (see Chapter 7). Ultrasound does help to exclude the single mass of an androgen-secreting tumour (see Chapter 7). Image kindly provided by Dr Sue Ingamells, University of Southampton.

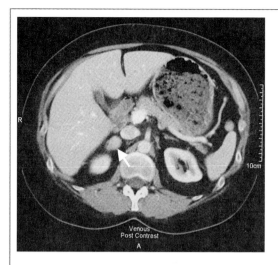

Figure 4.7 Abdominal computed tomography (CT) with contrast. This patient presented with Cushing syndrome (see Figure 6.9). The right adrenal mass on the CT (arrow) was a cortisol-secreting adenoma.

(Figure 4.6). The major advantage of ultrasound is its simplicity, safety and non-invasiveness. Machines are portable. It is helpful as an initial imaging investigation of many endocrine organs. For instance, the thyroid has a characteristic appearance in Graves disease because of its increased vascularity (see Chapter 8). The ovaries can be delineated transabdominally, or with specific consent, transvaginally, when the shorter distance between probe and ovary and fewer reflective surfaces create higher resolution images (Figure 4.6).

Computed tomography and magnetic resonance imaging

Computed tomography (CT) and magnetic resonance imaging (MRI) provide excellent depiction of the body's internal organs and tissues. The principle of CT is the same as for X-ray. X-rays pass differently through the various organs and tissues of the body. For instance, bone is not penetrated very well so a plain X-ray image is obtained as if the skeleton has cast a shadow. In CT scanning, the

patient lies on a table that slides through a motorized ring, which rotates and emits X-rays. Data are acquired on penetration from different angles (i.e. as if multiple plain X-rays had been taken), which are then constructed by computer into a single transverse 'slice' through the body (Figure 4.7). The brain is encased by the skull, hence its imaging by CT is limited.

In comparison to CT, MRI does not rely on X-rays and is particularly useful at imaging intracranial structures, such as the pituitary (Figure 4.8). It is also very useful for screening purposes when a patient will need life-long monitoring, e.g. to assess tumour formation in MEN. Repeat CT would provide a large cumulative radiation dose, itself a risk factor for tumour formation, which is avoided by MRI. The key components of MRI are magnets. At their centre is a hollow tube, into which the patient passes on a horizontal table. Once inside the tube, the patient is in a very strong magnetic field (this is the reason why MRI is dangerous to patients with metallic implants such as pacemakers or aneurysm clips). Within the magnetic field, some of the body's hydrogen atoms resonate after absorbing energy from a pulse of radio waves. Once the pulse ends, the resonating atoms give up energy as they return to their original state. These emission data are collected and differ slightly for different tissues, allowing the construction of high-definition images. By altering time (T) constants, different images can be generated. For instance, in T1-weighted images, cerebrospinal fluid (CSF) appears dark (Figure 4.8a), whereas in T2-weighted images, CSF appears white (Figure 4.8b).

Contrast agents are very useful for both CT and MRI scanning (Figure 4.7). In MRI, agents such as gadolinium can subtly alter the data acquired, for instance allowing the identification of an adenoma within normal anterior pituitary tissue.

Nuclear medicine and uptake marker scans

Simple X-rays, CT and MRI depict tissues and organs but provide limited insight into the cells that compose these structures or their function. In later life, many organs develop benign tumours of little or no significance. For instance, incidental adrenal tumours (incidentalomas) can affect ~5% of the

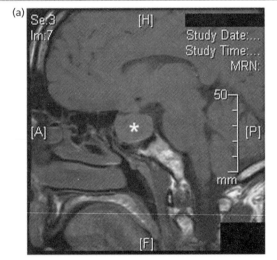

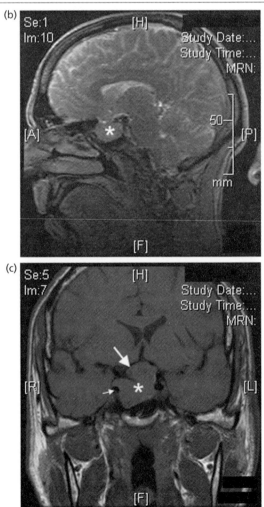

Figure 4.8 Magnetic resonance imaging of a pituitary tumour. (a) T1-weighted sagittal image. (b) T2-weighted sagittal image (cerebrospinal fluid appears white). (c) T1-weighted frontal image. A large irregularly-shaped pituitary tumour (*) has compressed the pituitary stalk (not visible) and raised and tilted the optic chiasm (large arrow) such that it appears draped on top of the tumour sloping down to the right. The tumour has also extended bilaterally into the cavernous sinus to encase partially the internal carotid arteries (small arrow marks the right internal carotid artery).

population after ~40 years. In a patient with hypertension, it would be important to distinguish these from a phaeochromocytoma that could be the curable cause of elevated blood pressure (see Chapter 6). Uptake markers (or 'tracers') specific to a particular cell type can provide valuable clues. For instance, meta-iodobenzylguanidine (mIBG) acts as an analogue of norepinephrine and is taken up by adrenal medulla cells. When labelled with radioactive iodine-123 (I^{123}) it can be used to distinguish a phaeochromocytoma from other tumours (Figure 4.9). At higher doses, it can even be used as targeted therapy, when instead of marking cells, it kills them. I^{123} or technetium-99m pertechnetate can also be used to delineate different causes of hyperthyroidism (see Chapter 8) when taken up by the thyroid gland. In Graves disease, the uptake is homogeneous; with a solitary 'toxic' adenoma, the uptake is restricted to the relevant nodule.

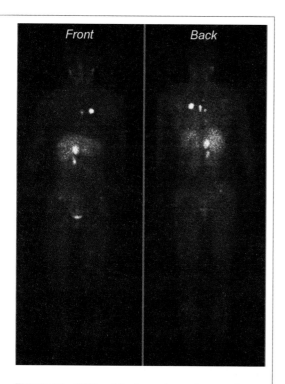

Figure 4.9 mIBG uptake by a phaeochromocytoma. A whole body I^{123} mIBG scan with imaging from the front and back shows a right phaeochromocytoma with pulmonary and bony metastases. This imaging is helpful to investigate potential metastatic disease prior to adrenalectomy. Image kindly provided by Dr Val Lewington, Royal Marsden Hospital.

Key points

- Diagnosing or excluding endocrine disorders relies on measuring the concentration of hormones and metabolites
- Immunoassays provide accurate, reliable laboratory measurement of many hormones and metabolites
- Techniques involving mass spectrometry are increasingly being used to measure hormones and metabolites
- Cellular and molecular biology can increasingly provide patient-specific diagnoses of congenital disorders or endocrine neoplasia syndromes; information that can predict and influence patient outcome and management
- Imaging investigations localize endocrine disorders and assist surgical intervention
- 'Incidentalomas' are common and conscientious effort is needed to correlate a biochemical endocrine abnormality to a tumour identified on imaging

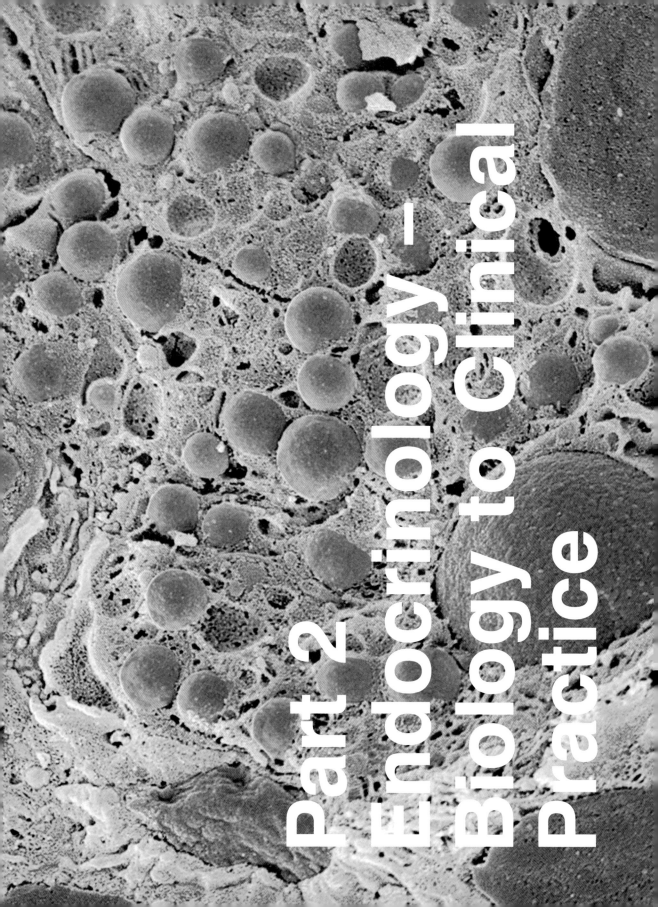

Part 2
Endocrinology – Biology to Clinical Practice

CHAPTER 5

The hypothalamus and pituitary gland

Key topics

- Embryology and anatomy   66
- Pituitary tumours as space-occupying lesions   67
- The hypothalamus   70
- The hypothalamic–anterior pituitary hormone axes   72
- The anterior pituitary hormones   73
- Hypopituitarism   90
- Hormones of the posterior pituitary   91
- Key points   96
- Answers to case histories   96

Learning objectives

- To appreciate the nature of the various hypothalamic–anterior pituitary–end-organ axes
- To understand the clinical disorders arising from excess or lack of anterior pituitary hormones
- To acquire familiarity with the hormones of the posterior pituitary and the associated clinical conditions
- To understand the nature of tumours within the pituitary gland and their clinical consequences

This chapter integrates the basic biology of the hypothalamus and the pituitary gland with important clinical conditions

Essential Endocrinology and Diabetes, Sixth Edition. Richard IG Holt, Neil A Hanley.
© 2012 Richard IG Holt and Neil A Hanley. Publlished 2012 by Blackwell Publishing Ltd.

To recap

■ Hormone production from the hypothalamus and pituitary gland is highly dependent upon negative feedback from the relevant endocrine end-organs. The principles underlying this and dynamic testing are introduced in Chapters 1 and 4 respectively

■ Hormones from the hypothalamus and pituitary gland are peptides; review their synthesis and modes of action in Chapters 2 and 3

Cross-reference

■ The hypothalamus and anterior pituitary function to regulate several endocrine end-organs: the adrenal cortex (see Chapter 6), ovary and testis (see Chapter 7), and thyroid (see Chapter 8)

■ Oxytocin is described here as a hormone from the posterior pituitary; its major function is to regulate birth and breast-feeding (see Chapter 7)

■ The hypothalamus regulates appetite, which is also covered in Chapter 15 on obesity

■ The hypothalamus plays critical roles in sensing hypoglycaemia, a major side-effect from insulin therapy in type 1 diabetes (see Chapter 12)

The hypothalamus and pituitary gland are critical for integrating the function of the central nervous and endocrine systems. The hypothalamus receives diverse endocrine inputs and signals to affect processes such as appetite, body temperature and circadian rhythms. It intimately regulates the pituitary gland's hormone secretion in a series of interconnected axes with endocrine end-organs, including the adrenal cortex, thyroid, testis and ovary. Each of the pituitary hormones is described in turn; the associated clinical disorders secondary to hormone excess or deficiency are mentioned here, or, where the phenotype is a consequence of the end-organ hormone, in the relevant end-organ chapter. For example, Chapter 6 describes the consequences of excess cortisol from the adrenal cortex in Cushing disease, even though the primary pathology is excessive adrenocorticotrophic hormone (ACTH) from an anterior pituitary corticotroph adenoma. The concluding section of this chapter describes the loss of multiple pituitary hormones ('hypopituitarism'). The structural consequences of pituitary tumours follow the description of pituitary anatomy and its surrounding landmarks.

Embryology and anatomy

The pituitary develops as two independent structures (anterior and posterior) from very different starting points (Figure 5.1). The anterior pituitary (also known as the adenohypophysis) is derived from the epithelial lining of the roof of the mouth. These cells are part of the foregut endoderm that goes on to form the pharynx, respiratory tract, thyroid, pancreas, liver and intestine as far as the proximal duodenum. In the mouth, proliferating epithelial cells fold upwards as Rathke's pouch and eventually detach from the oral lining prior to closure of the bony palate. At the same time, central nervous system (CNS) cells proliferate in the floor of the third ventricle (a region called the infundibulum) and migrate downwards to form the posterior pituitary (also known as the neurohypophysis). The downward movement creates the stalk of the pituitary, below which the anterior and posterior components become apposed within the bony casing of the pituitary fossa (also called the sella turcica, part of the sphenoid bone) (Figure 5.2). Sometimes, remnants of Rathke's pouch result in fluid-filled

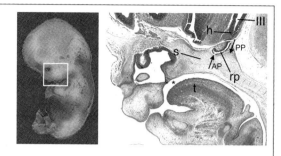

Figure 5.1 The human pituitary gland forms at ~8 weeks of development. The boxed region is enlarged to the right. The arrows show the respective migration of the cells that form the anterior (AP) and posterior pituitary (PP). III, third ventricle; h, hypothalamus; rp, Rathke's pouch; s, sphenoid bone; t, tongue; *, oral cavity.

cysts that, like pituitary tumours, cause detrimental effects from local pressure (see next section).

Above the pituitary, clusters of neurosecretory cells form the various hypothalamic nuclei (Figure 5.2); hormones secreted from these cells regulate hormones released from the pituitary (Table 5.1). Other functions include the control of temperature and appetite.

The anterior component forms three-quarters of the adult pituitary weight (~0.5 g), which doubles during pregnancy and puberty. Hypothalamic hormones released into the capillary plexus at the median eminence flow down the portal veins to the anterior pituitary (Figure 5.2). In turn, this stimulates specific anterior pituitary cell types to secrete their own hormones from storage granules.

The posterior pituitary receives hormone-containing granules transported down the hypothalamic neurones continually at a rate of 8 mm/h. Upon stimulation, these hormones are released from the nerve terminals into the adjacent fenestrated capillaries. Thus, the posterior pituitary functions largely as a store. Consequently, as some of the vasopressin fibres terminate in the median eminence of the hypothalamus (Figure 5.2), a patient with destruction of the posterior pituitary commonly recovers vasopressin function.

Pituitary tumours as space-occupying lesions

The commonest space-occupying lesions in the pituitary fossa are benign adenomas. If arising from endocrine cell types, the patient may present with features of the relevant hormone excess. These syndromes are dealt with later on. Here, we consider the physical consequences of pituitary tumours. Given the confined nature of the pituitary fossa and surrounding important structures (Box 5.1), knowledge of anatomy is important.

Non-functioning adenomas

The commonest pituitary adenoma does not secrete known active hormones and is termed a 'non-functioning' adenoma. Foci of pituitary adenoma are recognized in up to 20% of post-mortem examinations. The reason for this incredibly high rate of benign tumour formation is unclear; attention has fallen on the pituitary's unusual location where it receives privileged access to high concentrations of hormones and growth factors directly from the hypothalamus. Molecular genetics has also advanced understanding. For instance, ~40% of GH-secreting adenomas contain a mutation in $G_s\alpha$ (review G-protein–coupled receptor signalling in Chapter 3). Despite this high rate of tumour initiation, pituitary carcinoma is exceptionally rare.

The distinction between microadenoma and macroadenoma (Box 5.1; diameter < or >1 cm) is arbitrary and in part reflects historical resolution of imaging techniques. Magnetic resonance imaging (MRI) is now the investigation of choice for visualizing the pituitary gland (see Figure 4.8) and is capable of resolving tumours of a few millimetres in diameter.

Tumours restricted to the pituitary fossa may compress nearby cells and cause various forms of hypopituitarism (i.e. deficiency of one or more, or all pituitary hormones). Adenomas can also expand beyond the pituitary fossa, eroding the sella turcica, and bulge in all directions (see Box 5.1; Figure 4.8). Upward growth can compress the optic chiasm where the optic nerves cross, relaying information from the eyes to the visual cortex. This creates a characteristic defect, where the first fibres to be

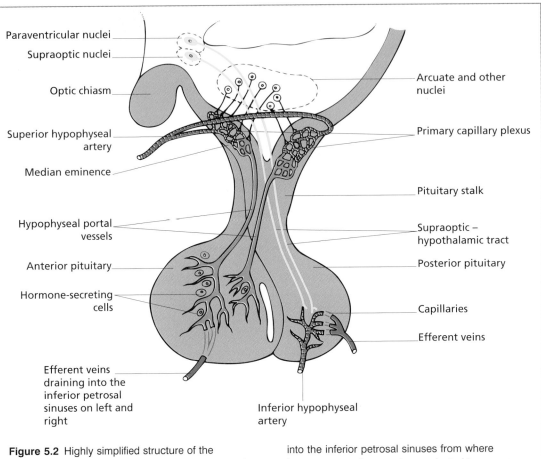

Paraventricular nuclei

Supraoptic nuclei

Optic chiasm

Superior hypophyseal artery

Median eminence

Hypophyseal portal vessels

Anterior pituitary

Hormone-secreting cells

Efferent veins draining into the inferior petrosal sinuses on left and right

Arcuate and other nuclei

Primary capillary plexus

Pituitary stalk

Supraoptic – hypothalamic tract

Posterior pituitary

Capillaries

Efferent veins

Inferior hypophyseal artery

Figure 5.2 Highly simplified structure of the hypothalamus and its neural and vascular connections with the pituitary. The superior hypophyseal artery branches to form the primary capillary plexus in the median eminence and the upper part of the pituitary stalk. From the primary plexus arise the hypophyseal portal vessels, which terminate in the anterior pituitary to form a secondary plexus of sinusoidal capillaries supplying the hormone-secreting anterior pituitary cell types. Efferent veins drain from the anterior pituitary into the inferior petrosal sinuses from where hormone sampling can be conducted to assess Cushing syndrome (see Chapter 6). The axons from the arcuate and other nuclei terminate close to the primary capillary plexus. Axons of the supraoptic and paraventricular nuclei traverse the pituitary stalk and terminate close to the capillaries of the inferior hypophyseal artery, which supplies the posterior pituitary. The entire pituitary gland is encased in the bony sella turcica.

affected are those crossing over ('decussating') from the inner portions of the retina. This leads to a bitemporal visual field loss, commonly as a hemianopia (the peripheral half of each visual field is lost). Figure 5.3 shows a more subtle defect. Sometimes the upper fields are lost first because the lower nerves are affected first by pressure from below. Visual field loss progresses insidiously and patients may present having already lost significant vision. A striking presentation is a road traffic accident where cars or pedestrians coming from either side were unappreciated.

Lateral extension into the cavernous sinus can cause ophthalmoplegia (paralysis of eye movement) from pressure on any of the three cranial nerves innervating the extraocular muscles of the eye

Table 5.1 Summary of anatomy and function of the hypothalamic nuclei

Nuclei			Function
Medial	Supraoptic	Paraventricular (PVN)	Secretes vasopressin and oxytocin; large neurones pass through the pituitary stalk as the 'supraoptic–hypothalamic tract' to the posterior pituitary where the nerve terminals contain storage granules Secretes corticotrophin-releasing hormone (CRH)
		Supraoptic (SON)	Vasopressin and oxytocin secretion (like PVN)
		Suprachiasmatic (SCN)	Biological clock functions (e.g. wake–sleep cycle); receives input from retina
	Tuberal	Ventromedial (VMN)	Satiety; lesions cause overeating ('hyperphagia') Mood
		Arcuate	Secretes multiple releasing hormones, somatostatin and dopamine from nerve terminals in the median eminence into capillary network for delivery to the anterior pituitary; overlapping function with PVN and other nuclei
	Mammillary	Mammillary	No known endocrine function; role in memory
		Posterior	Thermoregulation Blood pressure
Lateral			Hunger; lesions cause anorexia Thirst

Hormone axes and functions are detailed in the relevant sections of this chapter and later organ-specific chapters. Not all nuclei play endocrine roles and some functions remain incompletely understood. However, general appreciation of the diverse function is important as disruption (e.g. from space-occupying lesions or radiation damage) can have pronounced effects for patients attending endocrinology clinics.

(Table 5.2). Involvement of each nerve can give rise to characteristic forms of diplopia (double vision), exacerbated by looking away from the action of the paralyzed muscle. Laterally, tumour can also envelop the internal carotid artery in the cavernous sinus, after which restricted access and the dangers of operating around major vessels makes curative surgery impossible.

🔍 Case history 5.1

A 65-year-old man had attended the optician for new reading glasses when a routine assessment revealed loss of the entire lateral half of the visual fields on both sides.

What is the precise description for this visual deficit?
What is the likely cause?
How would it be best imaged?
If imaging of the pituitary gland is abnormal, why should this person be referred urgently to an endocrinologist?

Answers, see p. 96

Box 5.1 Pituitary tumours

Two issues must be considered:
- Potential hormone excess from the tumour cell type (see following sections)
- Physical pressure on local structures and other pituitary cell types:
  - Cranial nerve palsies (see below and Table 5.2)
  - Loss of pituitary hormones, either individually or in combination, causing hypopituitarism (see later sections)

Local anatomy at risk from expanding pituitary tumours
- Superiorly – optic chiasm:
  - Compression causes loss of vision (commonly bitemporal; Figure 5.3)
- Laterally – cavernous sinuses:
  - Compression of cranial nerves III, IV and VI (Table 5.2)
  - Encasing of the internal carotid artery; does no harm but prevents curative surgery
- Antero-inferiorly – sphenoid sinus (the route for transsphenoidal surgery):
  - Cerebrospinal fluid (CSF) rhinorrhoea secondary to tumour erosion is rare

Categorization of tumour size
- >1 cm diameter = macroadenoma
- <1 cm diameter = microadenoma

Other more generalized symptoms of pituitary masses include headache (especially frontal/retro-orbital) from stretching of the meninges or obstruction to CSF drainage. Very rarely, tumours extend anteriorly through the sphenoid sinus to cause CSF leakage through the nose ('CSF rhinorrhoea').

Not all pituitary masses are adenomas. The differential diagnosis includes metastasis, meningioma, lymphoma, sarcoid, histiocytosis, or an unusual tumour called a craniopharyngioma that more commonly presents to the paediatric endocrinologist. Histologically, this tumour is benign, but it is still invasive. It most likely arises from the epithelial cells that lined Rathke's pouch and can cause coincident diabetes insipidus (deficiency of vasopressin, see later).

Treating pituitary tumours

Pharmacological treatment is available for some hormone-secreting tumours (see sections on growth hormone and prolactin). For all others, and where drug treatment proves inadequate, there are three choices (Box 5.2).

Compression of the optic chiasm is a neurosurgical emergency. Even profound visual loss can recover quickly by relieving pressure on the chiasm. In this scenario, surgery is advantageous over radiotherapy, which is less invasive, but would damage optic neurones, can take up to 10 years for its complete effect, mildly increases the risk of cerebrovascular ischaemic events and frequently results in hypopituitarism because of the death of other hormone-secreting cell types.

The hypothalamus

The hypothalamus is a critical part of the brain linking diverse aspects of the endocrine system to the CNS and *vice versa* in health and disease. For example, depression is associated with altered function of the hypothalamic–anterior pituitary adrenocortical axis. In many situations it functions as a rheostat (e.g. like the thermostat on a heating system), regulating the stimulation or suppression of a variety of processes such as hunger or thirst. It lies below the thalamus and above the pituitary gland as a series of nuclei categorized anatomically as medial (plus subdivisions) and lateral (see Table 5.1). Many of the nuclei interact with peripheral endocrine organs either dependent on or independent of the hormone axes of the anterior pituitary (see next section). The hypothalamic role in appetite control is covered in Chapter 15. It is also involved in the body's counter-regulatory hormone response to hypoglycaemia (Chapter 12).

The hypothalamus is responsible for temperature control and the regulation of several circadian rhythms and 'biological clock' functions (e.g. the

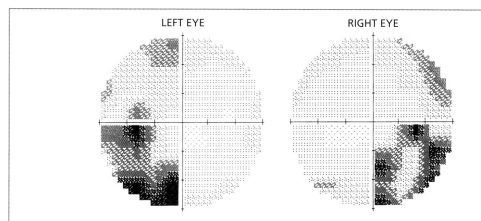

Figure 5.3 Visual field assessment. There is a bitemporal loss of the lower quadrants (black areas) caused by a pituitary tumour compressing the optic chiasm. More commonly the upper quadrants are lost first; however, such clinical variation is not unusual.

Table 5.2 Cranial nerves in the cavernous sinus

Cranial nerve	Function	Consequences of compression
Oculomotor nerve (III)	Innervation of suprapalpebral muscles	Ptosis (most obvious feature)
	Associated with parasympathetic nerve fibres from the Edinger–Westphal nucleus	Fixed, dilated pupil and loss of accommodation
	Innervation of all extraocular muscles except those supplied by IV and VI	Downward and outward-looking vision (unopposed actions of superior oblique and lateral rectus)
		Double vision (if ptotic eye lid is raised)
Trochlear nerve (IV)	Innervation of the superior oblique muscle	Weak downward and inward gaze
		Double vision on walking down stairs
Abducent nerve (VI)	Innervation of the lateral rectus muscle	Inward (medial)-looking gaze
		Double vision most pronounced on looking to affected side

wake–sleep cycle). Occasionally, despite careful monitoring of radiation dose, some patients consider that these latter functions become disturbed after external beam radiotherapy targeted at the pituitary gland.

In regulating thirst, the hypothalamus receives endocrine signals from circulating atrial natriuretic peptide (ANP) and angiotensin amongst other hormones, and has neurones that are receptive to sodium concentration and osmolality. These inputs

---

Box 5.2 Summary of non-pharmacological treatment of pituitary tumours

Observation
- Repeat MRI and monitor anterior pituitary hormone function:
  - Increasingly common as 'incidentalomas' are discovered on MRI performed for headaches and other CNS symptoms and signs
  - Can be sensible for tumours not compressing the optic chiasm

Surgery
- Transsphenoidal surgery:
  - From behind the upper lip or via the nose, the sphenoid sinus is crossed and the pituitary accessed via making a window in the sella turcica
  - Used for emergency decompression of the optic chiasm (except for prolactinomas – see later)

- Transfrontal surgery:
  - Less common but can be considered for particularly large tumours

Radiotherapy
- External beam radiotherapy:
  - Three beams at different angles are focused on the tumour region, but avoiding the optic chiasm
  - Common second-line modality when tumours re-grow after surgery
- Stereotactic radiotherapy:
  - Many beams at different angles produce a very high dose at a precise focal point
  - Considered for very discrete tumours in an attempt to retain surrounding pituitary function
  - Not used as the first-line radiotherapy treatment

---

then regulate vasopressin secretion (see section on the posterior pituitary) and the sensation of thirst.

The hypothalamic–anterior pituitary hormone axes

There is a special relationship between an anterior pituitary cell type, its hypothalamic regulator(s) and its secreted hormone(s), which in several instances goes on to regulate major endocrine end-organs (Table 5.3).

Hypothalamic-releasing hormones are mostly small peptides with pulsatile secretion and short circulating half-lives. *In vivo* action is very fast via specific anterior pituitary cell-surface G-protein–coupled receptors linked to second messenger pathways (review Chapter 3). Hypothalamic hormones may also be inhibitory; e.g. the actions of growth hormone-releasing hormone (GHRH) on somatotrophs and thyrotrophin-releasing hormone (TRH) on lactotrophs are inhibited by the hormones somatostatin and dopamine respectively. Clinically, hypothalamic hormones are rarely measured, although they can be injected as an infrequent

test of anterior pituitary function, e.g. to assess the magnitude and speed of rise in thyroid-stimulating hormone (TSH) concentration in response to intravenous TRH.

Regulation of hypothalamic and anterior pituitary hormone release can be complex. Axis-specific and associated clinical details are given in the relevant 'end-organ' chapters on the adrenal cortex, testis, ovary and thyroid. Generally, the common basic principle of negative feedback can be used to make biochemical diagnoses in the clinic (Figure 5.4 and review Chapter 1). Negative feedback influences transcription and translation of hormone-encoding genes, the release of stored hormone granules and the number of receptors on the target cell. For example, increased thyroid hormone reduces TRH production, the number of TRH receptors on anterior pituitary thyrotrophs and TSH production. Low thyroid hormone concentration has the opposite effects. This means that serum hormone concentrations from the end-organ, the hypothalamus (rarely measured) and anterior pituitary (frequently or always measured) can be used to diagnose if and where a clinical problem lies in the axis. For instance, lack of thyroid hormone because

Table 5.3 Hormone-secreting cell types of the anterior pituitary

Anterior pituitary cell type	Hormone secreted	Size (number of amino acids)	Target organ	Hypothalamic regulator (+ or – effect)
Somatotroph	Growth hormone (GH)	191	Diverse	GH-releasing hormone (GHRH, +) and somatostatin (SS, –)
Lactotroph	Prolactin (PRL)	199	Breast	Dopamine (–) and thyrotrophin-releasing hormone (TRH, +)
Corticotroph	Adrenocorticotrophic hormone (ACTH)	39	Adrenal cortex	Corticotrophin-releasing hormone (CRH, +)
Thyrotroph	Thyroid-stimulating hormone (TSH)	204	Thyroid	TRH (+)
Gonadotroph	Follicle-stimulating hormone (FSH) and luteinizing hormone (LH)	Both 204	Ovary or testis	Gonadotrophin-releasing hormone (GnRH, +)

of primary hypothyroidism (i.e. underactivity emanating from the thyroid) results in raised TSH (and TRH); low thyroid hormone with low or *normal* TSH indicates hypothalamic or anterior pituitary disease (tertiary or secondary hypothyroidism, although a distinction between the two is rarely made). The principle is the same for the other hormone axes.

Pulsatility of hypothalamic hormone release can also affect anterior pituitary responsiveness. Constant gonadotrophin-releasing hormone (GnRH) desensitizes the gonadotroph, leading to loss of luteinizing hormone (LH) and follicle-stimulating hormone (FSH) secretion, and, consequently, testicular or ovarian quiescence. Thus, continuous intravenous GnRH can be used as a contraceptive or as pharmacological castration in hormone-dependent prostrate or breast cancer. In contrast, pulses of GnRH every 90 min can be used to restore fertility in patients with hypothalamic dysfunction.

In addition to autonomous regulation, transient neural inputs from higher centres modulate endocrine axes via the hypothalamus. Several endocrine responses to environmental changes, such as psychological stress, exercise and temperature, are mediated in this way. Several anterior pituitary hormones exhibit a circadian rhythm, the regulation of which probably involves the suprachiasmatic nucleus and the pineal gland. In mammals, the pineal gland appears to transduce neural information on the day/night light cycle from the retina into a circadian rhythm of melatonin secretion. These poorly understood phenomena appear increasingly important: for instance, the type B receptor for melatonin has recently been associated with risk of type 2 diabetes; and shift workers have disturbed endocrinology with increased mortality and morbidity.

The anterior pituitary hormones

Growth hormone

GH is the most abundant hormone of the adult anterior pituitary, secreted by the somatotrophs, which account for up to 10% of the pituitary's dry weight. The major form of human GH is a protein of 191 amino acids, two disulphide bridges and a

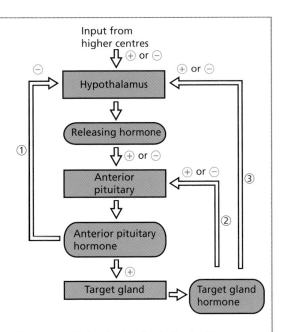

Figure 5.4 Endocrine feedback circuits. The diagram shows interactions between higher brain centres, the hypothalamus, anterior pituitary and peripheral endocrine glands. The controlling factors can be stimulatory (⊕) or inhibitory (⊖). Three feedback loops are shown: ① from anterior pituitary to hypothalamus; ② from the end-organ to the anterior pituitary; and ③ from the end-organ to the hypothalamus.

molecular weight of 22 kDa, although there are other minor variants. The structure of GH is species specific. Human GH differs markedly from that of non-primates. This is thought to reflect the dramatic evolution of the *GH/PRL* gene family with the appearance of primates. One practical consequence is the obligatory use of human GH, now produced recombinantly, to treat children and adults with GH deficiency.

Effects

The net actions of GH are both metabolic and anabolic (Figure 5.5). The latter are mediated predominantly through the generation of the mitogenic polypeptide insulin-like growth factor I (IGF-I), which acts either locally or in an endocrine manner.

IGF-I is produced in many tissues, including large amounts in the liver. In turn, the actions of IGF-I are regulated by a family of at least six highly specific IGF-binding proteins (IGFBPs). Most (> 95%) serum IGF-I is bound in a complex with IGFBP-3 and a protein called acid labile subunit (ALS). The production of IGFBP-3 and ALS is also increased by GH.

Metabolic actions
Intermediate metabolism
The direct metabolic effects of GH tend to synergize with cortisol and generally antagonize insulin, giving rise to the 'diabetogenic' properties of excess GH. GH leads to a stimulation of lipolysis and increases fasting free fatty acid (FFA) concentrations. During times of fasting or energy restriction, this lipolytic effect of GH is enhanced, while the effect is suppressed by co-administration of food or glucose. In the long term, and important clinically, GH leads to a reduction in fat mass.

GH and IGF-I both have roles in normal glucose homeostasis. GH increases fasting hepatic glucose output, by increasing hepatic gluconeogenesis and glycogenolysis, and decreases peripheral glucose utilization through the inhibition of glycogen synthesis and glucose oxidation. These effects are antagonistic to those of insulin and acute reductions in GH secretion are associated with enhanced insulin sensitivity. Longer term reductions in GH are associated with the development of insulin resistance in association with changes in body composition. In contrast to GH, IGF-I, as suggested by its name, acts like insulin to lower blood glucose by stimulating peripheral glucose uptake, glycolysis and glycogen synthesis, while having a minimal effect on hepatic glucose production.

Energy expenditure
GH causes an increase in basal metabolic rate through a number of mechanisms, including an increase in lean body mass, increased FFA oxidation and enhanced peripheral tri-iodothyronine production (see Chapter 8).

Anabolic actions
GH output increases with size to sustain growth during childhood. An individual destined to become

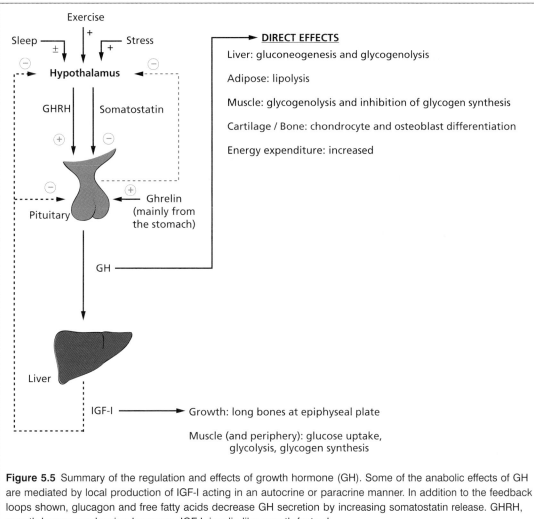

Figure 5.5 Summary of the regulation and effects of growth hormone (GH). Some of the anabolic effects of GH are mediated by local production of IGF-I acting in an autocrine or paracrine manner. In addition to the feedback loops shown, glucagon and free fatty acids decrease GH secretion by increasing somatostatin release. GHRH, growth hormone-releasing hormone; IGF-I, insulin-like growth factor I.

tall secretes GH at higher circulating concentrations than smaller peers. The consequence is faster than average growth and, year-by-year, height gain. There is a marked rise in circulating GH levels at puberty.

The anabolic effects of GH on protein metabolism are mainly mediated by IGF-I. This promotes growth of long bones at the epiphyseal plates, where there are actively proliferating cartilage cells. This 'growth spurt' at and following puberty ceases once the epiphyses of the long bones fuse at the end of adolescence – the reason why too much GH after this time leads to the progressively dysmorphic growth of acromegaly compared to the proportionate growth of gigantism (see Box 5.4). GH also has

profound effects on bone turnover. It is likely that these effects are largely indirect, as serum IGF-I correlates well with estimates of bone mineral density. In addition, GH and IGF-I may modify intestinal calcium absorption and serum levels of active vitamin D (see Chapter 9).

Acute administration of GH modestly stimulates muscle and whole-body protein synthesis, leading to nitrogen retention and increased lean body mass. The converse effects are seen with decline in GH secretion with ageing, features of which can be partially reversed by GH administration. As well as GH, IGF-I concentration also declines with advancing age. Accordingly, age- and sex-matched normal ranges are necessary for the appropriate interpretation of serum IGF-I assays. Without these details, there is a risk of incorrectly diagnosing overactivity or underactivity of the GH–IGF-I axis.

Sodium and water homeostasis

The mechanisms enabling the body to regulate sodium and water homeostasis are complex. Although incompletely understood, there is evidence that GH induces sodium and fluid retention, possibly by increasing glomerular filtration rate. The main clinical implication of this phenomenon is the side-effect of swollen hands or feet or pitting oedema reported by adults receiving GH replacement therapy or with acromegaly.

Mechanism of action of GH and IGFs

GH signals within the cell via the JAK–STAT pathway (see Figures 3.7 and 3.8). GH receptors have been detected within the first year of life in all known target tissues. The number of receptors in a target tissue (e.g. the liver) is changed both by peripheral factors, such as sex hormones, and down-regulated by GH itself. As suggested by the name, the indirect effects of GH via IGF-I are often 'insulin-like'. They can be antagonized by cortisol and are mediated intracellularly by pathways very similar to those for insulin signalling (review Chapter 3 and Figure 3.6).

Growth hormone regulation

Input from the hypothalamus and higher brain centres

GH secretion is stimulated by sleep and exercise and inhibited by food ingestion. During deep sleep, bursts of secretion occur every 1–2 h (Figure 5.6). Stress (e.g. excitement, cold, anaesthesia, surgery or haemorrhage) produces a rapid increase in serum GH. Although negative feedback has been proposed for IGF-I (see Figure 5.5), the GH axis lacks a single end-organ secreting a hormone with a clear negative feedback role. Contrast this with cortisol from the adrenal cortex, which suppresses corticotrophic-releasing hormone (CRH) and ACTH secretion.

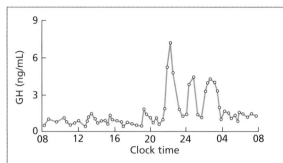

Figure 5.6 A 24-h profile of serum growth hormone (GH) in a normal 7-year-old child. Irregular pulses occur, which are greatest during sleep.

Box 5.3 Assessing the GH–IGF-I axis

- GH release is pulsatile (Figure 5.6):
  - Random serum GH is a poor marker of clinical GH status
  - Either dynamic testing (see later) or a series of serum measurements is needed
- Circulating IGF-I concentration is relatively constant:
  - Random serum IGF-I is a useful marker of clinical GH status

---

Instead, regulation of GH production comes from the dynamic, opposing interplay between hypothalamic GHRH (a positive influence) and somatostatin (negative) (see Figure 5.5). GH pulses are virtually simultaneous with peaks of GHRH and low somatostatin secretion; conversely, GH falls as somatostatin concentration rises. The pulsatile release of GH and its relatively short half-life of ~15 min mean that random serum measurements are usually barely detectable [<0.4 ng/mL (<1 mU/L)]. A circulating GH-binding protein slightly increases the half-life, but its physiological significance is unclear. This intermittent nature of circulating GH, compared to reasonably constant levels of serum IGF-I, is important in assessing clinical GH status (Box 5.3).

Input from other hypothalamic–anterior pituitary–end-organ axes

GH production from somatotrophs is dependent upon an adequate supply of thyroid hormone, which explains why hypothyroid children suffer from stunted growth. Glucocorticoids, as either endogenous cortisol or synthetic steroids given for inflammatory disorders such as asthma or rheumatoid arthritis, suppress GH secretion. Children with Cushing syndrome stop growing. By contrast, oestrogens sensitize the pituitary to the action of GHRH, so that basal and stimulated GH concentrations are slightly higher in women and rise earlier during female puberty.

Metabolic regulation

In addition to the regulation of GH by hypothalamic GHRH and somatostatin, ghrelin is secreted mainly by the stomach and acts as a potent GH secretagogue. It also stimulates hunger, acting oppositely from leptin (see Chapter 15).

FFA and GH form a negative feedback loop; GH induces lipolysis and a rise in FFA, which, in turn, inhibits further GH secretion by increasing somatostatin. FFA also increases following a meal and GH release is inhibited at the same time as insulin secretion rises, which suppresses lipolysis. As the individual moves back into the fasting state, FFA concentrations fall, GH secretion returns and falling insulin concentration removes the brake on lipolysis. Longer periods of fasting and chronic malnutrition are associated with increased amplitude and frequency of GH secretion. In contrast, obesity is associated with increased GH clearance and reduced GH secretion. The metabolic regulation of GH secretion is utilized clinically in the oral glucose tolerance test (OGTT) and insulin tolerance test (ITT) for assessment of GH status (Figure 5.7 and Table 5.4).

Clinical disorders

Growth hormone excess – acromegaly and gigantism

GH excess is rare, affecting approximately 60 people per million (Box 5.4). It most commonly arises from tumours of the pituitary somatotroph. In line with all pituitary tumours, these are virtually always benign adenomas rather than carcinomas.

Symptoms and signs

The phenotypic appearance of excessive bone growth differs depending on whether the patient

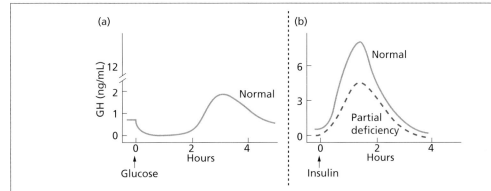

Figure 5.7 Dynamic tests of growth hormone (GH) status. (a) In an oral glucose tolerance test (OGTT) GH release is normally suppressed, although it can rebound as blood glucose returns to normal (as shown at 2–3h). In acromegaly, GH release does not suppress and may even rise paradoxically. (b) In an insulin tolerance test (ITT), insulin reduces blood glucose, which stimulates GH release in normal subjects. This response is blunted in partial GH deficiency and lacking in patients with complete deficiency; it is also diminished in some people with longstanding type 1 diabetes. The precise diagnostic values are shown in Table 5.4.

Table 5.4 Dynamic tests of growth hormone (GH) status

Test	Results
75 g oral glucose tolerance test (OGTT)	Rapid suppression of GH secretion to a nadir of <0.3 ng/mL (<0.8 mU/L) if normal
	Remains high in acromegaly or gigantism
Insulin tolerance test (ITT) [serum glucose ≤2.2 mmol/L (40 mg/dL)]	Stimulation of GH secretion: >6.7 ng/mL (>17 mU/L), normal 3–6.7 ng/mL (~8–17 mU/L), partial deficiency <3 ng/mL (<8 mU/L), severe GH deficiency
Amino acid infusion (commonly arginine)	Stimulation of GH secretion (useful in patients where insulin-induced hypoglycaemia is undesirable, e.g. in children)

Box 5.4 Growth hormone excess: a constellation of signs and symptoms caused by bony and soft tissue overgrowth, and metabolic disturbance

- *Gigantism*: occurs prior to epiphyseal closure and causes relatively proportionate increased stature
- *Acromegaly*: occurs after epiphyseal closure and causes progressive, cosmetic disfigurement because of disproportionate growth

---

presents prior to or after epiphyseal fusion. Before epiphyseal fusion, the excess GH promotes increased linear velocity, which remains relatively proportionate and results in extremely tall final stature – well over 2 m. Gigantism is relatively easy to recognize. After epiphyseal fusion, linear growth is no longer possible, leading to disproportionate growth and the features of acromegaly (Figure 5.8). A patient with a GH-secreting adenoma that started before puberty and only presents after epiphyseal fusion will carry features of both phenotypes. In isolation, acromegaly is more difficult to diagnose. The features are insidious, frequently causing a 10-year gap between the retrospective onset of symptoms and diagnosis (Box 5.5 and Case history 5.1). Making the diagnosis is important as acromegaly increases mortality two- to three-fold, mainly because of its cardiovascular complications.

Inspection of the patient will usually reveal many of the features of bony and soft tissue overgrowth (Figure 5.8). However, examination should also include the cardiovascular system as blood pressure might be increased and there might be signs of congestive cardiac failure (e.g. ankle oedema, basal lung crepitations).

Investigation and diagnosis

Three approaches can diagnose GH excess: serum IGF-I measurement elevated above the age- and sex-adjusted normal range; repeatedly detectable GH in a series of serum measurements illustrating autonomous production rather than the normal pulsatile secretion; and failure for GH to suppress [remaining >0.3 ng/mL (>0.8 mU/L) using newer immunoradiometric or chemiluscent assays following 75 g oral glucose (OGTT; Figure 5.7 and Table 5.4)]. In all but exceptionally rare ectopic GHRH secretion, the cause is a GH-secreting pituitary adenoma. By MRI these tumours are usually greater than 1 cm in diameter (i.e. a macroadenoma) and may have extended and eroded beyond the pituitary fossa at the time of diagnosis (see earlier anatomical complications of pituitary tumours).

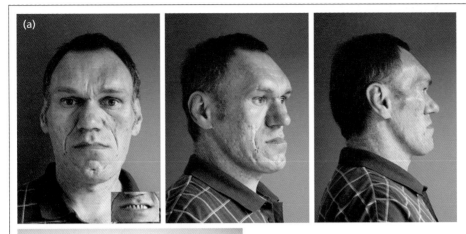

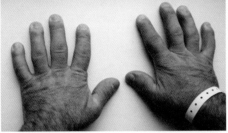

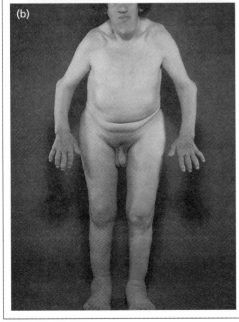

Figure 5.8 Two patients with acromegaly. (a) Patient 1. Note the large facial features, frontal bossing, prognathia causing under-bite (the lower teeth are further forward than the upper teeth) and dental separation, greasy skin quality, and thickened 'spade-like' hands. (b) Patient 2. Note enlargement of the hands and feet. The joints are abnormal and there is thickening of soft tissues with fluid retention, manifest here by ankle oedema, although this might also be a consequence of right-sided heart failure.

Box 5.5 Symptoms and signs of growth hormone excess

Musculoskeletal (acromegaly unless indicated)
- Increased stature (gigantism)
- Protruding mandible ('prognathia'), teeth separation on lower jaw
- Big tongue ('macroglossia')
- Enlarged forehead ('frontal bossing')
- Large hands and feet (carpal tunnel syndrome, tight rings, increasing shoe size)
- Osteoarthritis from abnormal joint loading

Cardiovascular
- Dilated cardiomyopathy, cardiomegaly, cardiac failure
- Hypertension

Metabolic
- Impaired glucose tolerance or potentially secondary diabetes (see Chapter 11)

Skin
- Irritating, thickened, greasy (increased sebum production)
- Excessive sweating

General
- Headaches
- Tiredness, often very disabling lowering quality of life and ability to work

Local tumour effects
- See earlier section on anatomy and pituitary space-occupying lesions

Treatment

Restoring normal GH status returns age-adjusted mortality to normal. The goal is a normal age-adjusted serum IGF-I and GH nadir on glucose loading of less than 0.3 ng/mL (0.8 mU/L). This is sometimes very difficult to achieve. There are several options (Table 5.5).

If the tumour is accessible in its entirety, trans-sphenoidal surgery can be curative. Serum GH falls promptly if successful; if it remains elevated, some neurosurgeons will re-operate straight away. If surgery is not curative (the goal may have been only to debulk an extensive tumour), medical therapy is possible. Normal somatotrophs respond to somatostatin via specific cell-surface receptors by reducing GH secretion. Most GH-secreting adenomas retain this feature to some extent so that they can be treated by potent somatostatin analogues delivered by monthly intramuscular injection. If these fail, dopamine agonists (see treatment of prolactinomas later) can sometimes be helpful, especially if the tumour co-secretes prolactin. Pegvisomant antagonizes GH action at the GH receptor. Although this is a beautiful example of drug design (see Figure 3.7), it remains prohibitively expensive for many patients in the UK and other countries.

A common management pathway sees a patient treated with a somatostatin analogue if trans-sphenoidal surgery is not curative. If this still fails to achieve normal GH status [e.g. normal serum IGF-I, nadir GH <0.3 ng/mL (<0.8 mU/L) on OGTT], external beam radiotherapy can be administered. Hypopituitarism is common after radiotherapy, requiring attentive follow-up; however, once radiotherapy has been effective (e.g. IGF-I in the age- and sex-adjusted normal range), somatostatin analogue therapy can be withdrawn.

There is much debate over whether GH promotes bowel tumour formation and/or growth. Colonoscopy, at least once at diagnosis, can be considered to look for colonic polyps with malignant potential. Long-term surveillance is contentious, but may have a role in patients who are not cured by the above modalities, i.e. where there is ongoing GH excess.

Growth hormone deficiency

Like GH excess, insufficient GH presents differently at different times of life. Prior to final height, it comes to the attention of the paediatric endocrinologist as failure to grow ('falling off' height centile charts; Figure 5.9). In adulthood, it presents insidiously, often in conjunction with other pitui-

Table 5.5 Treatments of acromegaly

Advantages	Disadvantages
Transsphenoidal surgery – common first-line	
Rapid effect	Invasive and requires general anaesthetic
Can restore vision in optic nerve compression	Non-curative for large, extrasellar tumours
Might be curative if complete resection	May cause hypopituitarism by damage to other cell types
Somatostatin analogue drugs – lower growth hormone (GH)	
Non-invasive	Monthly intramuscular injection (most commonly)
May shrink large extrasellar tumours	Expensive, may lower chance of curative surgery for intrapituitary lesions
Decreases GH in ~60% of patients	Gastrointestinal side-effects (commonly diarrhoea)
	Unlikely to be curative, i.e. continuous therapy needed
Radiotherapy – a good second or third line	
Non-invasive	Slow to act – may take up to 10 years
Likely to shrink tumour and reduce GH levels	Likely to cause hypopituitarism by destroying other pituitary cell types
Might be curative	Mildly increases risk of cerebrovascular disease

Case history 5.2

A 40-year-old woman had attended her family doctor for a cervical smear. She saw a new doctor, her previous doctor having known her since childhood. The new doctor was concerned by the patient's coarse facial appearance and asked some questions. The woman was surprised to be asked about her shoe size but confirmed that most of her shoes were now a size larger than 10 years ago.

What diagnosis is being considered?
What other questions should be asked?
What specific features of the examination should be sought?
What tests would confirm the doctor's suspicion?

Answers, see p. 97

tary hormone deficiencies following surgery or radiotherapy to the anterior pituitary (Box 5.6).

Any pituitary space-occupying lesion can cause loss of somatotrophs and GH deficiency. In childhood, this may be a craniopharyngioma; in adults, most likely a non-functioning adenoma. Other childhood causes include congenital deficiency (Figure 3.9; review Box 3.6) or cranial irradiation for CNS tumours or haematological malignancy. In adults, loss of GH secretion is part of physiological

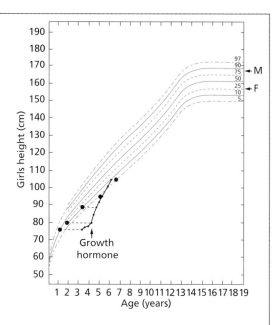

Figure 5.9 Short stature due to growth hormone (GH) deficiency and the effect of GH replacement. The height of a girl is shown compared to the reference growth charts, where the population is split into centiles (i.e. 50% of girls' heights lie below the 50th centile line, 5% below the 5th, etc.). Her height for chronological age (·) is greatly reduced, but skeletal maturity (or bone age) is also delayed. As a consequence, height plotted for bone age (•) falls within the centiles of normality. Bone age is determined by radiological examination of the left hand. Comparison is made with standard radiographs to assess skeletal maturity. Serum GH was undetectable in a basal sample and no secretion could be elicited by dynamic testing. Secretion of other anterior pituitary hormones was normal. After GH replacement was initiated, there was rapid catch-up of both height and skeletal maturity. M and F represent maternal and paternal height respectively.

> **Box 5.6 Symptoms and signs of growth hormone deficiency**
>
> - Decreased stature/cessation of growth (childhood)
> - Decreased exercise tolerance
> - Decreased muscle mass and strength
> - Increased body fat/decreased lean body mass
> - Centripetal fat distribution, increased waist:hip ratio
> - Hypertension and ischaemic heart disease
> - Decreased left ventricular mass
> - Dyslipidaemia [increased low-density lipoprotein (LDL)–cholesterol]
> - Osteoporosis
> - Poor quality of life

ageing and may be partly responsible for some of the changes in body composition associated with ageing, but does not usually produce obvious clinical symptoms.

If GH is lacking, try to stimulate it; lack of GH is diagnosed by stimulation testing alongside identifying a low serum IGF-I value (see Figure 5.7 and Table 5.4). It is treated by the daily subcutaneous injection of recombinant GH (oral peptides would be degraded in the intestine). In children with true GH deficiency, this results in a spectacular clinical effect, with a small child growing slowly into a normally sized adult. It is also used by paediatric endocrinologists to treat short stature of other causes (e.g. Turner syndrome/45,XO). Administration of GH in adequate dose will make any child grow more quickly in the short term, but does not necessarily increase final height.

The benefit of treatment in adulthood remains contentious amongst clinicians as improvements for individual patients can be minimal. Treatment is also relatively expensive and invasive; thus, it is important to demonstrate clear patient benefit from GH replacement. At present, UK guidelines include a quality-of-life questionnaire generating an Assessment of Growth Hormone Deficiency in Adults (AGHDA) score and clear biochemical evidence of GH deficiency (see Table 5.4). From the clinician's perspective, improvement in fasting lipid analysis would also be persuasive for continuing replacement therapy. In clinical trials, studies have reported extensive benefits:

- Improvements in fat mass
- Decreased waist-to-hip ratio and lower visceral fat
- Increased lean body mass
- Increased bone mineral density

- Increased muscle mass and strength
- Increased maximal exercise performance
- Increased VO$_2$max, maximum power output, maximum heart rate and anaerobic threshold
- Increased left ventricular mass, stroke volume, cardiac output and resting heart rate with decreased diastolic blood pressure
- Increased red cell mass
- Increased emotional reaction and improved social isolation scores
- Increased perceived quality of life
- Increased self-esteem
- Decreased sleep requirement

Prolactin

Human prolactin (PRL) is secreted by the lactotroph cells in the anterior pituitary and comprises 199 amino acids with three disulphide bonds. By weight, outside of pregnancy or breast-feeding, the PRL content of the normal human pituitary gland is ~1% that of GH.

Effects and mechanism of action

Prolactin plays some role in stimulating growth of the alveolar component of breast tissue during adolescence. However, its major action is to stimulate breast milk production (lactation) (Figure 5.10; also see the endocrinology of pregnancy in Chapter 7, Box 7.16). Following childbirth and the consequent decrease in maternal serum oestrogen and progesterone, PRL in the presence of cortisol initiates and maintains lactation. Its loss results in the immediate cessation of milk secretion. PRL also inhibits synthesis and release of LH and FSH by the anterior pituitary gonadotrophs. This causes a physiological secondary amenorrhoea (see Box 7.17) that acts as a natural contraceptive in the post-partum period. In birds, the hormone stimulates nest-building activity and crop-milk production; in reptiles, amphibians and some fish, it acts as an osmoregulator. These wider functions and the conservation of PRL-like molecules across species have led to other actions being attributed to PRL in both male and female humans. However, for many of these proposed functions, the physiological significance remains unclear (Figure 5.10). Like GH, PRL signals through specific receptors that dimerize and recruit tyrosine kinase signalling pathways (review Chapter 3 and Figure 3.8).

Regulation of production

The principles and features of PRL regulation are similar to those of GH. PRL from lactotrophs is under tonic inhibition by dopamine, with TRH providing a stimulatory input (Figure 5.10). Stress increases serum PRL. Although the peaks are not as discrete as for GH, PRL is also released episodically with highest levels during sleep. The most profound changes in serum PRL occur during pregnancy and lactation. The concentration increases progressively, up to 10-fold, through pregnancy, possibly in part because of rising oestrogen levels. It remains elevated during lactation under the stimulus of suckling, an example of a positive feedback loop: prolactin stimulates milk production, consumed by suckling, which in turn by a neural reflex stimulates further prolactin release. The loop is only broken once the baby stops suckling.

Clinical disorders

Hyperprolactinaemia
Symptoms and signs
Increased serum PRL causes oligomenorrhoea or secondary amenorrhoea (see Box 7.17), or subfertility in women of reproductive age by inhibiting the normal pulsatile secretion of LH and FSH, and the mid-cycle LH surge, leading to anovulation. When present, inappropriate breast milk production (galactorrhoea) is striking. Hyperprolactinaemia occurs with sufficient frequency to be relevant to the primary care physician. The underlying cause is commonly a microprolactinoma. Other causes are listed in Box 5.7 (Case history 5.3).

In contrast, men and post-menopausal women tend to present later when the underlying pathology is more likely to be a larger macroadenoma, and presenting symptoms and signs may reflect the consequences of a space-occupying lesion (see Box 5.1). Men with hyperprolactinaemia may also present with gynaecomastia or features of secondary hypogonadism (see Box 7.10).

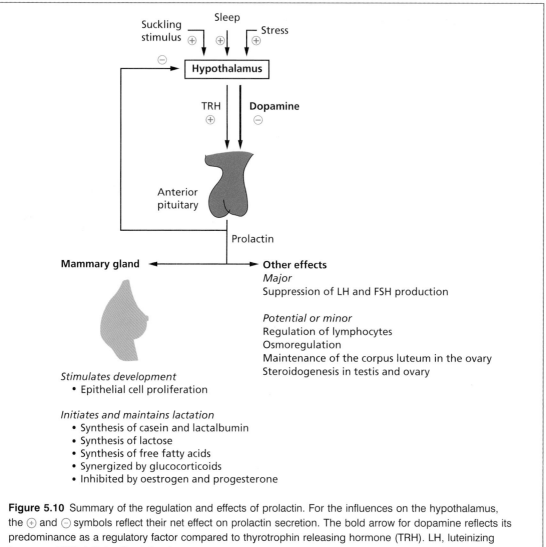

Figure 5.10 Summary of the regulation and effects of prolactin. For the influences on the hypothalamus, the ⊕ and ⊖ symbols reflect their net effect on prolactin secretion. The bold arrow for dopamine reflects its predominance as a regulatory factor compared to thyrotrophin releasing hormone (TRH). LH, luteinizing hormone; FSH, follicle stimulating hormone.

Investigation and diagnosis

Diagnosing hyperprolactinaemia requires several blood samples to avoid the risk of raised PRL secondary to stress from a single painful venesection leading to a false diagnosis. Also, on occasion, large forms of PRL, called macroprolactin (do not confuse the word with macroprolactinoma), are detected by some PRL assays. Although inactive biologically, macroPRL creates the false impression of hyperprolactinaemia. If suspected, additional laboratory methods can remove it from the assay. These issues aside, the major challenge is to tease apart the differential diagnosis when serum PRL is repeatedly above the normal range [i.e. >~500 mU/L (~25 ng/mL)] (Box 5.7).

The exclusion of pregnancy is mandatory to avoid further unnecessary investigation. Otherwise, the extent of the raised prolactin concentration gives a clue to the underlying diagnosis. PRL secretion from microprolactinomas and macroprolactinomas forms a continuum above the upper limit of the normal range. However, when PRL is only relatively modestly increased [500–2000 mU/L (~25–100 ng/mL)], other diagnoses need consideration, such as

Box 5.7 Hyperprolactinaemia

Commonly presents in women with amenorrhoea ± galactorrhoea
Confirm hyperprolactinaemia on several stress-free blood tests

Differential diagnosis
- Pregnancy
- Prolactin moderately raised [500–2000 mU/L (~25–100 ng/mL)]:
  - ○ Primary hypothyroidism (↑ TRH drive to PRL secretion)
  - ○ Stress
  - ○ Drug treatment [e.g. dopamine receptor antagonists antiemetics, antipsychotics, antidepressants, certain antihypertensives (α-methyldopa, reserpine), opioids and H₂ antagonists]
  - ○ Chronic renal failure (reduced clearance) and cirrhosis
  - ○ Idiopathic (PRL levels frequently return to normal)
  - ○ Stalk disconnection
  - ○ Acromegaly
  - ○ Chest wall injury
  - ○ Nipple stimulation
- High prolactin [>3000 mU/L (>~150 ng/mL)]:
  - ○ Microprolactinoma
- Very high prolactin [>6000 mU/L (>~300 ng/mL)]:
  - ○ Macroprolactinoma

Treatment
- Dopamine agonist (e.g. cabergoline)
- Surgery and radiotherapy rarely needed

primary hypothyroidism causing inadequate feedback of thyroid hormone on TRH, raised TRH and lactotroph (as well as thyrotroph) stimulation. Renal disease can compromise clearance, slightly elevating circulating PRL levels. Therefore, serum urea and electrolyte assays, and tests for pregnancy and thyroid function should be performed.

A drug history is important as some pharmacological agents can stimulate PRL release. For example, any drug that inhibits dopamine synthesis (e.g. L-methyldopa) or action (e.g. dopamine recep-

tor antagonists used as antiemetics) can increase serum PRL and cause galactorrhoea.

Having excluded other causes, the aetiology is likely to be a pituitary tumour, most frequently a microprolactinoma, which is the commonest scenario in women of reproductive age. With pituitary pathology, especially larger macroprolactinomas, other anterior pituitary axes need to be assessed as they may be underactive. On occasion, acromegaly may be suspected as some pituitary tumours can secrete both GH and PRL, possibly reflecting the shared developmental origin of the somatotroph and lactotroph. There is also the possibility of stalk disconnection syndrome where a pituitary tumour (especially if superiorly positioned), previous surgery or trauma can block hypothalamic dopaminergic neurones from reaching the lactotrophs, causing a mild rise in PRL. However, serum PRL concentration above 2000 mU/L (~100 ng/mL) most likely indicates a prolactinoma. Thereafter, serum levels tend to correlate with size and can exceed 100,000 mU/L (~5000 ng/mL) in large tumours. MRI will delineate the size of the pituitary tumour and any impact on the surrounding structures. Where there is extensive growth close to the optic chiasm, formal visual field assessment is very important.

Treatment

The major reasons for treating hyperprolactinaemia are to prevent inappropriate lactation, restore fertility and prevent bone demineralization from inadequate oestrogen in women or testosterone in men (see Chapter 7).

Treatment is by cause. If secondary to offending drugs, these should be withdrawn or changed wherever possible. This is frequently difficult with antipsychotic medication and treatment changes should be discussed with the mental health team. Primary hypothyroidism is treated with thyroxine.

Prolactinomas are exquisitely sensitive to dopamine agonists. Therefore, prolactinomas of all sizes should be treated with medical therapy in the first instance, even in the presence of optic chiasm compression and visual field loss. Surgery and/or radiotherapy are only very rarely required. Upon dopamine agonist treatment, PRL falls, tumour cells shrink quickly and sight is commonly restored.

Historically, bromocriptine has been used; however, it is frequently associated with nausea because of its action on other dopamine receptor sub-types. Better alternatives now include cabergoline, taken orally, usually twice weekly. By treating for 5 years, the majority of microprolactinomas are cured, i.e. PRL remains in the normal range permanently after withdrawal of therapy. This is not true of large macroprolactinomas, which are more likely to require on-going treatment. In recent years, there has been concern over drugs derived from ergot alkaloids, like cabergoline, causing sclerotic heart valve pathology. However, the data emanate from use in Parkinson disease at much higher dose than commonly prescribed for hyperprolactinaemia (e.g. cabergoline 250 μg twice weekly).

The management of prolactinomas in pregnancy can potentially be difficult. Although there is little evidence of a teratogenic effect, dopamine agonists are usually stopped. However, the lactotroph population normally increases significantly during pregnancy and there is a risk of excessive tumour growth, especially from macroadenomas. Headaches and visual disturbance are very important symptoms. One strategy is to conduct visual field analyses in each trimester. In addition, within a specialist setting, observing serum PRL measurements broadly commensurate with the stage of pregnancy is reassuring that very large tumour growth has not occurred. If necessary, MRI and potential reinstitution of dopamine agonist therapy can be considered.

Breast cancer

Epidemiological studies have linked higher levels of PRL with increased risk of breast cancer, treatment failure and worse survival, but whether therapeutic lowering of PRL alters these outcomes is unknown.

Hypoprolactinaemia

Low serum prolactin from loss of lactotrophs in hypopituitarism has no known clinical consequence beyond failure of lactation and thus inability to breast-feed. This demonstrates the questionable significance of PRL in humans other than on lactation and gonadotrophin production.

🔍 Case history 5.3

A 16-year-old girl was referred to the gynaecologist with a history of primary amenorrhoea, tiredness and poor growth. She was receiving no medication. She was not sexually active. She was short. Investigations showed raised PRL [2000 mU/L (~100 ng/mL)] and MRI revealed an enlarged pituitary. Her renal function was normal. A diagnosis of prolactinoma was made and she was treated with cabergoline. She started to have periods but did not grow. Repeat imaging of her pituitary showed no change. At this point she was referred to the endocrinologist who performed further investigations and realized that the initial diagnosis was wrong. Her treatment was altered and she started to grow. Her pubertal development continued and, furthermore, there was complete resolution of the abnormality on MRI.

What are the possible causes of
    hyperprolactinaemia?
What investigation made the diagnosis?
Why did the pituitary enlargement on MRI
    regress with treatment?

Answers, see p. 97

Adrenocorticotrophic hormone

ACTH is a short peptide of 39 amino acids. Residues 1–24 are highly conserved and confer full activity, such that synthetic ACTH(1–24) is used clinically to test adrenocortical function (see Chapter 6). ACTH comes from the *pro-opiomelanocortin* gene (*POMC*), which encodes the POMC protein that is cleaved enzymatically into many potential products (Figure 5.11). These include several forms of melanocyte-stimulating hormone (MSH) and β-endorphin with morphine-like activities that may inhibit pain signals to the brain. The enzyme that cleaves POMC to yield

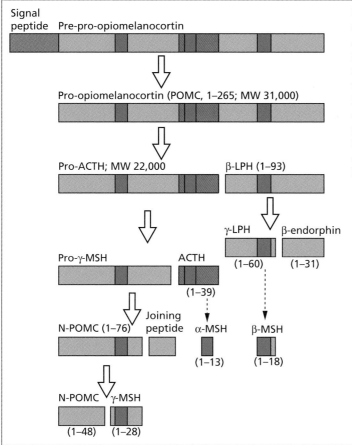

Figure 5.11 The cleavage of pro-opiomelanocortin (POMC). Adrenocorticotrophic hormone (ACTH) prior to and after cleavage is shown in red. Dark blue areas represent different forms of melanocyte-stimulating hormone (MSH). The number of amino acids in each peptide unit is shown in parentheses. LPH, lipotrophic hormone; N-POMC, the amino-terminal sequence of POMC. MW, molecular weight in kilodaltons.

ACTH is called prohormone convertase 1/3 (officially abbreviated as PCSK1), which also catalyzes the cleavage of insulin and C-peptide from proinsulin in pancreatic β-cells (see Chapter 11).

Effects and mechanism of action

The major clinical action of ACTH is at the adrenal cortex, where it stimulates several of the enzymatic reactions that convert cholesterol to either cortisol or adrenal sex steroid precursors (see Chapter 6). The hormone acts on the adrenocortical cell surface via a specific G-protein–coupled receptor, the type 2 melanocortin receptor (MC2R), to increase intracellular levels of cAMP (review Chapter 3). ACTH also binds the MC1R in the skin to cause pigmentation; a feature that acts as a surrogate marker of corticotroph overactivity in

adrenocortical insufficiency (see below and Chapter 6). The cleavage of POMC by PC1/3 to generate ACTH is also important in hypothalamic neurones as its failure is a rare monogenic cause of obesity (see Chapter 15).

Regulation of production

ACTH production is stimulated by CRH from the hypothalamus and inhibited by cortisol from the adrenal cortex in a negative feedback loop. Specific details of axis regulation and its circadian rhythm are discussed in Chapter 6 (see Figure 6.4). Vasopressin potentiates CRH action and may be particularly important during fetal life. Like PRL and GH, ACTH (and consequently cortisol) rises with stress, mediated by neural inputs from other parts of the brain. This includes stress from hypoglycaemia, such that insulin administration to lower serum glucose is a clinical test of corticotroph function and potential ACTH deficiency (see 'insulin tolerance test' in the next section).

Clinical disorders

Excess ACTH and Cushing disease

An excess of cortisol is called Cushing syndrome (see Chapter 6). When secondary to too much ACTH from a corticotroph adenoma, the disorder is called Cushing *disease*, after Harvey Cushing who described the original disorder. The corticotroph overactivity stimulates adrenal cortices bilaterally, which become enlarged, and cortisol increases to pathological levels. Clinically, the challenge is to recognize and diagnose glucocorticoid excess (i.e. Cushing syndrome); then to decipher whether the source is adrenal in origin (e.g. an adrenocortical adenoma; see Figure 4.7) or due to too much ACTH from either the anterior pituitary (Cushing disease) or secreted ectopically from rare tumours, such as small cell carcinoma of the lung (see Table 10.6). The tests, approach and treatment are described in Chapter 6.

In Cushing disease, the negative feedback from cortisol is unable to control ACTH secretion; however, it still exerts some effect. In particularly difficult operative cases and where pituitary radiotherapy has failed, a last resort is to remove the adrenal glands to solve the problem of excess cortisol. On occasion, this ultimate removal of negative feedback causes uncontrolled invasive growth of the corticotroph adenoma and is called Nelson syndrome.

Interestingly, some non-functioning adenomas with no recognizable hormone secretion, when removed, display cellular immunoreactivity for ACTH. These tumours pursue a slightly more aggressive course of recurrence and re-growth, requiring close surveillance with MRI and consideration of radiotherapy (see Box 5.2).

Excess ACTH as a result of adrenocortical insufficiency

Increased corticotroph activity is a physiological response to diminished negative feedback from cortisol in primary hypoadrenalism. Increased *POMC* expression leads to raised levels of ACTH and characteristic hyperpigmentation of the skin, especially in unusual places like scars, skin creases and inside the mouth (see Figure 5.11).

ACTH deficiency

In ACTH deficiency, biosynthesis of cortisol (and sex steroid precursors) by the adrenal cortex is lost, causing secondary hypoadrenalism (see Chapter 6). Historically, the diagnosis of hypoadrenalism as a result of pituitary dysfunction has been made using the ITT (see GH deficiency earlier; Table 5.4). Insulin is injected to produce hypoglycaemia [blood glucose <2.2 mmol/L (<40 mg/dL)], which, under normal circumstances, stimulates a large stress response, and a prompt rise in ACTH and thus cortisol. The test is unpleasant and not without danger, requiring continuous medical supervision. It is contraindicated in patients with cardiovascular disease. The ITT is still used as it allows simultaneous assessment of both ACTH and GH responses. However, ACTH deficiency for longer than a few months leads to atrophy of the adrenal cortex, which can also be revealed by an inadequate cortisol response to synthetic ACTH(1–24) (see Chapter 6). This latter test, which is easier to perform, may fail to diagnose recent corticotroph underactivity where the adrenal cortex has started to fail but can still respond to pharmacological stimulation.

Thyroid-stimulating hormone

TSH is a glycoprotein composed of two subunits (α and β; see Figure 2.4). The α-subunit is shared by TSH, LH and FSH, with hormone specificity conferred by different, distinctive β-subunits. TSH is synthesized in the thyrotrophs, which constitute ~10% of the cells in the anterior pituitary.

Effects and mechanism of action

TSH is the major physiological regulator of the thyroid gland, stimulating the biosynthesis and secretion of thyroid hormones (see Chapter 8). The hormone acts on the thyroid follicular cell surface via its specific cell-surface G-protein–coupled receptor to increase intracellular cAMP levels (review Chapter 3; see Figure 8.4).

Regulation of production

TSH production is stimulated by TRH and acts to stimulate the biosynthesis and release of thyroid hormones – thyroxine (T_4) and tri-iodothyronine (T_3). Basal TSH secretion depends on tonic TRH release; rare hypothalamic lesions or transection of the pituitary stalk result in TSH deficiency and subsequent hypothyroidism. Negative feedback by thyroid hormone at the anterior pituitary decreases the effectiveness of TRH, in part by reducing TRH receptor number on the cell surface of the thyrotrophs. Somatostatin also inhibits TSH secretion from the anterior pituitary.

Clinical disorders

Excess TSH
Excess TSH is almost always a normal compensation to thyroid underactivity and is used as a screen for hypothyroidism in newborn babies (see Chapter 8). Tumours that secrete TSH ('TSHomas') are very rare. They are usually sporadic macroadenomas and present with hyperthyroidism with inappropriately detectable TSH. The serum α-subunit is usually raised. The differential diagnosis is thyroid hormone resistance syndrome as a result of mutations in the thyroid hormone receptor. The latter condition is usually inherited and may be identified by the family history and genetic testing.

TSH deficiency
Any condition resulting in hypopituitarism (see later) can cause TSH deficiency and clinical hypothyroidism (see Chapter 8).

Gonadotrophins – luteinizing hormone and follicle-stimulating hormone

LH and FSH are secreted from the gonadotrophs, which make up 10–15% of cells in the anterior pituitary. As for TSH, the glycoproteins LH and FSH are composed of a common α-subunit and individualized β–subunit. Variation of the carbohydrate post-translational modification (i.e. the 'glyco-' part; review Chapter 3) leads to substantial subtle variation (microheterogeneity).

Effects and mechanism of action

LH and FSH regulate gonadal function in males (testosterone biosynthesis and spermatogenesis in the testis) and females (oestrogen and progesterone biosynthesis in the ovary, and the menstrual cycle). All of these complex functions are described in detail in Chapter 7. Both hormones act through cell-surface G-protein–coupled receptors linked to cAMP second messenger signalling.

Regulation of production

The production of gonadotrophins is stimulated by the hypothalamic 10-amino acid hormone, GnRH, which binds to its G-protein–coupled receptor on the cell surface of the gonadotroph and is linked to cAMP second messenger signalling. Factors such as stress and prolactin act negatively (see Figure 5.10). Like the hypothalamic–anterior pituitary axes regulating the adrenal cortex and thyroid, hormones secreted by the testis and ovary (steroid sex hormones and inhibins) exert negative feedback on the production of both GnRH and gonadotrophins (see Chapter 7, Figures 7.8 and 7.12).

Clinical disorders

Excess gonadotrophins
Increased levels of both gonadotrophins almost always reflect loss of negative feedback from the testis or ovary. Usually, primary testicular or ovarian failure yields serum LH and FSH levels several fold higher than the upper limit of normal. The commonest cause of this gonadotrophin overactivity is physiological after the menopause when ovarian depletion of ova ends cyclical hormone production in women. Excess gonadotrophin secondary to increased GnRH stimulation is rare. In contrast, inappropriately timed rather than excessive production causes central precocious puberty (see

Chapter 7). A pituitary adenoma secreting functional LH or FSH is incredibly rare. Commonly, however, non-functioning pituitary adenomas may stain by immunohistochemistry for the α-subunit, perhaps giving an indication of the developmental lineage, but little else.

Deficiency of the gonadotrophins

During childhood, it is normal for the gonadotrophins to be low and relatively unresponsive to GnRH; however, continued gonadotroph inactivity will delay puberty (see Chapter 7). This can be tested by GnRH stimulation when serum LH and FSH are measured 30 and 60 min later. A normal response is a two- to three-fold increase from basal serum levels. After puberty, loss of gonadotrophins causes secondary hypogonadism. In women, this is very common at some stage of the reproductive years as cyclical gonadotrophin secretion is very vulnerable to 'stress', such as major exercise (e.g. marathon running), excessive dieting or, most commonly, emotional anxiety of relatively minor proportions. A rise in prolactin levels is also sufficient to suppress LH and FSH production (see earlier). Several syndromes from mutations in any one of a number of genes also result in loss of gonadotrophins because of absent GnRH. Kallman syndrome is a combination of absent GnRH-secreting neurones and lack of smell (anosmia).

Clinically, it is important to realize that, in the face of significant hypogonadal symptoms and signs, and low levels of sex hormones, gonadotrophins within the normal range are inappropriately low. In women, where significant fluctuation of gonadotrophins accompanies the normal menstrual cycle, this can be more difficult to identify. It tends to manifest as amenorrhoea with low or undetectable serum oestrogen. In both sexes the disorder is described as 'hypogonadotrophic hypogonadism' (Box 5.8; see Chapter 7).

Hypopituitarism

Syndromes of pituitary hormone excess tend to be restricted to one particular hormone. In contrast, deficiency commonly affects several of the anterior

---

> ### Box 5.8 Hypogonadotrophic hypogonadism
>
> Low or 'normal' gonadotrophins + hypogonadal symptoms, signs and biochemistry
> = hypogonadotrophic hypogonadism

---

pituitary hormones and, potentially, those of the posterior pituitary (see next section). This is termed 'hypopituitarism' and when all hormones are inadequate, 'panhypopituitarism'. In adult endocrinology, hypopituitarism is most commonly encountered as a result of compression from non-functioning pituitary adenomas or their treatment by surgery or radiotherapy. In paediatric practice, congenital absence or malformation of the pituitary gland, or inactivating mutations affecting the synthesis of a particular hormone are more relevant.

Clinical issues relating to the lack of individual anterior pituitary hormones are covered in preceding sections. The clinical approach to hypopituitarism where multiple hormones may be missing is brought together here and in Box 5.9. Each hormone that is potentially missing and its consequences demands consideration. History taking and examination need to include all the features of hormone deficiency described in each of the preceding sections, e.g. hypogonadism, hypothyroidism and hypoadrenalism. For instance, diagnosing deficiency of LH and FSH, but missing concomitant ACTH deficiency might lead to a patient's death from hypoadrenalism (see Chapter 6 and Case history 5.4).

Mutations in several genes cause pituitary hypoplasia (Box 5.9). Those responsible for early formation of the pituitary gland tend to cause broader loss of anterior pituitary cell types and can include malformation of other nearby structures (e.g. absent corpus callosum and optic nerve underdevelopment in septo-optic dysplasia due to *HESX1* mutations). In contrast to the other lineages, isolated TSH deficiency is rarely a problem. Because corticotrophs are set aside relatively early during anterior pituitary differentiation, ACTH tends to be spared in cases of congenital hypopituitarism. However, isolated

Box 5.9 Hypopituitarism

Clinical suspicion requires investigation of all the hormone axes

Pituitary destruction
- Adenoma or other tumours (craniopharyngioma, meningioma, metastasis)
- Previous surgery
- Radiotherapy
- Infarction

Congenital pituitary disorders
- Pituitary hypoplasia or aplasia
  - E.g. mutations in *POU1F1*, *PROP1*, *HESX1*, *LHX2*
  - Mutations in *TPIT* tend to affect only the corticotroph lineage

Others
- Impaired secretion of hypothalamic hormones (e.g. loss of GnRH neurones in Kallman syndrome; see Chapter 7)
- Disconnection of the hypothalamic–pituitary axis (e.g. stalk tumour, trauma or infection)

ACTH deficiency is caused by inactivating mutations in *TPIT*.

In adults, the hypothalamic–pituitary axes are particularly vulnerable to irradiation. Loss of pituitary hormones, especially GH, can become almost inevitable after cranial radiotherapy, but may take up to 10 years to manifest. In contrast, gonadotrophin secretion is particularly vulnerable to trauma such as surgery. Infarction of the pituitary is rare, although one well-described condition, Sheehan syndrome, reflects hypotension following major post-partum haemorrhage. The sudden vascular insufficiency to a hypertrophied gland (i.e. following pregnancy) leads to sudden death of pituitary tissue. Major headache and the symptoms and signs of sudden hormone loss (e.g. failure of lactation, hypoadrenalism) are clues.

Having defined which hormone axes are underactive, replacement of the appropriate hormones needs consideration. In hypopituitarism, it is man-

datory to replace missing cortisol using hydrocortisone (see Chapter 6) and thyroid hormone using thyroxine (see Chapter 8). Depending on age and sex, gonadal hormones (in men and pre-menopausal women; see Chapter 7) and GH (during childhood, adolescence and in some adults; see earlier) may also be appropriate.

Case history 5.4

A patient has been diagnosed with acromegaly and referred to an endocrinologist. Visual field assessment reveals bitemporal hemianopia. MRI demonstrates a large pituitary mass extending to and compressing the optic chiasm. Serum PRL was 1200 mU/L (57 ng/mL), TSH was undetectable, fT$_4$ was 5.3 pmol/L (0.4 ng/dL) and an ACTH stimulation test gave a serum cortisol value at 30 min of 305 nmol/L (10.9 µg/dL).

What do these biochemistry results indicate?
What urgent treatments are needed and in what order?

Answers, see p. 97

Hormones of the posterior pituitary

The two hormones synthesized in the hypothalamus and released from the posterior pituitary are oxytocin and vasopressin (see Table 5.1). Although structurally similar, being composed of nine amino acids, they have markedly different physiological roles (review Figure 1.3).

Vasopressin

Clinically, vasopressin is also known as 'antidiuretic hormone' (ADH) and has also been called 'arginine vasopressin'. The biology of vasopressin is summarized in Box 5.10.

Box 5.10 Summary of vasopressin biology

Physiology
- Circulates largely unbound ⇨ rapidly metabolized in the liver and filtered by the kidney ⇨ $t_{1/2}$ ~15 min

Function
- Regulates water excretion by the kidney – its main action at normal circulating vasopressin levels:
  - Acts on the distal convoluted tubule ⇨ increased permeability to water ⇨ water resorption ⇨ increased urine concentration
- Potent vasoconstrictor

Cellular mechanism of action
- Distinct cell-surface G-protein–coupled receptor (V) sub-types and second messengers:
  - V_1 (two further sub-types) ⇨ phosphatidylinositol (PI) metabolism and raised intracellular Ca^{2+} ⇨ vascular smooth muscle contraction
  - V_2 ⇨ cAMP ⇨ renal water excretion (receptor antagonized by 'vaptan' class of drugs)

Box 5.11 Regulation of vasopressin

Serum osmolality (S_{OSM})
- High (e.g. dehydration) ⇨ increased vasopressin release ⇨ increased water retention ⇨ decreased S_{OSM}
- Low (e.g. water intoxication) ⇨ decreased vasopressin release ⇨ decreased water retention ⇨ increased S_{OSM}

Volume
- Fall in blood volume ≥8% (e.g. haemorrhage) ⇨ increased vasopressin release ⇨ vasoconstriction

O_2 and CO_2 tension
- Decreased arterial O_2 partial pressure (P_aO_2) ⇨ increased vasopressin release
- Increased arterial CO_2 partial pressure (P_aCO_2) ⇨ increased vasopressin release

---

Effects and mechanism of action

In the kidney, the presence of vasopressin and the high osmolality of the renal interstitium lead to water movement out of the final section of the distal convoluted tubule along the osmotic gradient. The effect can be truly remarkable. For example, a child weighing 30 kg needs to excrete a solute load of ~800 mOsm in 24 h: at its most dilute (~50 mOsm/kg), this load requires 16 L of urine; under maximal vasopressin stimulation, it can be achieved with little over 700 mL (~1100 mOsm/kg).

Vasopressin is a potent vasoconstrictor and has been utilized either directly or in synthetic analogue form to achieve haemostasis, e.g. in severe gastrointestinal bleeding or post-partum haemorrhage. It also acts on vascular tone at normal physiological levels. During fetal development, vasopressin serves as an additional stimulus for ACTH release from corticotrophs.

Regulation of production

The main physiological regulator of vasopressin release is serum osmolality detected by osmoreceptors in the hypothalamus (see earlier for functions of the hypothalamus). Circulating volume is detected by baroreceptors in the carotid sinus and aortic arch, and by plasma volume receptors in the left atrium.

In addition to the factors listed in Box 5.11, angiotensin II, epinephrine, cortisol and the female sex steroids, oestrogen and progesterone, can also modulate vasopressin release. The latter may explain the fluid retention that can occur in the latter part of the menstrual cycle. As with other hypothalamic hormones, the CNS plays an important part in the regulation of vasopressin. Pain and trauma associated with surgery cause a marked increase in the circulating vasopressin concentration, as do nausea and vomiting. The activity of the neurohypophyseal system is also influenced by environmental temperature; a rise in temperature stimulates vasopressin release prior to any change in plasma osmolality.

Clinical disorders

Excess vasopressin/syndrome of inappropriate antidiuretic hormone

The syndrome of inappropriate ADH (SIADH) refers to the release of vasopressin when normal regulatory mechanisms should restrict its secretion into the circulation (Case history 5.5). This is a difficult and dangerous clinical situation (Box 5.12) where hyponatraemia and low osmolality can cause irreversible brain damage and death.

Symptoms and signs

Headache and apathy progress to nausea, vomiting, abnormal neurological signs and impaired consciousness. In very severe cases, there may be coma, convulsions and death. Generalized oedema is not a feature because free water is evenly distributed across all body compartments.

Investigation, diagnosis and treatment

The cardinal features of SIADH are low serum osmolality, hyponatraemia and inappropriately high urine osmolality. Other common causes of hyponatraemia, especially in the elderly, are congestive cardiac failure and diuretic use. In SIADH, identifying the underlying cause is important (Box 5.12). Vaptans are new non-peptide drugs that can be given orally in chronic SIADH. They antagonize the V_2 receptor lowering the number of aquaporin water channels in the renal collecting duct thus reducing water re-absorption from the urine.

Box 5.12 Excess vasopressin/SIADH

Definition
- Hyponatraemia + low serum osmolality (<270 mOsm/kg) + inappropriately high urine osmolality

Causes
- Tumours (e.g. small cell cancer of the lung)
- Any brain disorders (trauma, infection, tumour)
- Pneumonia
- Cytotoxic therapy (chemotherapy or radiotherapy)
- Narcotics and analgesics
- Hypothyroidism
- Hypoadrenalism

Treatment
- Identify and treat underlying cause where possible
- Restrict fluid intake (up to 1 L/day) and replace sodium lost in the urine
- Vaptans act as V_2 receptor antagonists
- Demeclocycline may induce partial diabetes insipidus (see below) but it is less commonly used now

---

Case history 5.5

A 74-year-old man presented to the emergency medical service with a 2-week history of a cough productive of bloody green sputum, fever, shortness of breath and pleuritic chest pain. He was a life-long smoker. Serum sodium was 124 mmol/L (124 mEq/L), potassium 3.6 mmol/L (3.6 mEq/L), urea 2.7 mmol/L (~7.6 mg/dL) and creatinine 73 μmol/L (~0.8 mg/dL). Serum osmolality was 258 mOsm/kg and urine osmolality was 560 mOsm/kg.

What is the most likely endocrine cause for the hyponatraemia and what acute condition underlies it?
What measures might be taken to rectify the situation?
What further investigations might be considered?

Answers, see p. 97

Deficiency of vasopressin/diabetes insipidus

Even when damage to the posterior pituitary occurs, vasopressin or oxytocin deficiency commonly does not arise so long as the hypothalamic neurones that transport the hormones remain intact (see earlier anatomy section). When deficiency of vasopressin or its action does occur, it results in diabetes insipidus (DI). Deficiency of vasopressin production by the hypothalamus and posterior pituitary is termed 'cranial DI', whereas deficient action at the V_2 receptor causes 'nephrogenic DI' (Table 5.6). In the former, the vast majority of vasopressin production needs to be lost ($\geq$90%) before water balance is necessarily affected. The term DI stems from when physicians used to taste urine and contrast it with the sweet urine of diabetes mellitus.

Symptoms and signs

Patients with DI pass extremely large and frequent volumes of low osmolality urine (potentially 20 L in 24 h). This polyuria and passing urine at night (nocturia) demonstrate that in DI the patient is unable to reduce urine flow. Clinically, problems only tend to arise when the patient also lacks sensation of thirst or is deprived of water, when plasma osmolality rises.

Investigation and diagnosis

Some centres have access to a vasopressin immunoassay, which allows the diagnosis to be made by monitoring serum vasopressin concentration after an infusion of hypertonic saline. Most endocrinologists still rely on the water deprivation test and the use of the vasopressin analogue, desmopressin (Table 5.6).

Treatment

Having diagnosed DI, it remains important to consider and investigate the underlying cause, which may be curable. Otherwise management of DI relies on intact thirst and access to adequate fluid. For cranial DI, replacement of vasopressin is all that is required. Desmopressin, either by intranasal spray, tablet or injection, is a synthetic analogue that acts predominantly on the V_2 receptor and therefore has minimal hypertensive side-effects. Desmopressin is sometimes also used in normal children who suffer from nocturnal enuresis (bed-wetting). Nephrogenic DI and psychogenic polydipsia can be harder to

treat effectively. In the latter, the high urine flow rate tends to dilute the solutes that create the counter-current exchange mechanism in the renal parenchyma such that the kidney loses its ability to concentrate urine.

🔍 Case history 5.6

A 58-year-old woman was referred by her family doctor because of complaints of passing urine every hour during both the day and night. Nothing else was volunteered in the history and the doctor had excluded diabetes mellitus. The patient had browsed the internet and felt she had diabetes insipidus. Serum sodium was 135 mmol/L (135 mEq/L), potassium 4.5 mmol/L (4.5 mEq/L), urea 4.3 mmol/L (~12.0 mg/dL) and creatinine 93 μmol/L (~1.1 mg/dL).

What other aspects of the history need direct questioning?
What test(s) is appropriate to confirm or refute a diagnosis of diabetes insipidus?
If diabetes insipidus is confirmed, in which two sites might the pathology lie?

Answers, see p. 97

Oxytocin

The major roles of oxytocin are during birth and breast-feeding (see Chapter 7). It is also emerging as a brain neurotransmitter with roles in modulating behaviour and overeating.

Effects and mechanism of action

Oxytocin has two main sites of action: the uterus and the mammary gland. It is the hormone of parturition, literally meaning 'quick birth'. It increases the contraction of the myometrium during labour

Table 5.6 Diabetes insipidus (DI).

In brief

Deficient vasopressin secretion or action ⇨ large volume of low osmolality urine ⇨ problems from high serum osmolality

Cranial DI	**Nephrogenic DI**
Causes	*Causes*
CNS tumours	Drugs (e.g. lithium, demeclocycline)
Head trauma	Familial X-linked recessive (i.e. males affected):
Infection (e.g. meningitis and encephalitis)	*V_2 receptor* gene mutation*
Familial autosomal dominant:	Autosomal recessive:
Vasopressin gene mutation*	*Aquaporin 2* gene mutation*
DIDMOAD syndrome (DI, diabetes mellitus, optic atrophy and deafness)	Chronic renal disease
'Idiopathic'	

Investigated by the water deprivation test

Conducted over 8 h during the day with repeated measurements of weight and serum (S_{OSM}) and urine (U_{OSM}) osmolality

Terminate test if body weight falls ≥5% (dangerous) and allow the patient to drink

DI diagnosed if:

- S_{OSM} rises to ≥293 mOsm/kg (normal: 283–293 mOsm/kg); U_{OSM} remains ≤300 mOsm/kg

Desmopressin (a synthetic vasopressin analogue) is given to distinguish between cranial and nephrogenic DI**:

- Cranial DI, urine now concentrates to ≥750 mOsm/kg
- Nephrogenic DI, urine still fails to concentrate, U_{OSM} remains ≤750 mOsm/kg

Hypokalaemia and hypercalcaemia can suggest nephrogenic DI

Psychogenic polydipsia (i.e. habitual excess water intake): S_{OSM} should remain ≤293 mOsm/kg, commonly with partial concentration of urine. If S_{OSM} remains normal and U_{OSM} fails to concentrate with continued urine output, suspect covert drinking

Treatment

Ensure an intact sense of thirst and free access to fluid

Desmopressin provides hormone replacement for cranial DI

*Syndromes arising from gene mutations are due to loss of function.
**If desmopressin has been administered at the end of the water deprivation test, restrict fluid intake to <500 mL over the next 8 h to avoid risk of profound hyponatraemia (e.g. in cranial DI or polydipsic patients).

causing expulsion of the fetus and the placenta. In this role progesterone appears to antagonize and oestrogen potentiate the uterine response to oxytocin. Post-partum in the mammary gland, oxytocin causes contraction of the myoepithelial cells surrounding the alveoli and ducts to expel milk from the breast.

Like vasopressin, oxytocin circulates largely unbound and so is removed rapidly by the kidney ($t_{1/2}$ ~5 min). Outside parturition and breast-feeding, it circulates in very low concentrations and is normally undetectable in the blood. Oxytocin binds to its cell-surface G-protein–coupled receptor and signals intracellularly via phosphatidylinositol metabolism and calcium (review Figure 3.16).

Regulation of production

The movement of the fetus down the birth canal is an example of positive feedback in endocrinology (review Chapter 1). Oxytocin stimulates uterine muscular contraction which moves the fetus into the distending vagina, which in turn sends neural inputs back to the brain to enhance oxytocin secretion. This positive feedback loop is only broken once the fetus is expelled. Other factors, such as the fall in progesterone and the presence of oestrogen, may play a minor part in regulating oxytocin release.

Similarly, positive feedback regulates oxytocin release during breast-feeding. Suckling of the nipple causes release of oxytocin and leads to ejection of milk. Even the sight and sound of an infant can stimulate milk ejection. Stimulation of oxytocin secretion ceases once the baby stops suckling.

Clinical disorders

Endocrine syndromes of oxytocin excess and deficiency have not been described. However, increased oxytocin appears to improve behaviour in autism spectrum disorder.

🔑 Key points

- GH, PRL, ACTH, FSH, LH and TSH are the major hormones of the anterior pituitary
- Oxytocin and vasopressin are the major hormones of the posterior pituitary
- Pituitary tumours, especially non-functioning adenomas, are very common
- Hormone overactivity secondary to tumour formation can cause well-recognized endocrine syndromes
- Always consider local structural damage and compression from pituitary tumours
- Underactivity of the anterior pituitary tends to affect multiple hormones

---

🔍 Answers to case histories

Case history 5.1

The patient has bitemporal hemianopia. This is caused by loss of function of optic nerve fibres; the only point where pressure can cause this distribution of visual field loss is at the optic chiasm.

The most likely pathology at this location is upward growth of a pituitary tumour.

The best imaging modality is MRI. In an emergency setting, CT can be useful, but the resolution from MRI is much better for intracranial structures.

If a pituitary space-occupying lesion is detected, the patient should be referred urgently to an endocrinologist for two reasons: first, a prolactinoma will almost certainly shrink with dopamine agonist therapy with restoration of vision (see clinical section on prolactin); and second, with pituitary tumours, it is critical to think of what hormone function may have been lost by local pressure on pituitary cell types. Most importantly, the patient may be hypoadrenal because of loss of ACTH secretion (see Chapter 6) and hypothyroid (see Chapter 8) from TSH deficiency. In an emergency setting (e.g. if the patient has presented unconscious and hypotensive and a large pituitary mass has been detected), hydrocortisone should be administered intravenously.

Case history 5.2

The diagnosis under consideration is acromegaly. Its insidious nature means that those who know the patient well frequently miss it.

Questions should address symptoms and signs relating to GH excess (see Box 5.5). In addition, are there any symptoms or signs from loss of other pituitary hormones (e.g. hypoadrenalism or hypothyroidism) or a local mass effect? A sensitive question would interrogate potential loss of the menstrual cycle. Facial photographs should be sought from the previous 10–20 years.

In addition to the features listed in Box 5.5, examination should look for potential visual field defects or diplopia.

Serum IGF-I should be measured. A 75g OGTT should be considered or a serum GH day series conducted.

Case history 5.3

The differential diagnosis of hyperprolactinaemia is given in Box 5.7. The presence of poor growth and tiredness suggests hypothyroidism.
A thyroid function test showed a markedly raised serum TSH with low T_4.

The lack of thyroid hormone feedback to the pituitary had led to an increase in TRH which, in turn, had promoted growth of lactotrophs. Once this stimulus was removed by restoration of thyroxine negative feedback on TRH, the pituitary enlargement regressed.

Case history 5.4

The patient has secondary hypothyroidism and hypoadrenalism from the pituitary mass. The PRL is minimally raised but is unlikely to

represent co-secretion of PRL by the tumour. It is more likely to indicate a small degree of stalk disconnection.

The patient should be placed on daily hydrocortisone, then thyroid hormone, and programmed for urgent transsphenoidal surgery to debulk the tumour and relieve pressure on the optic chiasm. Vision might be permanently lost if surgery is delayed. Surgery is highly unlikely to be curative and suitable secondary treatments include somatostatin analogues and/or radiotherapy.

Case history 5.5

The man has SIADH. Although Addison disease might be considered in view of the hyponatraemia, the plasma osmolality is low. The SIADH is secondary to pneumonia, although an underlying lung malignancy cannot be excluded as a contributory factor.

After taking samples of sputum and blood for microbiology, antibiotics should be started and fluid intake restricted to ~1 L over the next 24 h with close attention paid to urine output and haemodynamic status, e.g. pulse and blood pressure. Tachycardia and hypotension would argue for high-dependency care.

Other investigations directly related to his symptoms include arterial blood gas assessment (with oxygen given if the patient is hypoxic), chest X-ray and sputum analysis for tuberculosis and malignancy.

In this case, fever settled rapidly with antibiotics, the patient remained haemodynamically stable, serum sodium rose within 12 h to 132 mmol/L (132 mEq/L) and, on continuing the same management, normalized 36 h later. Other symptoms gradually improved. No evidence was obtained for lung malignancy and electrolytes were normal at discharge.

Case history 5.6

The history needs to focus on the CNS for previous trauma or infection and specific symptoms such as headache. Questions need to exclude renal damage. A drug history and family history are required for agents or inherited syndromes that cause DI.

The patient should be admitted for a water deprivation test. This test needs strict monitoring as it can be dangerous (see Table 5.6) and patients with psychogenic polydipsia are known to cheat (taps may need to be isolated from mains water). An alternative if available might be serum vasopressin measurement following hypertonic saline.

DI is either 'cranial' (relating to the hypothalamus and posterior pituitary) or 'nephrogenic' (distal convoluted tubule of the kidney), reflecting deficient vasopressin production or action.

CHAPTER 6

The adrenal gland

Key topics

- The adrenal cortex   100
- The adrenal medulla   119
- Key points   124
- Answers to case histories   124

Learning objectives

- To appreciate the separate development of the adrenal cortex and medulla as two organs in a single gland
- Adrenal cortex:
  - To understand the zone-specific biosynthesis and function of mineralocorticoids, glucocorticoids and sex steroid precursors
  - To recognize the clinical consequences of underactivity, overactivity or disordered function of the adrenal cortex
- Adrenal medulla:
  - To understand the biosynthesis and function of adrenomedullary hormones
  - To recognize the clinical consequences of catecholamine over-production from tumours

This chapter integrates the basic biology of the adrenal gland with the clinical conditions that affect it

Essential Endocrinology and Diabetes, Sixth Edition. Richard IG Holt, Neil A Hanley.
© 2012 Richard IG Holt and Neil A Hanley. Published 2012 by Blackwell Publishing Ltd.

To recap

■ As preparation for understanding the role of the adrenal gland, review the synthesis of steroid hormones and hormones derived from tyrosine described in Chapter 2

■ To understand the effects of hormones from the adrenal gland, begin by reviewing hormone action, especially that of steroid hormones, described in Chapter 3

Cross-reference

■ The adrenal cortex is regulated by the anterior pituitary corticotroph such that the body's cortisol status reflects whether the corticotroph is physiologically normal, underactive or overactive (see Chapter 5)

■ Endocrine neoplasia syndromes can involve the adrenal gland resulting in cortisol excess (ectopic hormone-secreting tumours) or phaeochromocytoma and paraganglioma (see Chapter 10)

The adrenal cortex

Embryology and anatomy

Understanding the development of the adrenal gland can be necessary to appreciate adrenal pathology (Box 6.1).

The adrenal cortex forms from epithelial cells that line the abdominal ('coelomic') cavity of the developing embryo during the fifth week of development (Figure 6.1). These cells generate concentric functional layers called the outer definitive and the inner fetal zones of the adrenal cortex. This pattern is distinctive to higher primates and only begins its reorganization after birth into the more characteristic layers of the adult adrenal cortex (Figure 6.2 and Box 6.2). The development of the adrenal medulla is described later.

The adrenal gland lies immediately superior to the kidney (hence the anatomical name, 'suprarenal' gland). This anatomy can be important clinically in hypersecretion or tumours. For instance, when sampling the veins that drain centripetally through the adrenal gland to measure hormone secretion, access on the left is via the renal vein and technically more challenging. The adrenal and kidney capsules are closely assimilated. Removal of the kidney ('nephrectomy') almost always includes ipsilateral adrenalectomy. In contrast, either adrenal can be removed, increasingly by laparoscopic approaches, without disturbing the adjacent kidney. However, embryological variations can present challenges to the endocrine surgeon. Additional or unusual blood vessels can supply and/or drain the organ, or embryological 'rests' of adrenocortical cells can lie outside the gland.

Biochemistry by zones

Although what determines and maintains the distinct adrenocortical zones remains unclear, knowledge of the different regions is important because they define, and are defined by, very different biochemical activity (Box 6.2). This compartmentalized function is all the more remarkable in light of the prevailing theory of adrenocortical ageing, whereby steroid secretion changes as cells migrate from the outer glomerulosa to the innermost reticularis where they undergo apoptosis.

The principles of steroidogenesis were introduced in Chapter 2. To recap, the steroid product depends on the complement of enzymes that catalyze the sequential modification of cholesterol (Figure 6.3 and Box 6.3). Many of these enzymes are members of the cytochrome P450 superfamily. Although the nomenclature for the corresponding

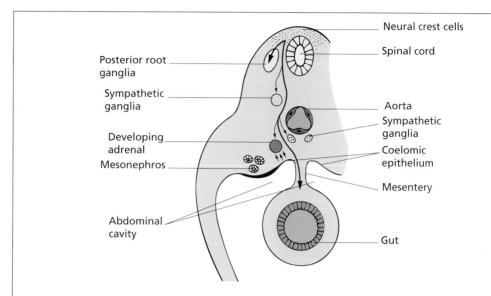

Figure 6.1 Development of the adrenal gland. The cortex is derived in part from the epithelium lining the abdominal cavity. Neural crest cells migrate from the back of the embryo; some give rise to dorsal root and sympathetic ganglia, while others invade the adrenal cortex to form the medulla. The rim of coelomic epithelium shown in black also gives rise to steroidogenic cells of the gonad.

Box 6.1 Clinical consequences of embryology

- The adrenal cortex and medulla develop separately – clinical disorders almost always affect either the cortex or medulla, but not both
- Forming the organ requires cell migration – adrenal disorders can occasionally cause trouble in unexpected places from embryological 'rests' of cells
- The cells forming the adrenal cortex also form the steroidogenic cell lineages in the gonad – disorders of steroid production can affect both organs simultaneously

genes has been unified, several names remain in common usage (Table 6.1). Awareness of these names is important as several of the genes are subject to mutation in congenital adrenal hyperplasia (CAH), one of the more common paediatric endocrine emergencies.

Function and regulation of the hormones

Aldosterone and cortisol serve as ligands for nuclear hormone receptors, which then function as transcription factors that influence target gene expression (review Chapter 3). It seems that both hormones also have more rapid non-genomic actions, although these are less well understood. The mechanism of action for dehydroepiandrosterone (DHEA) remains unclear, other than serving as an extra-gonadal precursor for sex hormone biosynthesis.

Cortisol

Cortisol is the major glucocorticoid in humans. Like all steroid hormones, it is not stored but synthesized according to acute changes in demand. Its release into the circulation influences cells in virtually every organ of the body. In the blood, cortisol is largely bound (>90%) to cortisol-binding globulin (CBG) and is assayed as total serum cortisol. Anything that alters the amount of CBG (e.g. oral contraceptive use or critical illness) alters total

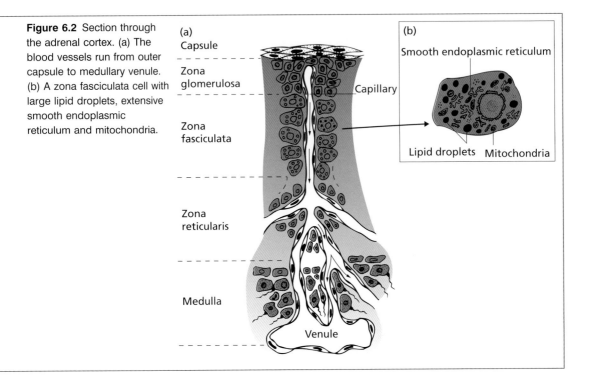

Figure 6.2 Section through the adrenal cortex. (a) The blood vessels run from outer capsule to medullary venule. (b) A zona fasciculata cell with large lipid droplets, extensive smooth endoplasmic reticulum and mitochondria.

(a) Capsule

Zona glomerulosa

Zona fasciculata

Zona reticularis

Medulla

Capillary

Venule

(b) Smooth endoplasmic reticulum

Lipid droplets   Mitochondria

Box 6.2 Zones of the adult adrenal cortex and their steroid hormone secretion

- *Zona glomerulosa*, nests of closely packed small cells creating the thinnest, outermost layer; secretes aldosterone
- *Zona fasciculata*, larger cells in columns making up ~three-quarters of the cortex; secretes cortisol and some sex steroid precursors
- *Zona reticularis*, 'net-like' arrangements of innermost cells, formed at 6–8 years to herald a poorly understood change called 'adrenarche'; secretes sex steroid precursors and some cortisol

cortisol measurement; an important clinical issue. Like thyroid hormones, it is only the free component that enters target cells. The free component also passes into urine – 'urinary free cortisol' (UFC) – where its collection and assay over 24 h has been used as a test of glucocorticoid excess (UFC is ~1% of cortisol production by the adrenal glands). Measuring salivary cortisol similarly avoids issues with fluctuating serum CBG.

Regulation of cortisol biosynthesis and secretion – the hypothalamic–pituitary–adrenal axis

The major regulation of the adrenal cortex comes from the anterior pituitary, via the production and circulation of adrenocorticotrophic hormone (ACTH), a cleavage product of the *pro-opiomelanocortin* (*POMC*) gene (review Chapter 5). In turn, ACTH is regulated by corticotrophin-releasing hormone (CRH) from the hypothalamus (Figure 6.4). By binding to cell-surface receptors and activating cAMP second messenger pathways, ACTH increases flux through the pathway from cholesterol to cortisol, particularly at the rate-limiting step catalyzed by CYP11A1. This happens acutely such that a rise in ACTH increases cortisol levels within 5 min. Cortisol provides feedback to the anterior pituitary and hypothalamus to

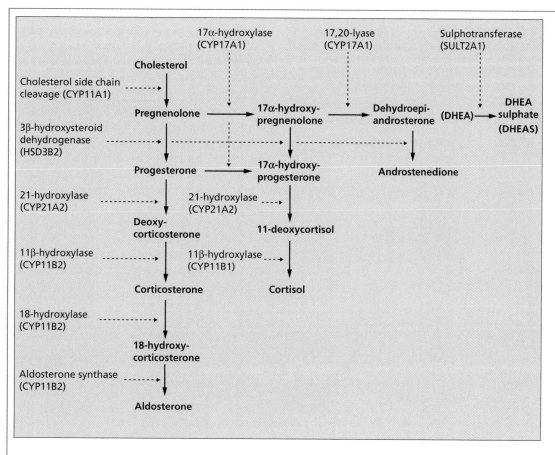

Figure 6.3 Biosynthesis of adrenocortical steroid hormones. HSD3B activity in the adrenal cortex arises from the type 2 isoform. The three steps from deoxycorticosterone to aldosterone are catalyzed by the same enzyme, CYP11B2 (also see Figure 2.6).

Box 6.3 Adrenocortical steroidogenesis can be summarized into a few key steps

- Transport of cholesterol into the mitochondrion by the steroid acute regulatory (StAR) protein
- The rate-limiting removal of the cholesterol side chain by CYP11A1
- Shuttling intermediaries between mitochondria and endoplasmic reticulum for further enzymatic modification
- Action of two key enzymes at branch points:
  - CYP17A1 prevents the biosynthesis of aldosterone and commits a steroid to cortisol or sex steroid precursor. Hence, CYP17A1 is absent from the zona glomerulosa
    - Early action of HSD3B2 steers steroid precursors away from the sex steroid precursors towards aldosterone or cortisol
- The presence and activity of CYP11B2 in the zona glomerulosa permitting aldosterone synthesis
- The presence and activity of CYP11B1 in the fasciculata (and less so the reticularis) zone allowing cortisol production

Table 6.1 Alternative names in common usage for steroidogenic enzymes

Gene name	Alternative common enzyme names and abbreviations
CYP11A1	Cholesterol side-chain cleavage enzyme (SCC) or desmolase
HSD3B2	Type 2 3β-hydroxysteroid dehydrogenase (Type 2 3β-HSD)
CYP21A2	21-hydroxylase
CYP11B1	11β-hydroxylase
CYP11B2	Aldosterone synthase
CYP17A1	17α-hydroxylase/17,20-lyase

inhibit CRH and ACTH production; thus, the hypothalamic–anterior pituitary–adrenal axis is established. Superimposed on this circuit is a circadian rhythm. Increased axis activity and cortisol levels (both in the serum and saliva) coincide with awakening in the morning, remain moderate during the day, then decline so that by late evening and during the night cortisol levels are low (Figure 6.5). Cortisol has a short half-life (~1–2 h in serum). Therefore, random measurement of a plasma or salivary cortisol is of limited clinical value. In diagnostic testing, samples tend to be collected at 9 AM (when they should be high) and late evening or midnight (when they should be low; see section on Cushing syndrome).

Damage to the anterior pituitary and loss of ACTH can lead to atrophy of the fasciculata and

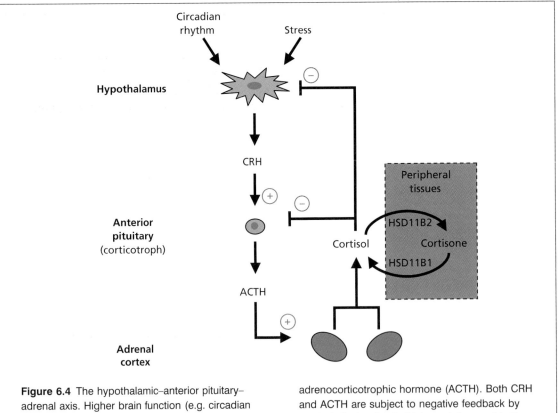

Figure 6.4 The hypothalamic–anterior pituitary–adrenal axis. Higher brain function (e.g. circadian rhythm and stress) influences corticotrophin-releasing hormone (CRH) synthesis and release, which acts on the corticotroph of the anterior pituitary to make adrenocorticotrophic hormone (ACTH). Both CRH and ACTH are subject to negative feedback by cortisol, the levels of which are influenced in the periphery and in target cells by the balance of 11β-hydroxysteroid dehydrogenase (HSD11B) activity.

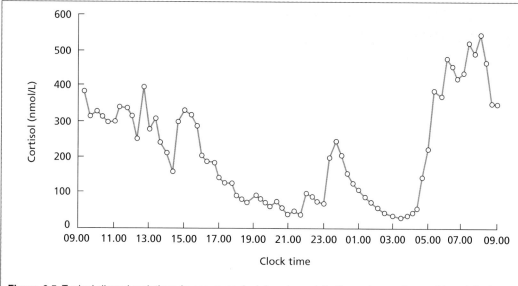

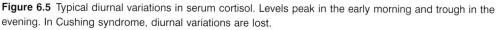

Figure 6.5 Typical diurnal variations in serum cortisol. Levels peak in the early morning and trough in the evening. In Cushing syndrome, diurnal variations are lost.

reticularis zones. In contrast, overactivity of the anterior pituitary induces a bilateral bulky increase in adrenocortical size. Unilateral growth also occurs following adrenalectomy of the contralateral gland.

Cortisol is metabolized in peripheral tissues to inactive cortisone, which can, in turn, be converted back to active hormone; the two enzymatic reactions being catalyzed by type 2 and type 1 11β-hydroxysteroid dehydrogenase (HSD11B2 and HSD11B1) respectively (Figure 6.4 and Box 6.4).

Functions
Intermediary metabolism
The net metabolic action of cortisol is to raise circulating free fatty acids and glucose, the latter stimulating glycogen synthesis (Box 6.5; see Figure 11.11). Excess cortisol also fosters an unfavourable serum lipid profile: raised total cholesterol and triglyceride with decreased high-density lipoprotein (HDL)–cholesterol. Cortisol has a permissive effect on epinephrine and glucagon, all of which creates a phenotype of 'insulin resistance' – the need for greater insulin secretion to maintain a normal blood glucose concentration (euglycaemia) (see Chapter 13 on type 2 diabetes). In the long-term, cortisol

---

> **Box 6.4 Important cortisol metabolism takes place in peripheral tissues and target cells**
>
> - Cortisol and cortisone are interconverted by isoforms of 11β-hydroxysteroid dehydrogenase (HSD11B):
>   - Type 2 (HSD11B2) inactivates cortisol to cortisone (the bulk of which occurs in the liver)
>   - Type 1 (HSD11B1) reactivates cortisone to cortisol
> - HSD11B1 is prevalent over HSD11B2 in visceral adipose tissue, making fat a significant source of cortisol:
>   - Centripetal obesity is associated with excess glucocorticoid

stimulates adipocyte differentiation, particularly in the viscera, predisposing to centripetal obesity.

Skin, muscle and bone
In skin, glucocorticoids inhibit keratinocyte proliferation and collagen synthesis. In muscle, the

catabolic effects reduce protein synthesis, resulting in atrophy. Similar catabolic effects in bone shift the balance of activity from osteoblast (the bone-forming cell type) to osteoclast (the bone-resorbing cell type), predisposing to osteoporosis (see Chapter 9). Taken together, there is a net flow of amino acids towards the liver.

Salt and water homeostasis and blood pressure

Glucocorticoids can potentially increase sodium resorption and potassium loss at the distal tubule through effects, not on the glucocorticoid receptor (GR), but thought to be via the mineralocorticoid receptor (MR). More proximally, cortisol increases glomerular filtration rate (GFR) and inhibits vasopressin to increase free water clearance. Cortisol raises blood pressure by several mechanisms, including increased sensitivity of the vasculature to catecholamines.

Growth and development

Cortisol is an important hormone during growth and development of the fetus. It stimulates the differentiation of cell types to their mature phenotype. This is particularly evident in the lung, where it stimulates the production of surfactant, which reduces alveolar surface tension. This is one of the final steps in preparing the fluid-filled fetal airways

for post-natal life. Too much glucocorticoid inhibits growth, in keeping with its largely catabolic effects on the musculoskeletal system. Cushing syndrome presents to the paediatric endocrinologist as cessation of linear growth.

Lactation

Post-partum, cortisol is required for the initiation of lactation by PRL. Its loss leads to a gradual reduction in milk secretion.

Central nervous system and psyche

The role of glucocorticoids in the brain is highly complex, matched by their potential to cause a range of emotional symptoms from euphoria to depression.

Anti-inflammatory effects

Glucocorticoid actions on inflammation and autoimmunity are among its most important, reflected by the use of potent synthetic steroids to treat a range of disorders. With glucocorticoid treatment, circulating T lymphocytes and eosinophils fall; however, neutrophils rise. This is a catch to remember for the patient with an acute exacerbation of asthma. Raised circulating neutrophil count does not necessarily mean infection; it may simply reflect glucocorticoid treatment. In tissues, for instance, the acutely inflamed joints of a patient with rheumatoid arthritis, glucocorticoids rapidly suppress inflammation by inhibiting cytokine production and antagonizing macrophage action.

Aldosterone

The synthesis of aldosterone in the zona glomerulosa is demarcated by the absence of CYP17A1 and the presence of CYP11B2. The hormone circulates in ~1000-fold lower concentration and with a shorter half-life (~20–30 min) than cortisol. In part, this results from a diminished affinity for serum carrier proteins. It acts via binding the MR to influence gene expression in the nucleus of target cells (review Chapter 3). The MR is not specific for aldosterone, binding cortisol with equal affinity. However, specificity is preserved by HSD11B2,

Box 6.6 Aldosterone is the body's major mineralocorticoid

- Promotes sodium resorption from the urine and potassium excretion
- Increases blood pressure

Aldosterone biosynthesis is regulated primarily by:
- Renin–angiotensin system (forming a negative feedback loop)
- Serum potassium concentration

which inactivates cortisol to cortisone, at the major sites of mineralocorticoid action, the distal tubule and collecting ducts of the kidney (Table 3.2). Here, aldosterone acts on the Na^+/K^+-ATPase transporter to increase sodium resorption in exchange for potassium excretion (Box 6.6). The net effect is to increase osmotic potential within the circulation, causing expansion of circulating volume. The direct effect of aldosterone to increase blood pressure comes from vasoconstriction.

Regulation of aldosterone secretion

The enzyme, renin, is synthesized predominantly in the kidney, in specialized cells of the juxtaglomerular apparatus. These cells surround the afferent arteriole before it enters the glomerulus (Figures 6.6 and 6.7) and form a sensing mechanism for intravascular volume whereby decreased volume stimulates renin biosynthesis. Renin acts upon its substrate, circulating angiotensinogen, to generate the decapeptide, angiotensin I, which is subsequently converted into angiotensin II (AII). This latter octapeptide binds to the type 2 angiotensin II receptor in the zona glomerulosa cells to stimulate aldosterone production. In addition, AII is a very potent 'pressor' agent, causing arteriolar vasoconstriction. Renin–angiotensin axes exist to some extent within individual organs, providing an element of paracrine adrenocortical regulation of aldosterone biosynthesis and secretion. High potassium also stimulates aldosterone biosynthesis (Figure 6.6). ACTH plays a minor role in regulating aldosterone synthesis, although too much or too little ACTH does not

impact on circulating aldosterone levels. More importantly, the cellular mass of the zona glomerulosa influences longer term mineralocorticoid production. Thus, 'westernized' high salt diets, which expand the intravascular volume and raise blood pressure, suppress the renin–angiotensin system, leading to a shrivelled zona glomerulosa.

Sex steroid precursors

DHEA and its downstream derivative, androstenedione, possess only weak androgenic activity; however, their conversion in other tissues can give rise in adults to both potent androgen (e.g. testosterone) and oestrogen (e.g. oestradiol) (review Figure 2.6). Therefore, these 19-carbon steroids are best termed 'sex steroid precursors' (rather than 'adrenal androgens'). Like cortisol, biosynthesis is primarily regulated by ACTH but emanates predominantly from the reticularis zone. The relative activity of CYP17A1 and HSD3B2 on 17α-hydroxypregnenolone determines the production of DHEA (and androstenedione) versus cortisol.

The function of the sex steroid precursors is debated. During the first trimester of pregnancy, the fetal adrenal gland actually secretes some potent androgen (including testosterone) even in females. During the second and third trimesters, huge amounts of DHEA and its sulphated derivative, DHEAS, are generated. However, these steroids are not essential and their roles remain poorly understood. Post-natally, little sex steroid precursor is produced until adrenarche at 7–8 years when the zona reticularis becomes functionally mature. Further metabolism of the precursors to active sex steroids stimulates linear growth in middle childhood, sometimes accompanied by some pubic and axillary hair growth. This physiology is important as it needs to be distinguished from precocious puberty, the hallmarks of which include breast development in females and testicular enlargement in males (see Table 7.5).

Clinical disorders

The major clinical disorders affecting the adrenal cortex arise from either too much or too little cortisol and aldosterone.

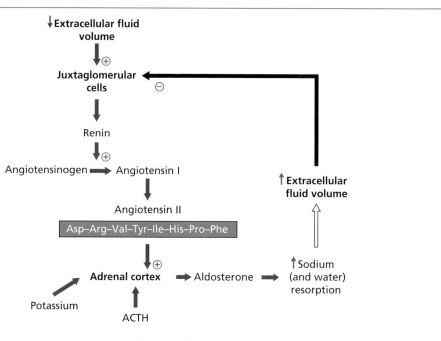

Figure 6.6 The renin–angiotensin–aldosterone axis. A fall in extracellular fluid (ECF) volume produces increased activity in renal nerves, reduced sodium flux in the macula densa and a fall in transmural pressure. These activate the juxtaglomerular apparatus to increase renin production, which catalyzes the beginning of the cascade that ends with angiotensin II-stimulated aldosterone secretion. This leads to increased sodium resorption with expanding ECF volume providing negative feedback on further renin production. High potassium, and to a lesser extent adrenocorticotrophic hormone (ACTH), also increase aldosterone production.

Hypoadrenalism

Primary hypoadrenalism arises from direct destruction of the adrenal cortex, whereas secondary disease arises from loss of the anterior pituitary corticotroph. In all circumstances there is shortage of cortisol and in primary disease additional deficiency of aldosterone.

Primary hypoadrenalism – Addison disease

Worldwide, the commonest cause of adrenocortical deficiency results from infection (either AIDS or tuberculosis). In the western world, autoimmune destruction of the cortex, first described by Thomas Addison in 1855, is prevalent. The disorder carries his eponymous title with the adjective 'Addisonian' referring to the clinical crisis from acute, severe cortisol (and aldosterone) deficiency. Other causes

of underactivity are more unusual, although developmental abnormalities should not be discounted in the paediatric setting (Case history 6.1).

Symptoms and signs

Symptoms and signs relate to:

- Diminished vascular volume and tone
- Renal sodium loss
- Bowel water and electrolyte loss
- Removal of negative feedback (causing pigmentation, see Chapter 5)
- Loss of cortisol action on hepatic and peripheral metabolism (Box 6.7).

The consequent classical laboratory findings are hyponatraemia (the vast majority) and hyperkalaemia (in most cases). Raised urea (a sign of con-

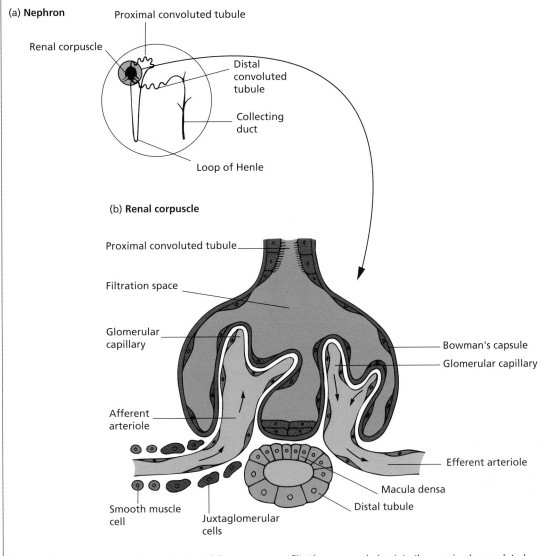

(a) **Nephron**

Proximal convoluted tubule

Renal corpuscle

Distal convoluted tubule

Collecting duct

Loop of Henle

(b) **Renal corpuscle**

Proximal convoluted tubule

Filtration space

Glomerular capillary

Afferent arteriole

Smooth muscle cell

Juxtaglomerular cells

Bowman's capsule

Glomerular capillary

Efferent arteriole

Macula densa

Distal tubule

Figure 6.7 The structure of a nephron and the juxtaglomerular apparatus. (a) A nephron. (b) Structure of a renal corpuscle, its blood supply and the juxtaglomerular apparatus. Between the afferent and efferent arterioles lies the glomerular capillaries, which are surrounded by Bowman's capsule. The filtration space drains into the proximal convoluted tubule. The juxtaglomerular cells, containing renin granules, replace the smooth muscle cells of the afferent arteriole and are positioned next to the closely packed macula densa cells of the distal tubule.

tracted intravascular volume) is a useful discriminator from inappropriate antidiuretic hormone syndrome (SIADH; hyponatraemia resulting from a diluted vascular space, see Chapter 5). Patients with autoimmune hypoadrenalism carry an increased risk of other autoimmune endocrinopathies (see Box 8.8).

Investigation

Plasma cortisol is variable, although a high enough level [e.g. >400 nmol/L (~14 μg/dL)] practically excludes Addisonian crisis. Similarly, serum cortisol <100 nmol/L (~3.6 μg/dL) in the morning becomes rather suspicious. ACTH tends to be high in

---

Box 6.7 Symptoms and signs of hypoadrenalism

- Weight loss and anorexia
- Fatigue and weakness
- Nausea, vomiting, abdominal pain and diarrhoea
- Generalized wasting and muscle cramps
- Hypoglycaemia (especially in children)
- Dizziness and postural hypotension
- Loss of body hair
- Pigmentation of light-exposed areas, pressure points, scars and buccal mucosa (in primary disease)
- Vitiligo (associated with autoimmune adrenalitis)
- Circulatory shock (in acute circumstances)

Box 6.8 A testing regimen for inadequate cortisol secretion

ACTH stimulation test ['short Synacthen test (SST)' in the UK; 'Cortrosyn stimulation test' in USA]
- Standard test: 250 μg IV or IM
- Measurements: pre-injection serum cortisol (and ACTH); serum cortisol 30 min post-injection
- Response: post-injection serum cortisol is >525 nmol/L (~19 μg/dL) in 95% of normal people

---

primary hypoadrenalism. *If under-activity is suspected, try to stimulate it*; the hallmark of diagnosis is dynamic testing. Serum cortisol is measured 30 min after intramuscular or intravenous injection of synthetic ACTH (Box 6.8), which contains the biologically active first 24 amino acids of ACTH. Tetracosactide is the generic name; however, it is better known by the trade names, 'Synacthen' in the UK and 'Cortrosyn' in the USA, leading to the 'short Synacthen test (SST)' and 'Cortrosyn stimulation test'. Although lower dose tests have been developed, the mainstay of adult endocrinology is to administer the full ampoule of 250 μg. Bearing in mind assay-to-assay variability and potential fluctuations in CBG, a serum cortisol level, 30 min later, greater than 525 nmol/L (~19 μg/dL) identifies the fifth percentile response (i.e. 95% of the population achieve higher values). In primary adrenocortical disease, plasma aldosterone may be low or normal; however, more tellingly, elevated renin (measured either as plasma activity and concentration) is indicative of adrenocortical failure.

Treatment

The mainstay of oral replacement therapy is hydrocortisone (the pharmacological name for cortisol – they are the same substance) and the synthetic

mineralocorticoid, fludrocortisone, according to the mantra '*if it is missing, replace it*'. Historically, endocrinologists have tended to over-replace cortisol with detrimental side-effects similar to those of Cushing syndrome (see next section). The standard adult replacement dose is 15–20 mg hydrocortisone/day – 10 mg on awakening, followed by either 5 or 10 mg mid-afternoon, or 5 mg at midday and a further 5 mg mid-to-late afternoon. This regimen is relatively effective at replicating the normal circadian rhythm: high levels in the morning, low levels by bedtime. Disturbance to this profile can present as either difficulty or tiredness executing daily tasks (inadequate cortisol) and inability to sleep at night (too much cortisol). Fludrocortisone is much longer acting and therefore is taken orally once daily (commonly 100 μg in adults).

To monitor hydrocortisone treatment, some endocrinologists advocate an intermittent series of serum measurements during the day (a 'cortisol day curve'), although no robust evidence supports its value. In contrast, mineralocorticoid replacement is frequently overlooked. Normalized renin (either serum concentration or plasma activity) from high values at diagnosis and normotension are valuable guides. Over-replacement tends to generate hypokalaemia and hypertension.

The major message for glucocorticoid replacement is that the patient is entirely dependent on tablets as the normal ability of the adrenal cortex to increase cortisol output during illness or stress is lost. Failure to advise the patient to double replace-

Box 6.9 Glucocorticoid replacement

- Double the dose during illness
- Carry a steroid alert card or bracelet

ment doses when unwell (i.e. illness sufficient to require bedrest) risks an Addisonian crisis, a critical lack of glucocorticoid presenting as circulatory collapse, hyponatraemia, hyperkalaemia and hypoglycaemia. This medical emergency demands immediate treatment with intravenous hydrocortisone as well as significant intravenous fluids to expand the contracted circulating volume. For these reasons, patients with adrenal insufficiency (either primary or secondary) should carry notification (Box 6.9).

Case history 6.1

A 35-year-old woman presented with tiredness and abdominal pain. She had fainted twice recently when unwell with vomiting and diarrhoea. Her sister takes thyroxine. On examination, she looked tanned with patches of skin depigmentation. Blood pressure was 90/60. Serum urea was slightly raised; however, creatinine was normal. Serum potassium was 5.5 mmol/L (5.5 mEq/L); serum sodium was low. Thyroid function tests were normal. The doctor also measured a full blood count. Haemoglobin was only 100 g/L with a mean cell volume (MCV) of 110 fl.

What is the likely diagnosis and what tests should be performed to confirm it?
What treatment should the patient be given?
What additional information should be provided?
What associated disorder should be considered to explain the haematological findings?

Answers, see p. 124

Secondary hypoadrenalism

If the anterior pituitary corticotrophs are underactive, ACTH-dependent processes in the adrenal gland also suffer. This translates as cortisol deficiency and loss of adrenal sex steroid precursors with retained aldosterone biosynthesis. The causes of corticotroph loss are covered in Chapter 5. However, the principles of glucocorticoid replacement therapy, and the consequences of its failure, are the same. Fludrocortisone is not required.

Hyperadrenalism

Adrenocortical overactivity most commonly produces either excess mineralocorticoid or excess glucocorticoid (± sex steroid precursors).

Glucocorticoid excess – 'Cushing syndrome'

An excess of glucocorticoid is called Cushing syndrome, named after Harvey Cushing, who in 1912 described the first case in a woman characterized by obesity and hirsuitism. Twenty years later, its hormonal basis was proposed. The commonest cause is exogenous glucocorticoid medication, e.g. as used in asthma. Discounting this, there are several endogenous causes of Cushing syndrome. However, despite greatly advanced knowledge, delays in detection remain problematic, the main hindrance being a failure of perception when presented with common, insidious symptoms. It most frequently occurs in women (Case history 6.2).

Symptoms and signs

The symptoms and signs of exaggerated cortisol action are shown in Box 6.10, and Figures 6.8 and 6.9. 'Buffalo hump' refers to the growth of a fat pad at the back of the neck.

Diagnosis

The first and most important step is to prove glucocorticoid excess; this diagnoses Cushing syndrome. Random plasma cortisol estimations are not useful as cortisol is a stress hormone and circulating levels vary during the day (see Figure 6.5).

Three screening tests are commonly used:

- Assessment of diurnal variation of cortisol
- 24-h urinary free cortisol measurement
- Low-dose dexamethasone suppression test.

For blood-based screening tests, ensure no confounding issues with CBG. For instance, in severely ill patients (e.g. those on intensive care), serum CBG may be decreased, and in female patients, testing must be conducted off the combined oral contraceptive pill, which increases CBG and thus total serum cortisol levels.

Autonomous production results in loss of diurnal variation with serum or salivary cortisol at

Box 6.10 Symptoms and signs of Cushing syndrome

- Muscle wasting, relatively thin limbs
- Easily bruised, thin skin; poor wound healing
- Striae (purple or 'violaceous' rather than white)
- Thin (osteoporotic) bones that easily fracture
- Diabetes mellitus
- Central obesity, rounded ('moon') face, 'buffalo hump'
- Susceptibility to infection
- Predisposition to gastric ulcer
- Hypertension
- Disturbance of menstrual cycle; symptoms overlapping with polycystic ovarian syndrome (see Chapter 7)
- Mood disturbance (depression, psychosis)

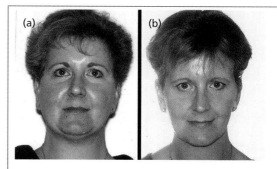

Figure 6.9 Cushing syndrome due to an adrenocortical adenoma secreting cortisol and sex steroisd precursors. The patient's face is shown prior to operation and 6 months after right adrenalectomy (the CT scan for the same patient is shown in Figure 4.7). The striking difference required the patient to renew her passport.

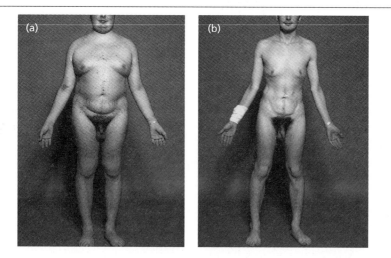

Figure 6.8 The effects of glucocorticoid excess in Cushing disease and the benefits of treatment. (a) Florid signs of excess cortisol in a 15-year-old boy: round face, greasy skin, severe acne, truncal obesity with stretch marks (striae) and bruising from a venepuncture site on the right arm. (b) Aged 16, 1 year after curative trans-sphenoidal surgery and an operation to remove excess abdominal skin.

midnight or bedtime failing to drop from daytime values (see Figure 6.5). Bedtime salivary collection avoids problems with CBG and can be done at home, avoiding the cortisol-raising stress and expense of hospitals (in-patient testing should be preceded by an acclimatization period of 1 or 2 days). In moderate-to-severe Cushing syndrome, cortisol is also raised several-fold in the urine. Patients are advised to collect all urine following the first micturition of the day and include the first sample from the following morning (i.e. capturing an entire 24-h period). Collection is relatively inconvenient to perform and is frequently incomplete. Subtle increases in cortisol excretion are seen in obesity and polycystic ovarian syndrome (PCOS). The third test is the low-dose dexamethasone suppression test (Table 6.2); a dynamic test based on the endocrine principle *'if overactivity is suspected, try to suppress it'*. Dexamethasone is a potent synthetic glucocorticoid, available orally, that inhibits physiological ACTH production from the anterior pituitary by negative feedback, decreasing cortisol production by the adrenal. There are two forms of the low-dose dexamethasone

test (Table 6.2). Occasionally, patients fail the 1-mg overnight test because they rapidly metabolize the dexamethasone; this should not occur using the formal 48-h test, which is otherwise more intrusive. Using either approach, Cushing syndrome is excluded if cortisol is less than 50 nmol/L (~1.8 µg/dL) the morning following the tablet(s). Additional factors can increase serum cortisol and complicate the differential diagnosis of Cushing syndrome. This is called 'pseudo-Cushing syndrome' (Box 6.11).

Alongside cortisol, DHEA and androstenedione, which can be converted into potent androgens causing hirsuitism and menstrual irregularities in women, may be elevated.

If cortisol remains high after low-dose dexamethasone testing, is raised in the urine and shows loss of diurnal variation (clinical endocrinologists commonly use a combination of screening tests), Cushing syndrome has been diagnosed. The next phase of investigation seeks to locate the causative site of the disease.

Diagnosing the cause and site of glucocorticoid excess

Primary adrenal Cushing syndrome is most commonly due to a benign adenoma of the zona fasciculata. The excess cortisol suppresses pituitary ACTH by negative feedback usually to undetectable levels (Box 6.12). In contrast, ACTH-secreting tumours may not increase serum ACTH above the normal

Table 6.2 Dexamethasone suppression tests
Low-dose dexamethasone suppression test
Diagnoses glucocorticoid excess
0.5 mg × 8 doses 6-hourly ending at 3 AM or single 1 mg dose at midnight
Positive diagnosis of Cushing syndrome: failure to suppress 9 AM serum cortisol the following morning to below 50 nmol/L (~1.8 µg/dL)
High-dose dexamethasone suppression test
Localizes glucocorticoid excess
2 mg × 8 doses 6-hourly ending at 3 AM
Anterior pituitary source: >50% suppression of 9 AM serum cortisol from pre- to post-test
Extra-pituitary ectopic source of ACTH (or adrenal tumour): <50% suppression of 9 AM serum cortisol from pre- to post-test

Box 6.11 Pseudo-Cushing syndrome

Causes
- Obesity
- Alcoholism
- Depression

Distinction from Cushing syndrome
- Diurnal variation is usually retained
- Cortisol falls on removal of alcohol abuse
- Cortisol tends to rise with insulin-induced hypoglycaemia

Box 6.12 Causes of Cushing syndrome

- Anterior pituitary tumour (Cushing disease): ACTH inappropriately normal or raised but can be suppressed by high dose dexamethasone
- Ectopic ACTH: extra-pituitary ACTH-secreting tumour: ACTH inappropriately normal or raised, less easily suppressed by high dose dexamethasone
- Adrenocortical tumour: baseline ACTH suppressed
- Exogenous glucocorticoids: baseline ACTH suppressed

reference range, but the hormone is inappropriately present for the level of circulating cortisol. The ACTH comes either from a corticotroph tumour of the anterior pituitary or from an ectopic source, e.g. small cell carcinoma of the lung (see Table 10.6). The high-dose dexamethasone suppression test has been used to distinguish between these options (Table 6.2). Baseline serum cortisol is assessed, followed by a total of 16 mg of dexamethasone over 48 h (2 mg 6 hourly). ACTH-secreting pituitary adenomas usually retain negative feedback in response to this high-dose dexamethasone sufficient to suppress serum cortisol by more than 50% from the baseline value. Cushing syndrome due to a corticotroph adenoma is referred to as 'Cushing *disease*'. Less effective suppression of serum cortisol (by less than 50%) suggests an ectopic source of ACTH. Although unreliable, serum ACTH levels tend to be higher from ectopic tumours than pituitary tumours. The high-dose dexamethasone suppression test lacks complete sensitivity and specificity; in experienced centres, venous sampling from the inferior petrosal sinus can be more effective for determining the origin of ACTH secretion, albeit with greater discomfort and risk from an invasive procedure, e.g. a very small percentage risk of stroke. Inferior petrosal sinus sampling (IPSS) is undertaken by interventional radiologists. The hormone is measured in left and right inferior petrosal sinus following CRH stimulation. A clear gra-

dient (3:1 or more) of ACTH from petrosal sinus to peripheral blood points to the anterior pituitary rather than an ectopic source and can also help to lateralize the tumour within the pituitary fossa. Because the normal pituitary gland would also show such a central:peripheral gradient, it is imperative that glucocorticoid excess is still present when IPSS is undertaken.

Having defined the excess and gained clues to location, it is now appropriate to image the anterior pituitary by MRI; the adrenal glands by MRI or CT; or continue the search for the ectopic source of ACTH (potentially by 'fine-cut' CT of the chest, PET scans where available or uptake scans that might identify a carcinoid tumour; review imaging in Chapter 4).

Treatment

Cushing syndrome causes premature mortality, predominantly from cardiovascular disease. The goal of treatment is to normalize glucocorticoid production and restore diurnal rhythm. For adrenal adenomas, unilateral adrenalectomy is undertaken. For pituitary adenomas, trans-sphenoidal surgery is commonplace in major centres but should be restricted to nominated surgeons (either ENT or neurosurgeons). The results of treating Cushing syndrome can be striking (see Figures 6.8 and 6.9).

In the immediate postoperative period, if the cause of excess glucocorticoid has been removed, the hypothalamic–anterior pituitary–adrenal axis should be so suppressed that endogenous cortisol cannot be detected. The body is so accustomed to high cortisol levels that the patient is commonly symptomatic of relative adrenal insufficiency on normal hydrocortisone replacement doses. Hydrocortisone therapy is needed for a sufficient period until the hypothalamic–anterior pituitary–adrenal axis returns to normal function. In those not fit for surgery, medical therapy, e.g. with metyrapone, can directly inhibit glucocorticoid secretion. For inoperable pituitary adenomas or following failed surgery, either because of location or size, pituitary radiotherapy remains a valuable option (review Chapter 5).

Case history 6.2

A 44-year-old woman had suffered symptoms that she attributed to PCOS by virtue of reading articles on the internet. She went to see the doctor because of feeling generally unwell, having put on 10 kg in weight and developing nocturia. She took no medication. The doctor suspected diabetes and, indeed, the patient's fasting blood glucose was 8.5 mmol/L (~153 mg/dL). However, the doctor was more struck by the patient's appearance of a flushed round face, poor facial skin quality and purple stretch marks on the abdomen. Blood pressure was 160/95 mmHg. The doctor arranged several tests that confirmed the diagnosis. Serum ACTH was then measured and was undetectable.

What is the initial diagnosis and what tests were used to make it?
Where is the causative lesion and what imaging investigations might be considered?

Answers, see p. 124

Primary mineralocorticoid excess – Conn syndrome

Tumours or bilateral idiopathic hyperplasia of the zona glomerulosa result in excess aldosterone with normal cortisol levels.

Symptoms and signs

Hyperaldosteronism most characteristically presents with hypokalaemic hypertension. In common with diagnosing any of the more unusual causes of hypertension, a high index of suspicion is required (Box 6.13). The electrolyte disturbance may be unmasked or exacerbated by concomitant potassium-losing diuretic therapy prescribed for the

---

Box 6.13 Think of unusual causes of hypertension, especially in younger patients

- Conn syndrome
- Phaeochromocytoma
- Renal artery stenosis
- Coarctation of the aorta

---

hypertension (e.g. thiazides). However, aldosterone excess also underlies a subset of normokalaemic hypertension. The symptoms tend to be vague. Hypertension may present with headaches and visual disturbances; hypokalaemia may cause muscle fatigue or tiredness (Case history 6.3). Initial biochemical screening becomes increasingly relevant in younger patients with marked hypertension, especially if it is resistant to multiple antihypertensive drugs and accompanied by hypokalaemia (either spontaneous or induced by diuretics). The incidence of Conn syndrome is seemingly higher in women in their third decade. If blood pressure is normal for age, other causes of hypokalaemia merit consideration (Box 6.14).

Diagnosis

The diagnosis of primary aldosterone excess requires assessment of the renin–angiotensin–aldosterone axis by screening and then diagnostic tests. Concomitant use of antihypertensive medications that affect the hormone axis is potentially confounding. MR antagonists need to be withdrawn for 4 weeks. It is debatable whether other agents, such as diuretics, β-blockers and ACE inhibitors, need to be stopped for initial screening because the hypertension can be dangerous and difficult to control without treatment. If initial testing is equivocal, medications may need to be withdrawn or substituted with drugs such as doxazasin, an α-adrenergic blocker. Serum potassium should be restored to the normal range with oral supplementation in the days prior to testing. Salt intake should be unrestricted to ensure the patient is sodium replete. For screening, plasma aldosterone and renin

Box 6.14 Causes of hypokalaemia

- Primary hyperaldosteronism
- Vomiting with metabolic alkalosis
- Diarrhoea or other fluid loss from the lower bowel:
  - Ileostomy
  - Villous adenoma of the rectum
- Diuretic use
- Hypomagnesaemia
- Insulin infusion
- Rare causes include renal tubular acidosis and various monogenic defects of renal tubule function:
  - Gitelman syndrome (usually normotensive)
  - Liddle syndrome (hypertensive)
  - Bartter syndrome (usually hypo- or normo-tensive)
  - Hypokalaemic periodic paralysis

(either plasma activity or serum concentration) are measured mid-morning (aldosterone levels fall during the day) with the patient having been seated for ~15 min, but having been out of bed for a couple of hours. Positive screening detects a high ratio of aldosterone to renin concentration or activity in the serum. Applied cut-offs vary and depend on assay units. For instance, measuring aldosterone in pmol/L and renin activity in nmol/L/h, a ratio of more than 2000 gives a very high likelihood of primary hyperaldosteronism. Some endocrinologists argue that the ratio is best interpreted only when serum aldosterone is above a certain threshold [e.g. ~200 pmol/L (~7 ng/dL)]. This avoids misleading high ratios simply due to a very low renin concentration. A normal or low ratio excludes primary aldosterone excess (see Box 6.13 for potential causes other than 'essential' hypertension).

If the aldosterone:renin ratio is raised, a variety of tests in the specialist setting confirm the diagnosis by observing a failure of aldosterone suppression in response to intravenous saline or fludrocortisone. Once a biochemical diagnosis has been made, the cause of excess aldosterone needs to be determined.

Aside from rare genetic causes, hyperaldosteronism usually arises from two pathologies: a discrete adenoma (Conn tumour) or bilateral hyperplasia that can often be discriminated by MRI or CT. If the patient is over 40 years old, when there is increased risk of an incidental non-functional adenoma, or if imaging is equivocal, adrenal vein sampling helps to localize the source of mineralocorticoid excess (but this is challenging; see earlier details on adrenal anatomy).

Treatment

A Conn tumour is ideally treated by unilateral adrenalectomy when hypertension can be cured or improved such that the number and dose of antihypertensives can be markedly reduced. Bilateral hyperplasia or adenomas in patients unfit for surgery are managed by drugs. Spironolactone has been used for many years as an MR antagonist. Indeed, a clue to diagnosis can come from its use followed by a rapid fall in previously refractory high blood pressure. Unfortunately, the drug also antagonizes the androgen receptor (AR), causing breast development (gynaecomastia) in men and necessitating contraceptive advice in fertile women to guard against feminizing a male fetus. The more specific but less potent antagonist, eplerenone, is available as an oral twice-daily preparation.

Tumours involving the zona reticularis

In addition to cortisol, tumours from the fasciculata and reticularis zones can secrete sex steroid precursors. These steroids are converted in the periphery to androgens and, potentially, oestrogens, causing virilization in women (deepened voice and clitoromegaly) or feminization in men (e.g. gynaecomastia). The tumours may be diagnosed by increased serum DHEA (some laboratories only measure DHEAS), androstenedione, testosterone and oestradiol according to sex, and assessment of glucocorticoid status. Where cortisol is normal, and only sex steroids and their precursors are raised, discrimination between an adrenal or gonadal source requires imaging by CT or MRI and potential catheterization and sampling of the adrenal and ovarian veins. The tumours are treated surgically with removal of the offending adrenal gland.

Case history 6.3

A physically active 23-year-old student is referred with a blood pressure of 158/94 mmHg. On examination, body mass index (BMI) is 20.5 kg/m². Serum sodium was 144 mmol/L (144 mEq/L) and serum potassium was 2.8 mmol/L (2.8 mEq/L).

What endocrine diagnosis should be suspected?
What biochemical screening test is required with what electrolyte preparation?
Outline the subsequent investigation plans if the screening test is positive.

Answers, see p. 125

Other tumours of the adrenal cortex
Adrenocortical carcinoma

The commonest malignant tumour of the adrenal cortex is metastatic. Primary adrenal carcinoma is rare. The vast majority is functional (80%), and most secrete a mixture of steroids characteristic of different zones and best detected by mass spectrometry. The clinical picture tends to be one of rapidly progressive Cushing syndrome and virilization accompanied by the more general effects of an aggressive tumour (e.g. weight loss, abdominal pain, anorexia and fever). Most tumours have metastasized by presentation so adrenalectomy is no longer curative. Mitotane, an adrenolytic drug, palliates symptoms and can reduce tumour growth, but survival is poor; historically, 20% or less of patients have survived 5 years. Newer trials with additional agents are underway.

Incidentalomas

An increasing problem is the management of tumours identified on CT or MRI performed for other reasons (Box 6.15). These 'incidentalomas' are common in individuals over 40 years, potentially affecting 5% of individuals (Case history 6.4).

Box 6.15 A pragmatic approach to adrenal incidentalomas?

- Exclude over-secretion of aldosterone, glucocorticoid, sex steroid precursors and catecholamines (see other sections)
- Assess likelihood that it is a metastasis:
  - Full history and examination
  - Is it poorly demarcated on CT or MRI?
  - Consider chest X-ray in smokers
- If >4 cm, risk of malignancy is increased, unilateral adrenalectomy advised
- If <4 cm, hormone-negative and not suspicious on imaging: follow-up with repeat investigation at 6 months and potentially annually thereafter if no change or discharge

Congenital adrenal hyperplasia

Congenital adrenal hyperplasia (CAH) is an autosomal recessive disorder (i.e. inactivating mutations in both copies of the gene are required for the phenotype). The causative genes encode enzymes in the pathway to cortisol (see Figure 6.3, plus others not shown for simplicity, such as cytochrome P450 oxidoreductase). This leads to cortisol deficiency, diminished negative feedback at the anterior pituitary and raised ACTH (see Figure 6.4). High ACTH and raised intermediaries 'upstream' of the inactive enzyme increase flux through the remaining intact steroidogenic pathways. For instance, inactivating mutations in *CYP21A2* account for 90% of CAH and cause decreased cortisol and raised 17α-hydroxyprogesterone; in the presence of high ACTH, pathways are stimulated to convert this build-up of CYP21A2 substrate to sex steroid precursors and potent androgens. In addition to the cortisol deficiency, this causes:

- Ambiguous genitalia in females at birth (Figure 6.10)
- Precocious puberty in males; and
- Hirsuitism, menstrual irregularities and subfertility in women.

Many patients also have inadequate aldosterone production ('salt wasting' CAH); some do not

---

Case history 6.4

A 74-year-old man is referred to the gastroenterology clinic with a 6-month history of right upper quadrant discomfort. His weight is steady, appetite maintained and there has been no change in bowel habit. He is a non-smoker. His past medical history includes diet-controlled type 2 diabetes diagnosed 4 years previously and mild hypertension for which he takes a thiazide diuretic. On examination, his BMI is $27.3 \, \text{kg/m}^2$ and blood pressure 154/82 mmHg. Otherwise there is nothing to find. Serum sodium is 142 mmol/L (142 mEq/L), serum potassium is 3.2 mmol/L (3.2 mEq/L), liver function tests are normal and HbA_{1c} is 7.2% (55 mmol/mol). Upper abdominal ultrasound scan is unremarkable. The doctor orders CT of the upper abdominal region, which is reported as showing no abnormality other than a 3.2-cm well-defined mass with uniform appearance in the right adrenal gland. The left adrenal gland appears normal. The gastroenterologist refers the patient to you as the endocrinologist.

What potential pathologies need to be considered to explain the findings in the adrenal gland?
What investigations for hormone secretion are warranted?
If hormone secretion appears normal from the adrenal gland, what follow-up would you suggest?

Answers, see p. 125

('simple virilizing' CAH). Partial inactivation of CYP21A2 can cause a late-onset form of CAH with milder post-pubertal features in women.

Neonates with hypotension and hyperkalaemia need investigation, especially when females are virilized (Case history 6.5). In CYP21A2 deficiency basal ACTH is high, serum cortisol is low and 17α-hydroxyprogesterone is commonly greater than 100 nmol/L (~3300 ng/dL). On ACTH stimulation testing (similar to testing for Addison disease; see Box 6.8), cortisol fails to rise significantly [i.e. <525 nmol/L (~19 μg/dL)], but in CYP21A2 deficiency serum, 17α-hydroxyprogesterone increases substantially [commonly >300 nmol/L (10,000 ng/dL)]. In rarer forms, mass spectrometry is useful to detect which intermediates are increased, hence which enzyme is inactive.

Treatment is with glucocorticoid (± mineralocorticoid) to replace missing steroid hormones, restore negative feedback on ACTH production and minimize androgen over-production. This can be complex: one extreme of treatment is bilateral adrenalectomy and life-long hydrocortisone and fludrocortisone replacement.

Case history 6.5

A 3-day old 46,XX neonate with virilized external genitalia develops profound hypotension and circulatory shock.

What is the most likely diagnosis?
What immediate therapy is required to replace a missing hormone?
What other hormone may be missing?

Answers, see p. 126

Therapeutic use of glucocorticoids

Glucocorticoids are used therapeutically throughout life. Dexamethasone is used in premature labour to stimulate fetal surfactant production. Post-natally, potent synthetic glucocorticoids are used in a range of autoimmune and inflammatory disorders for their immunosuppressive and anti-inflammatory properties. However, the morbidity and mortality

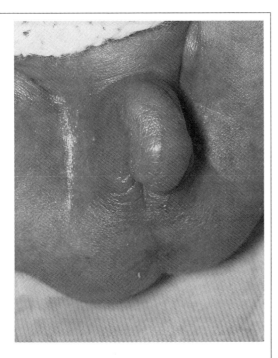

Figure 6.10 Ambiguous genitalia of a 46,XX infant with congenital adrenal hyperplasia. Virilization *in utero* presented at birth with clitoral hypertrophy, fusion of the labia and a urogenital opening at the base of the phallus.

from Cushing syndrome illustrates that these agents should only be used short-term and at the lowest possible dose.

The adrenal medulla

The adrenal medulla comprises chromaffin cells, which are like post-ganglionic neurones. However, rather than possessing distant nerve terminals, they respond to synaptic activation by releasing pre-formed catecholamine hormones into the circulation (Figure 6.11). Norepinephrine (noradrenaline) comprises 20% of circulating catecholamine, with an additional biochemical step generating the remaining 80% as epinephrine (adrenaline). The hormones are stored intracellularly in secretory granules complexed with proteins called chromogranins. The latter serve as clinical biomarkers of endocrine tumours characterized by periodic release

of stored hormones into the circulation (sometimes called 'neuroendocrine tumours'), such as phaeochromocytoma, paragangliomas, carcinoids and gut endocrine tumours (see later in this chapter and Chapter 10).

Embryology and anatomy

In contrast to the outer cortex, the adrenal medulla is derived from the neuroectoderm ('neural crest') cells that migrate in a forward direction from the peri-vertebral to the peri-aortic region (see Figure 6.1). Here, these cells predominantly give rise to the autonomic chain of ganglia that innervate much of the gut and blood vessels. However, some specialize by invading the adrenal to form the chromaffin cells of the adrenal medulla; both structures are innervated by pre-ganglionic sympathetic neurones that emanate from nerve roots T7–L3. Realizing this common neural crest origin, it becomes easy to understand why the clinical presentation of phaeochromocytoma (tumour of the adrenal medulla) and paraganglioma (tumour of the autonomic chain of ganglia) can be very similar (see later clinical section).

Catecholamine biosynthesis and metabolism

The biosynthesis of catecholamines occurs in four steps (Figure 6.12, upper half). The hydroxylation of tyrosine is rate-limiting and subject to negative feedback by the downstream hormone products, norepinephrine and dopamine. The two steps to dopamine also occur in the substantia nigra of the brain stem – the cells that are lost in Parkinson disease. The last step converting norepinephrine to epinephrine reflects the unusual embryology of the adrenal medulla. Expression of phenylethanolamine *N*-methyl transferase (PNMT) is induced and depends upon high concentrations of glucocorticoid that are only present in the adrenal medulla because of the centripetal drainage of venous blood from the outer adrenal cortex. Stimulation of the chromaffin cell by pre-ganglionic neurones is mediated by acetylcholine, and to a lesser extent serotonin and histamine. Catecholamines are released and diffuse the short distance into the adjacent blood vessels (Figure 6.11).

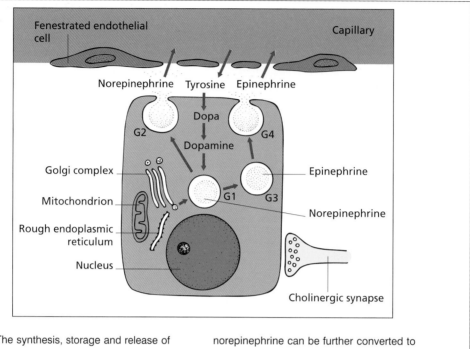

Figure 6.11 The synthesis, storage and release of catecholamines from the chromaffin cell of the adrenal medulla. The components of the storage granules (G), including the chromogranins, are synthesized on the rough endoplasmic reticulum and packaged in the Golgi complex. Dopamine enters a granule (G1) and is converted to norepinephrine, which can then be released exocytotically (G2). Alternatively, norepinephrine can be further converted to epinephrine (G3) and released by exocytosis (G4). Each cell has a cholinergic synapse where acetylcholine initiates the train of events leading to exocytosis. Individual chromaffin cells usually only secrete either norepinephrine or epinephrine, but phaeochromocytomas usually over-secrete both hormones.

Ending the effect of catecholamines relies on several different mechanisms (Figure 6.12, lower half). The most efficient method sees norepinephrine taken up by post-ganglionic sympathetic nerve terminals, where it can be metabolized by monoamine oxidase (MAO). Similar mechanisms in platelets take up mainly epinephrine. Circulating catecholamines are also metabolized in neuronal and other sites (e.g. the liver) and metabolites excreted in urine (Figure 6.12).

Physiology

Epinephrine and norepinephrine are major stress hormones responsible for the body's 'fright, fight and flight' responses following provocation (Table 6.3). Subtle differences in their action reflect relative affinities for the different adrenoreceptors, predominantly α and β sub-types 1 and 2. Norepinephrine stimulates α and β1 receptors, and thus does not cause bronchodilation, a β2 response. In contrast, the distribution of α and β2 receptors in skeletal muscle beds can actually cause vasodilation (i.e. increased muscle blood flow) compared to vasoconstriction in the gut. Thus, the combined effects of both catecholamines raise blood pressure, divert nutrients away from non-essential organs and promote their delivery to muscles that are active in the 'fight or flight' response to danger.

Both hormones also raise blood glucose by stimulating glycogenolysis in liver and muscle, and hepatic gluconeogenesis. Fatty acid release is

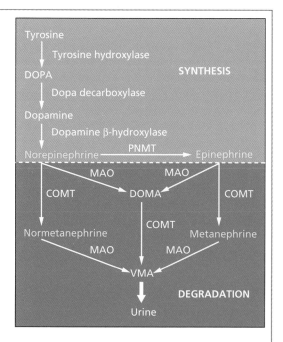

Figure 6.12 The synthesis (upper half) and degradation (lower half) of catecholamines. DOPA, 3,4-dihydroxyphenylalanine; dopamine, 3,4-dihydroxy phenylethylamine; PNMT, phenylethanolamine *N*-methyl transferase; MAO, monoamine oxidase; COMT, catechol-*O*-methyl-transferase; DOMA, 3,4-dihydroxymandelic acid; VMA, vanillylmandelic acid (3-methoxy-4-hydroxymandelic acid). Components measured clinically in the urine are shown in yellow.

Table 6.3 The effects of catecholamines	
Epinephrine	**Norepinephrine**
Systolic blood pressure and heart rate rise	Systolic and diastolic blood pressure rise (increasing mean arterial pressure)
Gut motility decreases	Heart rate decreases
Circulation diverted to limb muscle beds and away from the gut	
Bronchodilation; reduction in mucus secretion	
Piloerection	
Mydriasis (pupil dilation)	

increased. These metabolic actions increase energy substrate availability, making catecholamines counter-regulatory hormones to insulin (see Chapter 12).

Clinical disorders

Catecholamines from the adrenal medulla are dispensable. In bilateral adrenalectomy, glucocorticoid replacement is mandatory, but catecholamine replacement is not required.

Phaeochromocytoma

The only important clinical disorder of the adrenal medulla is overactivity caused by a tumour of the chromaffin cells called 'phaeochromocytoma' (Case history 6.6). Similar excessive episodic release of catecholamines results from some para-gangliomas (previously sometimes called 'ectopic phaeochromocytomas').

Symptoms and signs

Catecholamine-secreting tumours are rare and can occur sporadically or as part of familial syndromes (see multiple endocrine neoplasia in Chapter 10). As a teaching aid, a '10% rule' has been described: 10% are malignant, 10% are ectopic to the adrenal gland and 10% are bilateral. These points serve as useful reminders that the vast majority of these tumours are benign and paragangliomas may occur outside the adrenal gland along the sympathetic chain. It used to be said that 10% were inherited, although, with the wider availability of molecular genetic testing and greater knowledge of causative mutations, this is an underestimation of the 25–30% of tumours with accompanying germline mutations (see below and Chapter 10). Excessive unregulated catecholamine release occurs at inappropriate times, resulting in unusual and distinctive

Box 6.16 The triad of classical symptoms in phaeochromocytoma

- Sweating
- Throbbing bilateral headaches
- Palpitations

symptoms (Box 6.16). Hypertension is the most common finding (90–100% of cases), which may be constant (in ~50%, especially children) or episodic.

The frequency of symptomatic events can vary from daily to monthly, which can make diagnosis difficult. If suspicion is high, investigation should be repeated at intervals. Sweating, tremor, angina, nausea and anxiety can also occur. Diabetes may have been recently diagnosed.

Diagnosis

Secretion is episodic. The commonest screening test to detect excess catecholamines is assay of urine collected over 24 h. Collections can be done on random days, starting after the first micturition of the day until the equivalent time the following day; or, with infrequent symptoms, starting immediately after an attack and continued for 24 h. Most laboratories will assay a range of substances: metanephrine and normetanephrine, their parent hormones epinephrine and norepinephrine, and possibly the precursor, dopamine (Figure 6.12). This combined approach is helpful as it is unusual for catecholamine-secreting tumours to over-secrete one of the parent hormones in isolation without the corresponding metabolite. Occasionally, very large phaeochromocytomas or paragangliomas (because they are extra-adrenal) escape the normal influence of cortisol on PNMT and secrete an increased proportion of norepinephrine. Once a biochemical diagnosis has been made, imaging, ideally by MRI, aids localization. In specialized centres, uptake scans with meta-iodobenzylguanidine (mIBG) is possible (see Figure 4.9). PET scanning is becoming available in research centres. Patients should be screened for diabetes or glucose intolerance (see Chapter 11).

Treatment

Treating phaeochromocytoma has two steps: blocking the effects of catecholamine excess using α- and β-adrenoreceptor blockers, and then surgical removal of the offending tumour. α-Blockade is the first step to avoid a potential hypertensive crisis from unopposed α-adrenoreceptor stimulation (i.e. if β-blockers had already prevented muscle vasodilatation). One example regimen is the introduction of increasing doses of phenoxybenzamine followed by metoprolol, if needed, in the run-up to surgery. This preparation is mandatory as manipulation of the tumour at operation can result in catastrophic release of stored catecholamines.

Follow-up including the identification of germline mutations

All tumours arise from genetic abnormalities in the affected cell type. However, in ~25–30% of catecholamine-secreting tumours, these mutations are present in the germline, meaning every cell in the body is affected and risk of recurrence or tumours in family members is hugely increased (Table 6.4). Suspicious features demanding a rigorous family history, additional examination, and, after counselling and consent, genetic testing are as follows:

- Bilateral tumours
- Paragangliomas
- Previous catecholamine-secreting tumours
- Young age at presentation
- Presence of other tumours.

Two syndromes of 'multiple endocrine neoplasia (MEN)' have been described in particular detail (see Chapter 10). Phaeochromocytoma most commonly associates with type 2 MEN. Catecholamine-secreting tumours are also part of Von Hippel–Lindau syndrome and neurofibromatosis type 1.

If genetic defects are found (Table 6.4), appropriate life-long clinical follow-up is required with assessment of first-degree relatives. Historically, this has relied on annual 24-h urine screening (as above for diagnosis). However, current guidelines argue for

Table 6.4 Genetic defects predisposing to catecholamine-secreting tumours

Gene	Associated syndrome	Other associations	Inheritance of germline mutations
RET	MEN2 (see Chapter 10)	Medullary thyroid cancer, primary hyperparathyroidism; Marfanoid appearance and mucosal neuromata (type B)	AD
SDHB	Familial paraganglioma	Paragangliomas, commonly malignant, anywhere along sympathetic chain; renal cell carcinoma	AD
SDHD	Familial paraganglioma	Paragangliomas, commonly benign, anywhere along sympathetic chain	AD
VHL	Von Hippel-Lindau	Haemangioblastomas of central nervous system, kidney and retina; renal cell carcinoma, café-au-lait spots, pancreatic cysts	AD
NF1	Neurofibromatosis type 1 (Von Recklinghausen syndrome)	Neurofibromata, optic nerve gliomas, axillary freckling, café-au-lait spots and skeletal abnormalities	AD

RET, RET proto-oncogene; SDHB, succinate dehydrogenase, subunit B; SDHD, succinate dehydrogenase, subunit D; VHL, Von Hippel-Lindau tumour suppressor, NF1, neurofibromatosis type 1; MEN2, multiple endocrine neoplasia type 2; AD, autosomal dominant.

more frequent analysis. In addition, plasma assays of catecholamine metabolites, especially normetanephrine, are proving a more sensitive means of detecting excess hormone and are especially useful in screening where excluding a tumour is the primary goal (i.e. a very low false-negative rate).

Even in seemingly sporadic phaeochromocytomas without known germline mutations, many centres regard it as important and prudent to perform annual follow-up with 24-h urine collection for catecholamine measurement.

Therapeutic uses of catecholamines

Based on their physiology, catecholamines, particularly epinephrine, are useful in clinical scenarios that range from the trivial to the profoundly serious. In intensive care medicine, catecholamine infusions can maintain blood pressure in septic shock. In everyday life, their vasoconstrictive action makes catecholamines useful nasal decongestants.

🔍 Case history 6.6

A 44-year-old man attended his doctor because of headaches. His partner attended the consultation and also commented on several occasions during the last few months when he had gone extremely pale and appeared ill at ease. Closer questioning elicited the presence of palpitations during these events, which lasted ~15 min. Examination was unremarkable except for a blood pressure of 180/110 mmHg. The man was not overweight, took plenty of exercise and had no significant past medical history.

What diagnosis should be considered?
What investigations are appropriate?

Answers, see p. 126

🔑 Key points

- The adrenal cortex and adrenal medulla develop as separate organs
- The adrenocortical hormones are aldosterone, cortisol and the sex steroid precursors
- Excess and deficiency of adrenocortical hormones cause important disorders, Cushing syndrome, Conn syndrome and Addison disease

- The major hormones from the adrenal medulla are the catecholamines, epinephrine and norepinephrine
- Phaeochromocytoma and paraganglioma are tumours that over-secrete adrenomedullary hormones

🔍 Answers to case histories

Case history 6.1

The patient has Addison disease as a result of autoimmune destruction of the adrenal cortex. Decreased circulating volume has caused hypotension associated with dehydration and raised serum urea. The pigmentation is caused by inadequate negative feedback from cortisol, leading to corticotroph overactivity and increased ACTH stimulating the MC1R. The pale areas are vitiligo, another autoimmune condition.

Addison disease is diagnosed by an ACTH stimulation test with serum cortisol measured at 30 min. Putting aside slight variation between assay platforms and fluctuations in serum CBG, a response of greater than 525 nmol/L (~19 µg/dL) occurs in 95% of the normal population; lower values increasingly raise suspicion of Addison disease. Serum ACTH at baseline would be expected to be elevated. Plasma renin concentration or activity may also be increased secondary to aldosterone deficiency.

Once diagnosed, the patient should be commenced on hydrocortisone and, potentially, fludrocortisone. If there is concern over Addisonian crisis, treatment should be started before diagnosis. The patient should be given a steroid alert card and informed

about steroid alert bracelets. Advice should be given to double hydrocortisone doses during illness. If unable to take tablets (e.g. if vomiting during an episode of gastroenteritis), the patient needs intravenous treatment. Hydrocortisone is absorbed ~30 min after consumption.

This patient has an increased risk of autoimmune disease affecting other endocrine organs and cell types. This is exemplified by the vitiligo and family history of thyroid disease. The haematology results are suspicious of pernicious anaemia. Autoimmune destruction of the parietal cells in the stomach that make intrinsic factor prevents vitamin B_{12} absorption. This causes defective red blood cell biosynthesis with the presence of large red cells in the circulation ('macrocytosis'). Hypothyroidism is another cause of macrocytosis; however, this was excluded. Serum vitamin B_{12} levels should be measured.

Case history 6.2

The patient has signs and symptoms of Cushing syndrome, which has precipitated diabetes mellitus, centripetal weight gain and the cardinal feature of purple abdominal 'striae'. On closer examination, thin bruised skin and proximal myopathy might be evident.

Initial investigations aim to demonstrate glucocorticoid excess; midnight serum or bedtime salivary cortisol estimation, low-dose dexamethasone suppression tests and 24-h urine collections on three occasions can all be used to confirm glucocorticoid excess.

In the absence of steroid medications, the undetectable ACTH means the Cushing syndrome is of adrenal origin. CT (or MRI) is appropriate (review Figure 4.7). CT scans can even suggest whether the lesion is lipid rich, consistent with a functional adrenocortical adenoma.

Case history 6.3

The patient has marked hypertension with spontaneous hypokalaemia. This points strongly to aldosterone excess, especially if there are no other causes of potassium loss such as diarrhoea or vomiting.

A serum aldosterone-to-renin ratio is required to investigate whether this is primary aldosterone excess, i.e. Conn syndrome. Prior to this, potassium should be replaced to restore serum values to the normal range and unrestricted salt intake should be recommended for the few days before testing. On the day of testing, the patient should be ambulant for ~2h after wakening, with blood drawn mid-morning after sitting down for ~15min.

If the screening test is positive, a confirmatory biochemical test, such as intravenous saline challenge or fludrocortisone suppression test, should be performed. If a biochemical diagnosis is made, CT (or MRI) of the adrenals should be performed. If there is a clear Conn adenoma, usually smaller than 2cm in diameter, accompanied by clear biochemistry results, then adrenal venous sampling is probably not needed in a young patient. Non-functioning incidentalomas are unlikely at this age. If imaging is equivocal, then the decision to proceed to venous sampling is guided by the likelihood of surgical intervention if a unilateral source of the aldosterone excess is found. In this case, surgery is highly likely to be curative for the hypertension and hypokalaemia in a young fit patient. This might not be the case in an 80-year-old with co-morbidities and in whom blood pressure is satisfactorily controlled on an MR antagonist. Adrenal venous sampling is undertaken by an interventional radiologist with cortisol and aldosterone measured on samples drawn from both adrenal veins and the inferior vena cava. Cortisol levels at least twice those of the peripheral circulation are proof that the catheter is/was correctly positioned in the adrenal vein (some centres have access to rapid assays allowing intraprocedural assessment).

Case history 6.4

The incidental abnormality in the right adrenal gland has the appearances of a solid mass rather than an abscess or cyst. The first question is whether the mass arises directly from the adrenal gland or whether it is metastastic. There is little to suggest the latter both in the history (e.g. no loss of weight or appetite; normal bowel habit) and the examination. If the mass arises from the adrenal gland then it could be cortical or medullary.

Before it is classified as a non-functional 'incidentaloma', several types of hormone excess need to be considered. It could be a phaeochromocytoma secreting catecholamines, which could underlie both the hypertension and the diabetes. 24-h urine collection for catecholamines would be a sensible screening test. If suspicion is high, demonstrating normal serum normetanephrine would be the most sensitive way to exclude phaeochromocytoma. The mass would be larger than average for a Conn tumour secreting aldosterone, but the patient is hypertensive and mildly hypokalaemic (the most likely cause of these findings is essential hypertension treated by thiazide diuretic). Measuring the aldosterone-to-renin ratio would screen for primary hyperaldosteronism. The hypertension, diabetes and slightly raised BMI could also be explained by cortisol excess. Cushing syndrome should be excluded by any of the screening tests described in the chapter. Finally, measurement of sex steroid precursors, androstenedione and DHEA (or DHEAS), should be undertaken.

This tumour diameter is less than 4 cm and therefore there is a low risk of malignancy. Follow-up strategies for incidental tumours with no detectable hormone secretion vary. One approach would be to repeat investigations after 6 months, which, if normal, could then be monitored annually. If excessive hormone secretion was not detected on two occasions, it is unlikely to develop subsequently. Some endocrinologists discharge such patients. Repeat imaging at 6 months looks for growth, which would press the case for surgical removal, most likely via the laparoscopic approach.

The patient can be reassured for now on the original symptom of discomfort. Reinforcement of good diabetes care is important. If future medical intervention became warranted, metformin would be the appropriate first-line agent. Assessment of fasting lipids would be prudent given diabetes and hypertension, with statin therapy warranted according to published risk tables (e.g. in the British National Formulary). A series of further blood pressure measurements would be sensible outside the hospital setting. If similar levels persisted, antihypertensive therapy should be optimized to lower blood pressure to less than 140/80 mmHg.

Case history 6.5

The most likely diagnosis is CAH caused by mutations in both copies of *CYP21A2*.

Intravenous hydrocortisone and intravenous fluids are required. Ideally, a blood sample should be taken beforehand for cortisol and ACTH, but immediate therapy is mandatory.

Aldosterone may also be lacking if this is salt wasting rather than a simple virilizing CAH. CYP21A2 catalyzes steps in the pathway to both cortisol and aldosterone.

Case history 6.6

The history and the finding of hypertension are suggestive of a catecholamine-secreting tumour.

24-h urine collection for excreted catecholamines and their metabolites should be undertaken on several occasions, ideally incorporating an episode. Given the convincing history, it would be reasonable to measure serum normetanephrine as a normal result practically excludes a catecholamine-secreting tumour. In addition, electrocardiography and echocardiography might be considered. The latter may show left ventricular hypertrophy. Only if catecholamine excretion is increased, should the adrenal glands be imaged by CT or MRI. Although more restricted in availability, mIBG scans delineate phaeochromocytoma tissue.

CHAPTER 7
Reproductive endocrinology

Key topics

- Embryology of the reproductive organs   128
- The male reproductive system   134
- The female reproductive system   142
- Pubertal disorders   159
- Subfertility   159
- Key points   162
- Answers to case histories   162

Learning objectives

- To appreciate reproductive endocrinology and its clinical disorders during different phases of life
- The male reproductive system:
    - To understand normal male development and the regulation and function of the testis
    - To recognize the clinical consequences of an underactive male reproductive axis
- The female reproductive system:
    - To understand normal female development and the regulation and function of the ovary
    - To understand the endocrinology of pregnancy and lactation
    - To recognize the clinical consequences of a dysregulated female reproductive axis
- To understand how to approach, counsel and treat the subfertile couple

This chapter integrates the basic biology of the reproductive system with the associated clinical conditions in males and females

Essential Endocrinology and Diabetes, Sixth Edition. Richard IG Holt, Neil A Hanley.
© 2012 Richard IG Holt and Neil A Hanley. Publlished 2012 by Blackwell Publishing Ltd.

To recap

- Gonadal regulation depends on both negative and positive feedback loops, the principles of which are introduced in Chapter 1
- Understanding gametogenesis requires knowledge of meiosis, covered in Chapter 2
- The most important gonadal hormones are steroids; review the general principles of steroid hormone biosynthesis described in Chapter 2
- The effects of gonadal steroid hormones are diverse; however, they are all based upon the same principles of steroid hormone action introduced in Chapter 3

Cross-reference

- Ovarian and testicular function is dependent upon the function of the hypothalamus and anterior pituitary gonadotroph, which is covered in Chapter 5
- Development of the gonad is intimately linked to that of the adrenal cortex (see Chapter 6), resulting in overlapping steroidogenic pathways that affect normal physiology and several clinical disorders (e.g. congenital adrenal hyperplasia or sex-steroid secreting tumours)

Embryology of the reproductive organs

Reproductive development *in utero* can be broken down into two processes: sex determination, whereby the bipotential gonad becomes either the testis or ovary; and sex differentiation, the male or female phenotype that unfolds according to the presence or absence of male hormones from the testis. Both are remarkable for normally showing complete dimorphism, i.e. one or the other but not both, without which our species would be a reproductive failure.

Sex determination

Chromosomal sex depends on whether the fertilizing spermatozoon bears an X or a Y chromosome. However, the translation of chromosomal sex into gonadal sex depends on events during the second month of gestation (Box 7.1). Initially, there is no morphological difference between 46,XX and 46,XY gonads (Figure 7.1a). However, at ~7 weeks of development, the cells of the male gonad start to express critical genes encoding transcription factors

> ### Box 7.1 The early development of sexual phenotype
>
> *At fertilization*
> - Spermatozoan with either an X or a Y chromosome determines sex by fusing with an X-bearing ovum
>
> *At ~4 weeks of development*
> - Proliferation of cells in the urogenital ridge creates the bipotential gonad
>
> *At ~7 weeks of gestation (sex determination)*
> - 46,XY gonad becomes a testis
> - 46,XX gonad remains as an ovary

(review Chapter 2), foremost amongst which are Sex-determining region of the Y chromosome (SRY) and SRY high mobility group box family member 9 (SOX9). These regulators orchestrate a range of gene expression that creates a testis. During this period, called 'sex determination', the cells of the 46,XX gonad undergo far less morphological

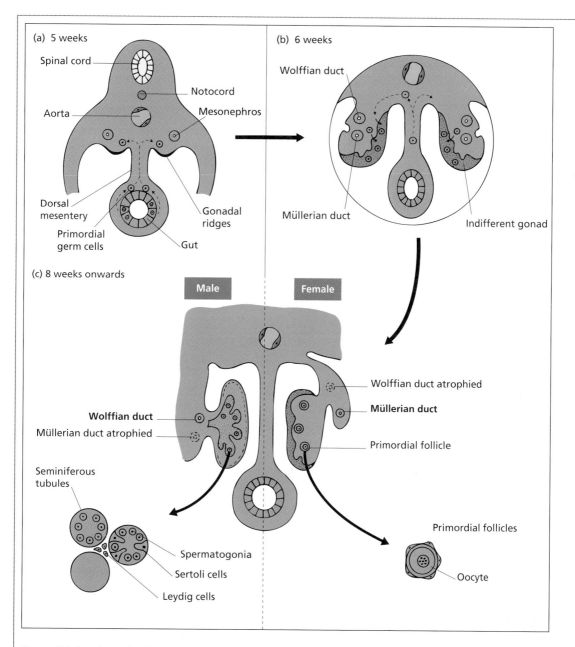

Figure 7.1 Sex determination and sexual differentiation. (a) Cross-section of a human embryo showing the primordial germ cells migrating via the gut mesentery to the developing gonads (dashed arrows). (b) The appearance of the Wolffian and Müllerian ducts at ~6 weeks with germ cells invading the bipotential gonad. (c) In the male (testis), seminiferous tubules differentiate and contain spermatogonia and Sertoli cells with Leydig cells interspersed between the tubules. The Müllerian duct regresses. In the female (ovary), primordial follicles develop and the Wolffian duct regresses.

change. Although genes have been discovered that influence ovarian development, the process is still defined by relative lack of activity.

Future gonadal function also relies on germ cells generating either spermatozoa or ova. Prior to and during sex determination, primordial germ cells migrate from the wall of the yolk sac through the gut mesentery into the gonad. In males, the formation of Sertoli cells within testicular cords induces mitotic arrest in germ cells. In females, proliferation, some atresia and, ultimately, entrance into the first stage of meiosis over the next few weeks determines the total number of ova for reproductive life.

Sexual differentiation

The differentiation of the sexual organs occurs from two pairs of ducts and the urogenital sinus. Male events progress rapidly so that major development is complete by the end of the first trimester. Without high levels of male hormones during this period, default female differentiation occurs.

The internal genitalia originate from the bilateral Müllerian (also called mesonephric) ducts that drain the primitive kidney (the mesonephros) and the Wolffian ducts that form along the length of each urogenital ridge (Figure 7.1b). In each sex, the pair of ducts that is not required regresses, while the other matures into recognizable parts of the adult anatomy (Box 7.2). In the male, anti-Müllerian hormone (AMH), also known as Müllerian inhibiting substance (MIS), from Sertoli cells causes regression of the Müllerian ducts (Figure 7.1c). In its place, androgen, thought to be testosterone, from the interstitial Leydig cells, virilizes the Wolffian ducts into the structures that transport and mature spermatozoa from the testicular cords to the seminal vesicles and prostate (Figure 7.2 and Box 7.2). In the female, the absence of AMH and the much lower androgen levels allow growth of the Müllerian ducts, while the Wolffian system regresses (Figures 7.1c and 7.2).

5α-dihydrotestosterone (DHT) is required for the urogenital sinus to deviate from female differentiation. DHT forms in target tissues by the action of type 2 5α-reductase (SRD5A2) on high levels of testosterone (review Table 3.2; see Figure 7.7). It virilizes the external genitalia by causing the ure-

---

Box 7.2 Differentiation of the internal genitalia

Female
- Müllerian duct derivatives:
  - Fallopian tubes (oviducts)
  - Uterus
  - Upper third of the vagina

Male
- Wolffian duct derivatives:
  - Rete testis
  - Epididymis
  - Vas deferens

---

thral folds to fuse in the midline, enclosing the terminal urethra, and the primitive genital tubercle to expand and elongate into the penis. The labioscrotal swellings migrate posteriorly and fuse together as the scrotum into which the testes finally descend (Figure 7.3). DHT also stimulates prostate formation.

In the female, relative lack of androgen lessens growth of the genital tubercle as the clitoris and retains patency between the urethral and labioscrotal folds as a vaginal opening flanked by the labia minora and majora (Figure 7.3).

After 12 weeks the testes descend under the dual hormonal influence of insulin-like 3 (INSL3) and androgen, while the latter also causes continued growth of the penis.

Disorders of sex development

The more severe the disruption or complete the sex reversal at birth, the earlier *in utero* the problem occurred. Clinical nomenclature used to be based on the very rare disorder of hermaphroditism—the presence of both testicular and ovarian tissue causing aspects of both male and female sexual development. These conditions are now classified as 46,XY or 46,XX disorders of sex development (DSD). Hermaphroditism is now termed 46,XX ovotesticular DSD. Completely disrupted gonad formation (streak gonads) in chromosomal males is 46,XY complete gonadal dysgenesis (CGD) (Box 7.3).

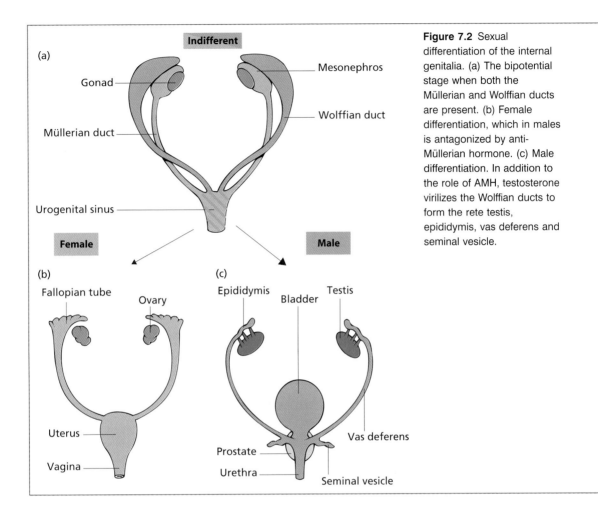

Figure 7.2 Sexual differentiation of the internal genitalia. (a) The bipotential stage when both the Müllerian and Wolffian ducts are present. (b) Female differentiation, which in males is antagonized by anti-Müllerian hormone. (c) Male differentiation. In addition to the role of AMH, testosterone virilizes the Wolffian ducts to form the rete testis, epididymis, vas deferens and seminal vesicle.

Disturbances at any point during sex determination or sexual differentiation carry clinical consequences. Mutation or altered dosage of the genes responsible for gonad formation, failure of hormone biosynthesis or loss of hormone action at the target receptor all potentially result in genital ambiguity or 'sex reversal' phenotypes; all of which causes major parental distress at birth and challenge the diagnostic skills of the paediatric endocrinologist.

Clinical features

Human society ascribes sex discretely, either male or female, with grades of intersex considered abnormal (Figure 7.4). This creates emotive clinical situations requiring empathy and careful diagnosis (Boxes 7.4 and 7.5).

46,XY Complete gonadal dysgenesis

Severe loss-of-function mutations in *SRY* or several other genes cause a complete failure of testicular development. Neonates present with normal female external genitalia and a uterus.

46,XY Disorder of sex development

Less severe mutations in the genes responsible for 46,XY CGD can cause 46,XY DSD presenting with ambiguous genitalia.

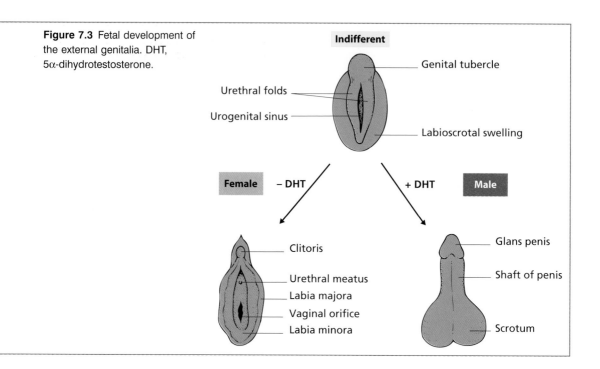

Figure 7.3 Fetal development of the external genitalia. DHT, 5α-dihydrotestosterone.

Box 7.3 Disorders of sex development

46,XY Complete gonadal dysgenesis
- Complete failure of testis formation
- Severe loss-of-function mutations in *SRY* and other genes

46,XY Disorder of sex development
- Failure of testicular determination (e.g. loss-of-function mutation in *SRY*)
- Failure of steroidogenesis (mutation inactivating enzyme in biosynthetic pathway to testosterone)
- Failure of DHT biosynthesis (mutation in *SRD5A2*)

- Androgen insensitivity (mutation in the gene encoding the androgen receptor)
- Maternal consumption of anti-androgenic drugs (e.g. spironolactone)

46,XX Disorder of sex development
- Congenital adrenal hyperplasia (CAH) due to 21-hydroxylase deficiency (see Figure 6.10)
- Maternal androgen excess (e.g. androgen-secreting tumour or anabolic steroid abuse)

Sex chromosome abnormalities
- Turner syndrome (45,XO)
- Klinefelter syndrome (47,XXY)

Deficiencies of any of the enzymes in the biosynthetic pathway to testosterone, its conversion to DHT or mutations of the androgen receptor (AR) can cause inadequate androgen action. Hypospadias resulting from incomplete closure of the urogenital sinus is a common consequence. The urethra opens onto the ventral surface rather than on or as well as the tip of the penis (review Figure 7.3). In severe hypospadias the scrotum may also fail to fuse in the midline.

Androgen deficiency causes incomplete testicular descent. Abdominal dysgenetic gonads carry a ~five-fold increased risk of tumourigenesis and require surgical removal. Testes in the inguinal canal should be manipulated into the scrotum and may have adequate future function.

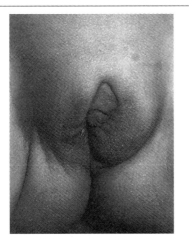

Figure 7.4 Genitalia of a 2-year-old with 46,XY disorder of sex development due to mutation of the *SRD5A2* gene encoding type 2 5α-reductase. Note the genital ambiguity and swelling in the left 'labium' due to a testis.

Box 7.5 Contentious issues in the management of disorders of sex development

- To what extent has the developing brain been virilized by inappropriate androgen in 46,XX DSD and with what future consequences on sexuality and behaviour? Knowledge is limited of 'normal' central nervous system virilization during 46,XY development
- To what extent should surgery reconstruct the external genitalia in 46,XX DSD, at what age and under whose consent?
  - Neonatal reduction of clitoral size could create a visually more 'normal' female appearance, but nullify future sexual sensation. Surgery is now undertaken at an older age when reconstruction is more sympathetic to future sexual needs and some form of direct patient consent can be gained

Box 7.4 Defining the diagnosis in disorders of sex development

- What is the extent of under-development or sex reversal?
  - Complete – early fetal influence
  - Incomplete – later fetal influence, e.g. clitoromegaly or hypospadias
- Are there associated clinical emergencies (salt-wasting hypoadrenalism in CAH, see Chapter 6)?
- Are there other congenital abnormalities?
- Is there a family history of similar events?

Answering two questions is particularly important
- What is the karyotype?
  - Is it 46,XY or 46,XX DSD? (or possibly 45,XO may be suspected)
- In 46,XY DSD, is there a uterus?
  - Yes – deficient action of both androgen and AMH
  - No – deficient androgen action but appropriate AMH

46,XX Disorder of sex development

Translocation of the *SRY* gene onto the X chromosome can cause testicular development in 46,XX individuals. Exposure of female fetuses with normal gonads to androgens before week 12 of pregnancy risks virilization with fusion of the urethral folds, posterior migration of the labioscrotal folds and growth of the phallus. Later exposure is less damaging, more limited to phallic growth as clitoromegaly. The most common 46,XX DSD is congenital adrenal hyperplasia (CAH) caused by 21-hydroxlase (CYP21) deficiency, which may present with Addisonian crisis (see Case History 7.1 and Chapter 6). As there is no abnormality in the ovary or internal genitalia, reproductive function may be possible after appropriate treatment.

Chromosomal disturbances without obvious phenotypes beyond the gonad may not present as DSD at birth but as later failure of puberty (e.g. Klinefelter syndrome/47,XXY), hypogonadism or premature ovarian failure (e.g. Turner syndrome/46,XO). Turner syndrome usually has other features (see later section on amenorrhoea with absent oestrogen).

Case history 7.1

The paediatric endocrinologist receives a request from the neonatal unit for 'routine review of a baby boy born the previous day with ambiguous external genitalia'. The parents are cousins and this is their first child. The call is followed later in the day by an urgent referral because the baby has become very unwell and is hypotensive. On arrival, a junior doctor is in the process of taking a blood sample from the baby.

What diagnosis was the endocrinologist considering and why were serum urea and electrolytes, ACTH, cortisol, 17α-hydroxyprogesterone, renin and aldosterone requested on the blood sample?

What emergency treatment is needed?

The blood results confirm the endocrinologist's suspicion. What is the baby's karyotype?

What mistake was made in ascribing a sex identity to the baby at birth?

Answers, see p. 162

The male reproductive system

Morphology and function of the testis

The testis can be thought of as two compartments: sperm-producing seminiferous tubules that develop from the testicular cords, largely determining testicular volume and requiring an operating temperature in the scrotum a few degrees below that of the body's core; and an interspersed interstitium containing lipid-laden, steroidogenic Leydig cells (Figure 7.5 and Box 7.6). The seminiferous tubules contain the germ cells and the Sertoli cells (Figure 7.6). Tight junctions between adjacent Sertoli cells produce two compartments: a basal compartment with spermatogonia (self-renewing stem cells), and an adluminal compartment for the spermatocytes,

---

Box 7.6 The testis has two important functions

- Synthesis of androgens – the male sex hormones
- Production of gametes – spermatogenesis

---

spermatids and spermatozoa. The tubules of each testis lead via the rete testis to the epididymis, where maturation of the spermatozoa occurs, and on to the vas deferens.

Spermatogenesis

The primordial germ cells that invade the embryonic gonad enter mitotic arrest as spermatogonia until puberty, after which they become reactivated by hormones (see following section on puberty). During mitosis (see Figure 2.1), the basal spermatogonial stem cell renews itself and gives rise to a diploid daughter cell (the primary spermatocyte) that moves into the adluminal compartment (Figure 7.6). Primary spermatocytes then undergo the first meiotic division to form haploid secondary spermatocytes (review Figure 2.1). The second meiotic division produces spermatids, which gradually mature into spermatozoa. An intimate association with the Sertoli ('nurse') cells is essential for this process. The spermatozoa are extruded into the lumen of the tubule and pass to the epididymis, following which they become mixed with the secretions of the seminal vesicles, prostate and bulbourethral glands at the time of ejaculation. Volumetric and microscopic analysis of the semen is an important part of assessing clinical testicular function because normal measurements strongly imply physiological follicle-stimulating hormone (FSH) and androgen secretion, and anatomical integrity (see next sections). Semen analysis can be part of investigating hypogonadism or subfertility (Box 7.7; see later clinical sections).

Androgen biosynthesis, secretion and metabolism

Androgen biosynthesis in the Leydig cell follows the same path by which cholesterol is converted to the

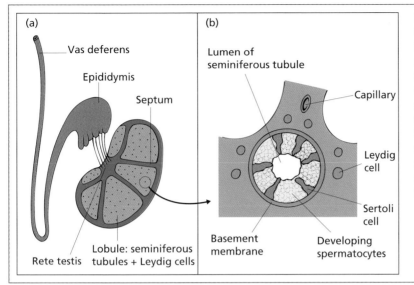

Figure 7.5 A testis in cross-section. (a) The testis is organized into lobules containing Leydig cells and seminiferous tubules, which drain into efferent ducts and, via the rete testis, into the epididymis. The circle in (a) is shown at higher magnification in (b). (b) The organization of the seminiferous tubules and the interstitial Leydig cells.

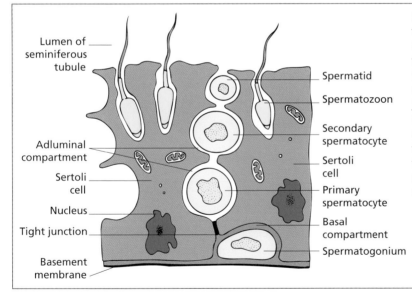

Figure 7.6 The structure of the seminiferous tubule. Sertoli cells span the thickness of the tubule from basement membrane to central lumen. Tight junctions between adjacent Sertoli cells separate the spermatogonial stem cells in the basal compartment from the later stages of spermatogenesis in the adluminal compartment.

weak androgen, androstenedione, in the adrenal cortex (review Figures 2.6 and 6.3). However, in the testis, the additional presence of type 3 17β-hydroxysteroid dehydrogenase (HSD17B3) generates the potent androgen, testosterone (Figure 7.7). The testis is the major site of androgen synthesis, with only a small contribution (<5%) by the adrenal. Testosterone acts in its own right as a potent andro-

gen hormone, virilizing the internal genitalia and acting anabolically on muscle cells. It is also required in high local concentration for normal numbers of fully motile, mature spermatozoa (one reason why spermatogenesis is not restored in men taking exogenous testosterone replacement for hypogonadism). In other target tissues the action of the microsomal enzyme 5α-reductase (SRD5A) forms the more

Box 7.7 Semen analysis (WHO standards)

- Critical to investigation of infertility (see last section of chapter)
- Very useful bioassay for normal testicular function
- Standards within 60 min of ejaculation:
  - Volume > 2.0 mL (usually 2–6 mL)
  - pH 7.2–8.0
  - Concentration > 20 million/mL
  - Total sperm count > 40 million
  - Morphology > 30% normal forms
  - Motility > 50% with forward progression (or >25% with rapid progression)
  - Vitality > 75%
  - White blood cells < 1 million/mL
- Useful clinical terms:
  - Normozoospermia: normal as defined above
  - Oligozoospermia: spermatozoa present but <20 million/mL
  - Azoospermia: no spermatozoa in ejaculate
  - Aspermia: no ejaculate

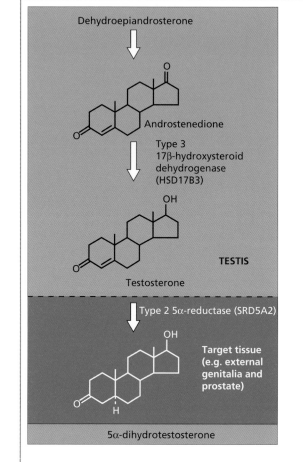

Figure 7.7 The biosynthesis of androgens in Leydig cells. Earlier steps can be reviewed in Figure 2.6.

potent DHT (Table 3.2 and Figure 7.7). There are two isoforms of SRD5A, type 1 (SRD5A1) and type 2 (SRD5A2) encoded by different genes. SRD5A2 functions in the external genitalia and prostate. DHT binds with greater affinity than testosterone to the AR. The DHT–AR complex then mediates androgen action by regulating the transcription of downstream target genes (review Figures 3.18 and 3.20). As well as forming DHT, testosterone may also be aromatized by the cytochrome P450 enzyme, CYP19, to oestradiol in target cells (see Figure 2.6 and Table 3.2); or, alternatively, metabolized to degradation products that are excreted in the urine. The conversion of testosterone to oestradiol is important for normal bone health in men.

Clinical laboratories measure total serum testosterone; DHT is less commonly assayed. In the circulation, testosterone is largely protein bound to albumin and sex hormone-binding globulin (SHBG) with only ~2% circulating free (i.e. directly capable of entering cells). In practice, the equilib-

rium dynamics of androgen binding to protein mean that ~50% of circulating testosterone has the potential to enter target cells ('bioavailable'). Testosterone secretion also has some diurnal variation, falling later in the day. Therefore, borderline low serum measurements from afternoon clinics should be repeated at 9 AM.

Regulation of testicular function – the hypothalamic–anterior pituitary – testicular axis

The testis is regulated by the two pituitary gonadotrophins, FSH and luteinizing hormone (LH), both of which act via cell surface G-protein–coupled receptors predominantly linked to adenylate cyclase second messenger systems (review Chapter 3). Testosterone biosynthesis is stimulated by pulsatile LH, particularly at the rate-limiting step of catalysis by the cholesterol side-chain cleavage enzyme (CYP11A1). LH-induced testosterone diffusing from the Leydig cells acts along with FSH on the Sertoli cells to stimulate spermatogenesis (Box 7.8).

The secretion of LH and FSH is regulated by gonadotrophin-releasing hormone (GnRH, also known as LHRH); a decapeptide released by the hypothalamus in pulses every 90 min (Figure 7.8). The pulsatility is important to the extent that continuous GnRH inhibits LH and FSH release and can be used clinically as a constant infusion to 'shut

down' the reproductive endocrine axis in both men (e.g. to provide chemical castration in prostate cancer) and women (to treat oestrogen-responsive breast cancer; see Chapter 10).

Testosterone inhibits the release of LH (more than FSH), with a minor contribution from peripherally converted oestradiol and DHT (Figure 7.8; review Figure 1.4). The secretion of FSH from gonadotrophs is selectively inhibited by the Sertoli cell hormone, inhibin. Inhibin comprises α- and β-peptide chains, linked by disulphide bonds. Different types of β-chain generate two forms of the whole protein, called inhibin A and inhibin B. Inhibin B is of major physiological relevance; it is produced by the testis under stimulation by FSH and creates a complete negative feedback loop.

Box 7.8 Major functions of the gonadotrophins

- FSH – spermatogenesis
- LH – androgen biosynthesis

Phases of testicular function and reproductive development after birth

Only by understanding normal development can abnormality be correctly diagnosed during the different phases of life.

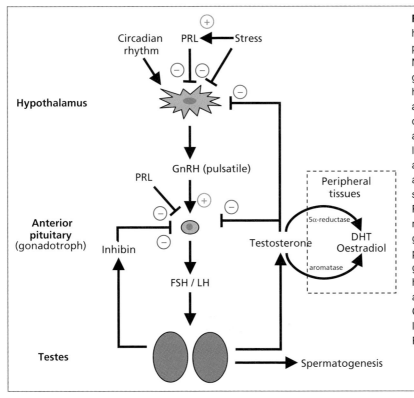

Figure 7.8 The hypothalamic–anterior pituitary–testicular axis. Negative feedback at the gonadotroph and hypothalamus is complex and involves: 5α-dihydrotestosterone (DHT) and testosterone on luteinizing hormone (LH); and inhibin, testosterone and oestrogen on follicle-stimulating hormone (FSH). Prolactin (PRL) exerts a negative influence on gonadotrophin release, probably via altering gonadotrophin-releasing hormone (GnRH) pulsatility and action. Stress inhibits GnRH release and action at least in part by stimulating PRL.

Neonatal life and childhood

During the first year of life, gonadotrophin levels rise, providing a surge in testosterone and inhibin secretion of uncertain significance. During childhood, gonadotrophin secretion is low because of the very sensitive negative feedback from the testis. However, occasional nocturnal pulses of LH and FSH occur in young children, the frequency and amplitude of which gradually increase with advancing years. By 9–11 years, children normally experience regular nocturnal pulses of gonadotrophins as a result of increased GnRH secretion and gonadotroph sensitivity. Ultimately, this stimulates sufficient sex steroid to initiate secondary sexual development and entrance into puberty. Note that minor signs of androgen action, such as some emergent axillary and pubic hair, are a normal reflection of adrenarche (review Chapter 6).

Puberty

Male pubertal development is categorized into five Tanner stages (Figure 7.9). Most of the changes reflect rising concentrations of testicular androgens from an increased number and size of Leydig cells (Box 7.9). However, in addition to penile growth, the onset of puberty can also be detected by an increase in testicular volume following maturation of the seminiferous tubules and the onset of spermatogenesis (Figure 7.9).

Adulthood and old age

The effects of puberty are largely permanent; a deepened ('broken') voice does not regress if a patient becomes hypogonadal. Other aspects, such as maintenance of muscle mass and sex drive, require an ongoing supply of androgen. Beard growth is only likely to slow rather than stop if androgen is lost later in life. In old age testosterone usually remains in the normal range. However, levels do fall slightly and circadian rhythm is diminished, which, when pronounced, has recently been described as a new syndrome of 'late-onset male hypogonadism'.

Clinical disorders

Hypogonadism

The major clinical disorder of the testis is underactivity – 'hypogonadism'. Its presentation in adults may occur as a result of primary (i.e. testicular),

---

Box 7.9 The effects of rising androgens at puberty

- Skeletal muscle growth
- Lengthening and development of the larynx/deepening of the voice
- Pubic hair and beard growth
- Sebaceous gland activity and odorous sweat
- Thickened and pigmented skin over external genitalia
- Increased size of the prostate, seminal vesicles and epididymis
- Epiphyseal fusion and termination of linear growth

Figure 7.9 The stages of pubertal development in males and females as defined by Tanner.

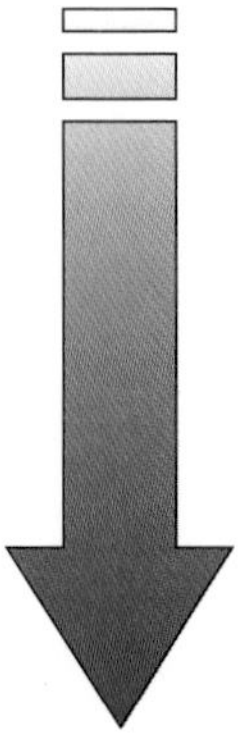

Stage 1: Preadolescent genitalia, no pubic hair or breast development

Stage 2: Scrotal reddening; testicular enlargement (♂)
Breast bud, increased areola diameter (♀)
Straight, pigmented pubic hair

Stage 3: Penile and testicular growth; scrotal darkening (♂)
Increase in breast and areola size, same contour (♀)
Darker, coarser, curlier hair

Stage 4: Penile (and glans) growth in length and breadth (♂)
Projection of areola and nipple (secondary mound) (♀)
Adult hair but restricted coverage

Stage 5: Adult genitalia and hair distribution
Projection of papilla, areola and breast of same contour (♀)

secondary (i.e. pituitary) or tertiary (i.e. hypothalamic) causes. In practice, the latter two can be largely categorized together (Case history 7.2).

Symptoms and signs

Understanding normal physiology and hormone action predicts the symptoms of hypogonadism (Box 7.10). The history should take special care to document two aspects of earlier development:

- Was virilization complete at birth (see earlier section on 46,XY DSD)?
  - For instance, hypospadias might indicate androgen deficiency *in utero*:
    - Did the patient have to sit to urinate as a child?
  - Was testicular descent complete or was surgical intervention necessary?
- The second important time point is puberty:
  - Did puberty begin and progress at the same time and rate as for his peers?

Box 7.10 Clinical features of male hypogonadism

Post-puberty
- Loss of libido
- Subfertility/abnormal semen analysis (see Box 7.7)
- Decreased muscle mass and exercise tolerance; tiredness
- Decreased shaving frequency
- Smooth skin, loss of pubic hair
- Small, soft testes, possibly not fully descended into scrotum
- Gynaecomastia
- Decreased bone mineralization, e.g. osteoporosis or osteopaenia

At (or dating back to) puberty
- Failure of voice to deepen
- Failure of testicular enlargement and penile growth
- Lack of scrotal pigmentation
- Eunuchoidism (arm span > height)
- Delayed bone age

Other questions should address potential trauma or infection, orchidectomy, previous chemotherapy or radiotherapy, alcohol intake and anabolic steroid abuse (present or past) (Box 7.11). Performance enhancing drug use is under-recognized and, while current use would not cause loss of muscle bulk (the opposite is the case), it would cause infertility and the testes to shrink through secondary hypogonadism. Wider questioning should consider other causes of secondary or tertiary hypogonadism and whether other pituitary hormones might be present in excess (e.g. prolactin) or absent (e.g. in panhypopituitarism) (review Chapter 5). Kallman syndrome results from inactivating mutation in a range of genes. There is aberrant migration of the GnRH-producing neurones and a failure of smell (anosmia). Other specific causes of secondary hypogonadism include haemochromatosis (does the patient also have diabetes?) or Prader–Willi syndrome (is there morbid obesity? See Chapter 15). Opiate use can also cause secondary hypogonadism.

Examination should assess the degree of virilization (Box 7.10), the existence and size of both testes correctly positioned in the scrotum, and signs from other hormone axes and organ systems that might potentially point to the diagnosis (e.g. Does the patient have acromegaly? Can the patient smell?).

Investigation and diagnosis

Primary hypogonadism is defined by low serum testosterone, most commonly assayed as total testosterone, and raised gonadotrophins. Sub-clinical (i.e. no symptoms), subtle or incipient primary hypogonadism might be reflected by serum testosterone in the lower half of the normal range with raised gonadotrophins. Equivocal testosterone values from afternoon clinics should be repeated at 9 AM to allow for diurnal variation. Serum total testosterone is also influenced by SHBG and albumin, measurement of which allows estimated calculation of free testosterone levels (several online calculators are freely available). These calculations can be important as low SHBG (e.g. in obesity or hypothyroidism) lowers total testosterone and can cause diagnostic confusion. In primary hypogonadism, raised LH more sensitively reflects loss of testosterone negative feedback; FSH is primarily regulated by inhibin B, but this Sertoli cell hormone is not frequently available as a clinical assay. After confirming primary hypogonadism, the cause needs to be determined (Box 7.11). Obtaining the karyotype may define chromosomal disorders.

In secondary or tertiary hypogonadism, normal gonadotrophin levels are inappropriate and pathological when accompanied by unequivocally low serum testosterone (i.e. the physiological response should be raised LH and FSH) (Box 7.12). All the other anterior pituitary hormone axes should be investigated and the pituitary delineated by magnetic resonance imaging (MRI; review Chapter 5 and see Figure 4.8). In younger patients, congenital deficiency needs to be excluded, as does craniopharyngioma, a histologically benign but erosive tumour derived from cells thought to have lined Rathke's pouch. Although rarely performed, a GnRH test, where GnRH is injected and LH and FSH are measured at baseline and after 30 min, distinguishes hypothalamic or tertiary (greater than two-fold increase in serum LH and FSH) from pituitary or secondary (little or no LH or FSH response) causes of hypogonadism.

Hypogonadism from pathology at any level of the hormone axis would be expected to cause an abnormal semen analysis (e.g. oligozoospermia or azoospermia; see Box 7.7). Conversely, a normal semen analysis should give reassurance in the face of dubious symptoms and signs and equivocal blood results. Gaining a prescription for testosterone replacement (see below) can be a motivation for individuals interested in performance enhancing drugs. Once hypogonadism is diagnosed, bone densitometry (a dual energy X-ray absorptiometry or 'DEXA' scan) assesses the consequence of androgen deficiency on bone mineralization (see Chapter 9).

Treatment

'If it is missing, replace it': give testosterone. As androgens are removed by first-pass metabolism through the liver, oral preparations are relatively ineffective at delivering testosterone to the systemic circulation. The mainstay has been depot intramuscular injection, which lasts between 3 and 4 weeks. Newer preparations last approximately 3 months, superseding much of the use of testosterone implants. Transdermal gel preparations are applied daily after washing and before dressing, followed by

---

Box 7.11 Causes of male primary hypogonadism/testicular failure

- Maldescended or undescended testes:
  - Common cause
  - 10% risk of malignancy
- Inflammation:
  - Mumps orchitis
  - Trauma
- Post-chemotherapy or post-radiotherapy – semen storage advisable pre-treatment for future fertility
- Drugs – rare side-effect of commonly used drugs such as HMGCoA reductase inhibitors ('statins')
- Anabolic steroid abuse
- Alcohol
- Chronic illness
- Autoimmune disorder
- Chromosomal disorders:
  - Klinefelter syndrome (47,XXY; 1:500 males), possible intellectual impairment
  - Others rare (47,XYY; 46,XX with *SRY* translocation)
- Idiopathic/unknown

Box 7.12 Distinguishing primary and secondary or tertiary male hypogonadism

- Low testosterone/high LH and FSH = testicular cause (primary)
- Low testosterone/normal or low LH and FSH = pituitary or hypothalamic cause (secondary or tertiary)

---

hand-washing. Transbuccal absorption is ineffective for most patients. Monitoring replacement therapy should aim for a serum testosterone in the normal range. Serum LH can become normalized. For monthly depot testosterone injection, total serum testosterone is commonly measured immediately prior to an injection. This 'trough' value should be at the low end of the normal range.

Supra-physiological androgen replacement carries risk. Polycythaemia (a raised red blood cell count) increases the risk of thrombosis, and stimulation of the prostate may promote prostatic hypertrophy or accelerate androgen-dependent prostatic cancer. Full blood count (FBC), haematocrit and serum prostate-specific antigen (PSA; an imperfect biomarker of prostate cancer) are measured at least annually at follow-up appointments.

When fertility is desired in secondary or tertiary hypogonadism, testosterone is exchanged for twice-weekly injections of human chorionic gonadotrophin (hCG) as a mimic for LH and, if needed to achieve spermatogenesis, human menopausal gonadotrophins (hMG; a mimic for FSH) (see last section of this chapter). Over the course of a few months, these hormones stimulate the quiescent testes into active steroidogenesis and spermatogenesis. This therapy is not the first-line method for replacing testosterone as it requires regular injection and is more expensive.

Case history 7.2

A 35-year-old man was referred to the endocrinologist after his partner had persuaded him to see his doctor. His partner had commented that the patient had no interest in sex, had lost interest in social life and was commonly asleep in the evenings. Total serum testosterone was 3 nmol/L (~86 ng/dL) with an SHBG in the upper part of the normal range. Levels of both gonadotrophins were three times the upper limit of normal. On further questioning, the man, who was tall, had never really felt much sex drive. He only needed to shave once a week to avoid facial hair growth. On examination, bilateral gynaecomastia was noted and both testes were small and soft.

Where is the site of pathology?
What chromosomal disorder might this be and how might this be investigated?
What treatment and advice are needed?
What abnormality might a DEXA scan indicate?

Answers, see p. 163

Testicular tumours

Testicular tumours occur at all ages. The type of tumour is age-dependent (Box 7.13). Incidence is raised in undescended or dysgenetic testes (~five-fold; see Chapter 10). Testicular germ cell tumours are associated with extra copies of the short (p) arm of chromosome 12, where several genes important for germ-cell proliferation are located (review Chapter 2). Tumours of Sertoli or Leydig cells are less common.

Tumours usually present as painless testicular enlargement; however, they metastasize early. Reticence regarding the need to consult a physician is common; the cyclist Lance Armstrong thought a grapefruit-sized swelling was a consequence of trauma from his saddle. Thus, education to self-examine is as important for men as breast-care is for women. For functional Leydig cell tumours, abnormal sex steroid production is usually obvious as virilization (e.g. precocious puberty) or feminization (e.g. gynaecomastia, see below). For non-seminomatous germ cell tumours, serum hCG and α-fetoprotein (AFP) are very useful as they fall with successful treatment and can be used as serum biomarkers.

Orchidectomy is important, if only for debulking tumour mass, and may need to be bilateral. Chemotherapy is very successful and combinations of vinblastine, bleomycin, etopiside and cisplatin cure most tumours. Prior cryopreservation of sperm allows future *in vitro* fertilization (IVF) if surgery and chemotherapy render the patient infertile (see final section). Androgen replacement may be needed for primary hypogonadism (see previous section).

Box 7.13 Testicular tumours of germ cell origin

Embryonal carcinoma or teratocarcinoma
• Tends to affect children
• hCG and AFP are useful serum markers

Seminoma
• Tends to occur in early adulthood or old age

Gynaecomastia

Gynaecomastia is defined as the development of breast tissue of greater than 2 cm diameter in males. It can be physiological or represent abnormal sex hormone production or metabolism (Table 7.1). Enlargement of breast tissue at birth because of oestrogens of either placental or maternal origin is

Table 7.1 Gynaecomastia	
Causes of gynaecomastia	**Investigations to consider**
Physiological	General investigations
Neonatal	Serum testosterone, LH, FSH, prolactin, thyroid function test, urea and creatinine
Pubertal	
Old age	
Any cause of hypogonadism, e.g. Klinefelter syndrome (47,XXY)	Karyotype analysis
Adrenal or testicular tumours, oestrogen or androgen (+ peripheral aromatase activity) secretion	Serum hCG, DHEA(S), androstenedione, oestrogen, imaging
Liver disease	Liver function tests
Inadequate clearance and altered metabolism of steroid hormones	
Alcohol	
Drugs	
Oestrogens, antiandrogens (spironolactone), cimetidine, ACE inhibitors	

LH, luteinizing hormone; FSH, follicle-stimulating hormone; hCG, human chorionic gonadotrophin; DHEA, dehydroepiandrosterone; DHEAS, DHEA sulphate; ACE, angiotensin-converting enzyme.

short-lived. A similar increase commonly follows puberty. It can be unilateral and painful, although it usually involutes by the end of the teenage years. Gynaecomastia can also occur in old age because of a variety of factors, including a rise in SHBG, reduced androgen availability or increased aromatization to oestrogen (review Figure 2.6). Normal physiological variation should only be diagnosed by exclusion, especially if onset is rapid and persistent. History (especially drug history), examination and investigation are important. Treatment is most commonly one of reassurance, withdrawal of offending medications (e.g. spironolactone) or cosmetic surgery.

The female reproductive system

Puberty in females heralds the beginning of the female menstrual cycle when usually one germ cell reaches full maturity at intervals of ~28 days. This cycle has limited lifespan as only ~400 germ cells reach full maturity and ovulation. The cycle is associated with coordinated changes in ovarian steroidogenesis that prime the reproductive tract for potential pregnancy.

Ovarian morphology and function

Oogenesis begins in the fetal ovary when, towards the end of the first trimester, germ cells start entering the first stage of meiosis and arrest in prophase (review Figure 2.1). Termed primary oocytes, they are surrounded by a layer of steroid-producing granulosa cells as primordial follicles (Figure 7.10). There are ~6–7 million primordial follicles at 20 weeks of gestation, after which their number declines inexorably. At birth, there are ~2 million and by puberty only 300,000. Menopause marks the depletion of all germ cells within the ovaries.

Follicle development, ovulation and early embryogenesis

At the beginning of a menstrual cycle, the granulosa cells in 10–20 primordial follicles proliferate to form primary and then secondary follicles (Figure 7.10). In any one menstrual cycle, only one follicle usually reaches full maturity as the dominant

Graafian follicle, when stromal cells become arranged around the outside to form the vascularized 'theca'. At mid-cycle, the follicle ruptures (ovulation) and the oocyte is captured by the fimbriated opening of the Fallopian tube, down which it is wafted by ciliated epithelial cells and peristaltic contractions towards the uterine cavity (see Figure 7.2b). During this course, if the ovum meets spermatozoa and is fertilized, embryogenesis starts such that, upon arrival in the uterine cavity, it has developed into a blastocyst ready for implantation into the endometrium. If the ovum is not fertilized, it dies. Hormonal regulation of this process is described below.

Formation of the corpus luteum

Thecal cells plus some granulosa cells of the ruptured follicle play a critical role in the second half of the menstrual cycle. They proliferate, enlarge and fill the collapsed antrum of the follicle as a solid, round mass of steroidogenic cells called the corpus luteum; so named because it is initially red, but matures to a yellowish colour (Figure 7.10). If fertilization and blastocyst implantation do not occur, the corpus luteum is only active for ~2 weeks, after which it stops synthesizing steroids and dies (luteolysis), leaving white atrophied tissue (the corpus albicans). However, if implantation occurs,

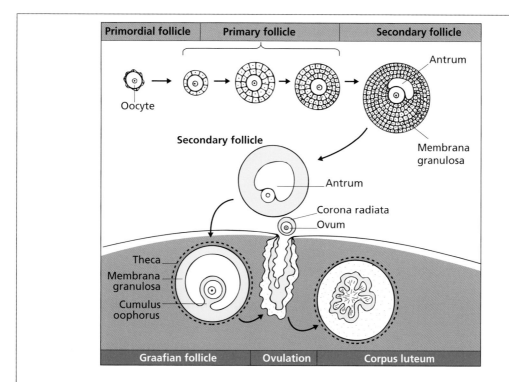

Figure 7.10 Follicle growth, maturation and ovulation. The entire process takes place close to the ovarian surface. The outer steroid-producing granulosa cells divide and grow to form a multi-layered membrana granulosa. The appearance of a liquid-filled antrum defines the transition from a primary to a secondary follicle. The antrum enlarges, creating a stalk of cells (the 'cumulus oophorus') that attaches the oocyte to the membrana granulosa. Stromal cells form the outer steroidogenic theca cell layer. The entire structure is now termed a Graafian follicle, which ruptures at ovulation, expelling the ovum surrounded by a layer of cells, the corona radiata. The collapsed follicle becomes the corpus luteum.

the corpus luteum grows and its hormone secretion maintains the uterine endometrium during the early weeks of pregnancy until, in humans, the placenta assumes steroidogenic function. The hormones involved in this process are described below.

Ovarian steroidogenesis and the hypothalamic–anterior pituitary–ovarian axis: the menstrual cycle

During the reproductive years, ovarian hormone production accompanies egg development in ~4-week cycles (Box 7.14 and Figure 7.11). In the absence of fertilization, the cycle is terminated by the restricted 2-week lifespan of the corpus luteum.

The most potent oestrogen in humans is oestradiol. Its biosynthesis relies on two somatic cell types within the developing follicle, the inner theca cells (theca interna) that synthesize testosterone, which is then aromatized by CYP19 (also called aromatase) to oestradiol in the granulosa cell (Figure 7.12 and review Figure 2.6). Oestrogen can also be generated by CYP19 acting on androstenedione to form oestrone that can be converted to oestradiol by HSD17B1. Progesterone biosynthesis is relatively straightforward. Removal of the cholesterol side chain generates pregnenolone in theca cells, which is converted to progesterone by HSD3B activity (review Figure 2.6).

The menstrual cycle is regulated by the hypothalamic–anterior pituitary–ovarian axis and intra-ovarian mechanisms (Figure 7.13).

The follicular phase: the control of follicle development

At the beginning of each cycle, pulsatile GnRH stimulates FSH secretion (see Chapter 5). Under FSH regulation, a cohort of ~20 primary follicles develops into secondary follicles, which produce oestradiol (Figures 7.10 and 7.12). In turn, oestradiol increases FSH receptors on the surface of the proliferating granulosa cells. Because of this regular, predictable start to the menstrual cycle, this is also the best time for clinical investigation of serum LH, FSH and oestradiol (Box 7.14). Oestradiol and inhibin secretion suppress FSH production from the anterior pituitary by negative feedback (Figure 7.13). As the concentration of FSH falls, only the ripening follicles with the highest concentration of FSH receptors are able to sustain development, while the rest atrophy. Thus, progressively, one dominant follicle is selected, around which theca cells develop under the influence of LH (Figure 7.10).

Ovulation

Mid-cycle is associated with a surge of LH and, to a lesser extent, FSH from the pituitary (Figure 7.11). The LH surge lasts ~36 h, stimulating factors that aid follicle rupture and final maturation of the oocyte. The principal cause for this gonadotrophin surge from the pituitary is a temporary switch in oestradiol feedback. At mid-cycle, as the dominant follicle ripens, oestrogen output increases and at ~day 12, a threshold is exceeded, which, if main-

---

Box 7.14 Ovarian hormone action and measurement during the menstrual cycle

A cycle of two halves
- Oestrogen: prepares the egg for release during the follicular phase (Figure 7.12)
- Progesterone: maintains early pregnancy (i.e. 'pro-gestation') in the luteal phase

Ovulatory cycles are usually 28 days but may vary slightly
- Variation in length reflects speed of egg preparation, i.e. follicular phase

- Luteal phase is relatively fixed at 14 days

This physiology determines the timing of clinical hormone measurement
- Day 1: first day of vaginal bleeding from preceding cycle
- Days 2–5: time to measure FSH, LH and oestradiol
- Day 21 (or mid-luteal phase if cycle ≠ 28 days): time to measure progesterone

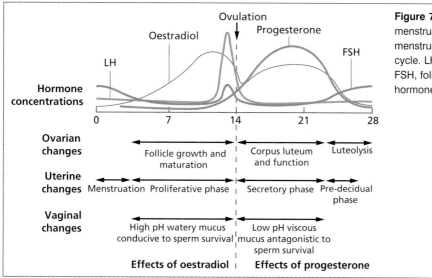

Figure 7.11 The 28-day menstrual cycle. The start of menstruation is day 1 of a new cycle. LH, luteinizing hormone; FSH, follicle-stimulating hormone.

tained for 36 h, turns feedback at the gonadotroph from negative to positive. Now, high levels of oestradiol drive further gonadotrophin secretion, creating the feed-forward surge that culminates in and is ended by ovulation.

The luteal phase: maintaining an early pregnancy

After ovulation, negative feedback at the gonadotroph is restored and lower levels of LH stimulate progesterone from the corpus luteum. This allows clinical measurement of progesterone at day 21, which, if > 30 nmol/L (~9.4 ng/mL), strongly implies ovulation has occurred (Box 7.14). The corpus luteum also secretes oestradiol, now providing negative feedback on LH and FSH (Figure 7.12). By ~day 25, the falling LH is no longer able to maintain adequate steroidogenesis. The fall in progesterone leads to endometrial degeneration and menstruation follows (see next section). This drop in oestradiol and progesterone also removes negative feedback from the pituitary, which, under the ongoing stimulus of GnRH pulses, resumes secretion of FSH and LH. So begins the next cycle.

If fertilization has occurred and a blastocyst has implanted (~day 20 of the menstrual cycle), the resulting embryonic trophoblast begins to secrete hCG, a glycoprotein hormone that acts

like LH at the LH receptor. hCG maintains the corpus luteum and, in the face of continuing oestradiol and progesterone, menstruation is postponed (covered in more detail later and in Figure 7.15).

Cyclical effects on the uterus and vagina

The changing ovarian steroid output causes cyclical alterations in the uterine endometrium and the rest of the female genital tract (Figures 7.11 and 7.14). Increased secretion of oestradiol at the start of a cycle stimulates repair and proliferation of the endometrium and expression of receptors for progesterone and oestradiol. After ovulation, raised progesterone prepares the endometrium for potential implantation. It doubles in thickness, and the simple tubular glands become tortuous and saccular. However, with luteolysis the endometrium breaks down and sloughs off as menstrual bleeding. The cyclical hormones also alter the consistency and pH of cervical mucus (Figure 7.11).

Phases of ovarian function and reproductive development after birth

Neonatal life and childhood

Ovarian function should be quiescent after birth and during childhood such that precocious puberty always needs investigation.

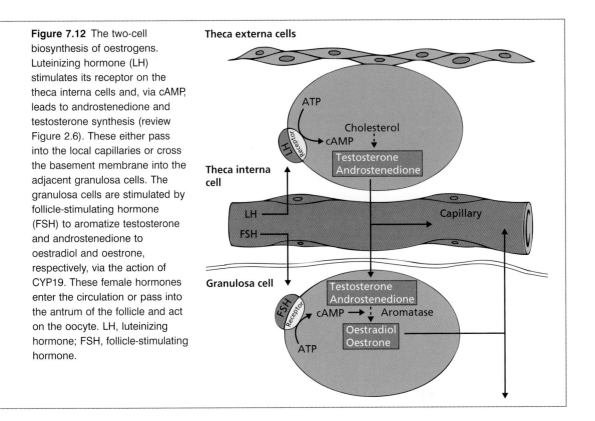

Figure 7.12 The two-cell biosynthesis of oestrogens. Luteinizing hormone (LH) stimulates its receptor on the theca interna cells and, via cAMP, leads to androstenedione and testosterone synthesis (review Figure 2.6). These either pass into the local capillaries or cross the basement membrane into the adjacent granulosa cells. The granulosa cells are stimulated by follicle-stimulating hormone (FSH) to aromatize testosterone and androstenedione to oestradiol and oestrone, respectively, via the action of CYP19. These female hormones enter the circulation or pass into the antrum of the follicle and act on the oocyte. LH, luteinizing hormone; FSH, follicle-stimulating hormone.

Puberty

Puberty sees the transition from a quiescent, immature state to a fully developed, fertile female (Table 7.2). Although the growth spurt starts first, the most obvious early pubertal sign is breast development (see Figure 7.9). Tanner stages 1–4 are dependent on oestrogen; stage 5 also requires progesterone. Coincident with breast development, pubic hair starts to grow. Pubic hair growth is largely under the influence of androgen from both adrenal sex steroid precursors and the ovary, and may have commenced at adrenarche (see Chapter 6). However, it usually progresses in parallel with oestrogen-stimulated breast development. There are also oestrogen-dependent changes in vaginal size, mucosal appearance and pH. The labia thicken and rugate, a process similar to that which occurs in male scrotal skin. Periods usually commence (menarche) during Tanner stage 4.

Puberty in females also marks a transition from nocturnal pulsatile secretion of gonadotrophins to the 24-h pulsatility that is necessary for fertility. The first few cycles after menarche are potentially anovulatory and slightly irregular, but a regular pattern should emerge relatively quickly. Failure to establish a regular cycle is suggestive of polycystic ovarian syndrome (see later).

Menopause

Fertility tends to decline progressively once a woman has entered her 30s. Thus, the menopause may be preceded by some years of less regular ovarian function. Cycles may release multiple ova interspersed with spells of anovulation. Low follicle counts during this pre-menopausal stage increase follicular phase gonadotrophin levels. Clinically, a raised serum FSH on day 3–5 or low serum levels of ovarian AMH indicates relatively poor 'ovarian reserve' and lower likelihood of successful IVF therapy. This normal sequence culminates in the menopause, defined as the last menstrual period, usually aged 50 or slightly later, after which the ovaries are depleted of follicles, serum oestrogen and inhibin fall, and circulating LH and FSH rise

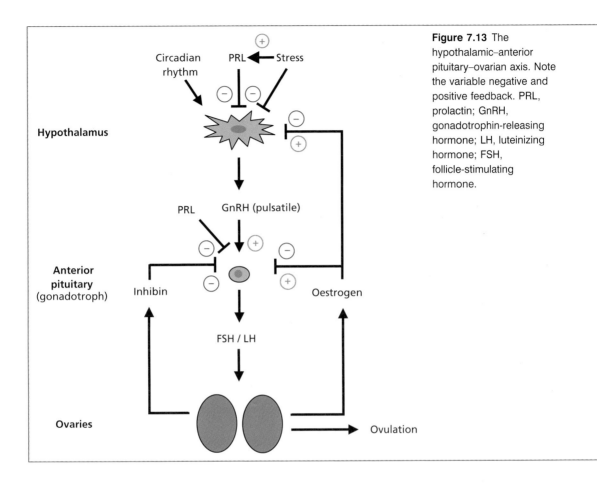

Figure 7.13 The hypothalamic–anterior pituitary–ovarian axis. Note the variable negative and positive feedback. PRL, prolactin; GnRH, gonadotrophin-releasing hormone; LH, luteinizing hormone; FSH, follicle-stimulating hormone.

several-fold, i.e. a normal pituitary response to primary hypogonadism.

The fall in oestradiol production causes atrophy of the vaginal mucosa and breasts and, for reasons that are not entirely clear but reflect the inhibitory action of oestrogen on osteoclasts (Chapter 9), bone mass begins to decline more rapidly. Acute loss of oestrogen causes characteristic episodes of hot 'flushes' (UK) or 'flashes' (USA). The only post-menopausal source of oestrogen is from CYP19 aromatizing adrenal androstenedione in peripheral locations to the weak oestrogen, oestrone.

The endocrinology of pregnancy

Human pregnancy is ~9 months divided into three trimesters, each of approximately 3 months. Review the earlier sections on spermatogenesis, follicle development, ovulation and early embryogenesis. The embryo develops until 56 days post-fertilization; thereafter it is a fetus. However, the dating of pregnancy (gestational age) is timed by obstetricians from the last menstrual period (LMP). Thus, for a 4-week menstrual cycle, LMP age = true fetal age + 2 weeks.

Fertilization and implantation

In humans, for one spermatozoon to fertilize the ovum, ~25–30 million are ejaculated into the vagina (Box 7.7). From here, they traverse the cervix and body of the uterus *en masse* (the 'sperm train') to reach the Fallopian tube and the ovum. Hydrolytic enzymes from the acrosomes of many spermatozoa loosen the corona radiata (Figure 7.10). However, as soon as one sperm has entered the ovum, a

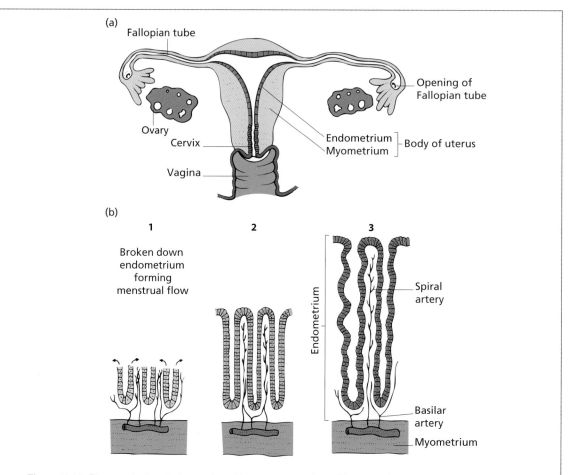

Figure 7.14 Changes in the uterine endometrium during the menstrual cycle. (a) The female reproductive organs. The body of the uterus consists of the inner endometrial layer and surrounding smooth muscle myometrium. (b) Uterine changes during the menstrual cycle. (1) Breakdown of the endometrium (days 1–3) when the outer two-thirds is shed to form the menstrual flow. The basal third of the endometrium persists and its cells divide and grow over the exposed tissue (arrows) to repair the endometrium. (2) During the oestrogenic proliferative phase (days 3–14), the uterine glands grow in length as the endometrium thickens. (3) During the secretory phase (days 14–28), uterine glands double in length and become tortuous and sacculated. Stromal oedema is maximal by day 21, the approximate time of blastocyst implantation. In the absence of pregnancy, during the last 2–3 days of this phase, the spiral blood vessels vasoconstrict and rupture. Lakes of blood form in the stromal tissue. Endometrial breakdown follows.

series of reactions block multiple penetrations ('polyspermy'). The window period for fertilization is relatively short, ~72 h, based on: favourable cervical mucus for sperm penetration; lifespan of spermatozoa in the female genital tract; and the presence of the ovum in the Fallopian tube, where local environmental conditions foster early embryogenesis (Box 7.15). If all goes well, the fertilized egg (zygote) undergoes serial rounds of mitosis creating a morula of ~16 cells followed by a blastocyst containing an inner cell mass (the embryo's future body) and trophectoderm (major part of the future placenta). The blastocyst implants into the endometrium a few days after fertilization.

Table 7.2 Different phases of ovarian function and its effects

Phase	Oestrogen	Progesterone
Puberty	Stimulates growth of the uterus and breast Shapes female figure via fat deposition Contributes to closure of epiphyses Exerts important effects on psychological development and sexual responsiveness	Aids transition from Tanner Stage 4 to 5
Menstrual cycle	Follicular phase: Causes endometrial proliferation; and secretion of clear, high pH cervical mucus – conducive to sperm survival Matures the vaginal epithelium Causes negative and temporary positive feedback at the hypothalamus and anterior pituitary	Luteal phase: Causes a rise in body temperature; development of secretory endometrium; and secretion of thick, low pH cervical mucus – not conducive to sperm survival Negative feedback at the hypothalamus and pituitary
Pregnancy	Causes growth of the breast duct system and myometrial hypertrophy together with fluid retention and increased uterine blood flow	Causes reduction of uterine contractions and reduced smooth muscle tone Causes a rise in body temperature and growth of the alveoli of the breasts
General cellular effects	Enhances receptors for progesterone (i.e. oestrogen is needed for progesterone to exert its intracellular actions)	Stimulates HSD17B isoforms which inactivate oestradiol to weak oestrone

HSD17B, type 3 17β-hydroxysteroid dehydrogenase.

Box 7.15 Local environmental factors for early embryo growth and implantation

- Healthy Fallopian and intrauterine nutritional/metabolic milieu (e.g. euglycaemia)
- Poorly controlled diabetes is associated with early miscarriage (see Chapter 14)
- Receptive endometrium for implantation

Failure of these attributes is likely to contribute to subfertility

Endocrine changes during pregnancy, parturition and lactation

Successful implantation leads to development of the trophoblast, which begins to secrete hCG into the maternal bloodstream. hCG is similar enough to LH to act via the LH receptor, and it maintains the corpus luteum and early pregnancy, and postpones the next cycle of ovulation (Figure 7.15). Its high levels during the first trimester also stimulate the thyroid (see Chapter 8) as hCG also mimics thyroid stimulating hormone (TSH; the α-chain is identical between hCG, LH, FSH and TSH). This offsetting of TSH action leads to lower serum TSH

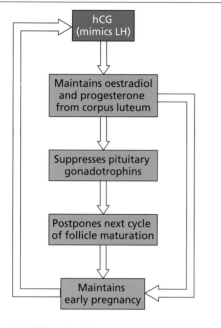

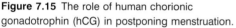

Figure 7.15 The role of human chorionic gonadotrophin (hCG) in postponing menstruation.

Box 7.16 Endocrine alterations during pregnancy, parturition and lactation

Pregnancy
- Maternal:
  - Hypertrophy/hyperplasia of lactotrophs synthesizing prolactin
  - hCG (partially mimics TSH) stimulation of thyroid hormone synthesis
  - Increased β-cell function and potential growth of pancreatic islets
  - Increased adrenal cortisol output
  - Increased heart rate; cardiac output rises by 30–50% because of alterations in the hormonal milieu and placental circulation
- Fetal growth and development:
  - Requires thyroid hormone (CNS development), insulin and GH–IGF axes
  - Maturation of the fetal lung (surfactant production) by cortisol near term

Parturition
- Local prostaglandins stimulate the early uterine contractions
- Oxytocin increases as the fetus descends the birth canal and distends the vagina (see Chapter 5)

Lactation
- High oestrogen and progesterone during pregnancy inhibit lactation
- Post-partum, lactation relies on continued prolactin and cortisol
- Oxytocin, released via the suckling reflex, stimulates milk ejection

---

levels (Box 7.16), which is physiological but needs to be remembered when interpreting thyroid function tests in the first trimester (see Table 8.1). In a small minority of women, higher hCG levels, as can arise in molar pregnancy (when there is only trophoblast and no embryo proper) or a twin pregnancy, causes a transient thyrotoxicosis. It also associates with excessive early morning vomiting (hyperemesis gravidarum). hCG excreted into the maternal urine forms the basis of most pregnancy tests. Levels can be detected by urine strip assays soon after menstruation / a period is delayed (~3 weeks of embryo development).

Towards the end of the first trimester, fetal steroidogenesis occurs across several organs, leading to the term, the 'feto-placental unit'. Placental secretion of progesterone takes over from the corpus luteum, which regresses. In the fetal adrenal cortex there is early cortisol biosynthesis, followed by the production of large amounts of dehydroepiandrosterone (DHEA) and its sulphated derivative, DHEAS (review Figures 2.6 and 7.16). A series of enzymatic reactions gives rise to different oestrogens: oestradiol, oestrone and oestriol, the latter

detected from the end of the first trimester onwards in maternal urine. Growth hormone (GH) and especially insulin-like growth factor (IGF) hormones are important for fetal growth. Similarly, fetal insulin secretion acts more to stimulate growth than control glucose levels, which are ordinarily regulated by the mother. However, if the mother has diabetes, the increased transfer of glucose to the fetus stimulates excessive insulin secretion, leading to overgrowth (macrosomia), difficult delivery (e.g.

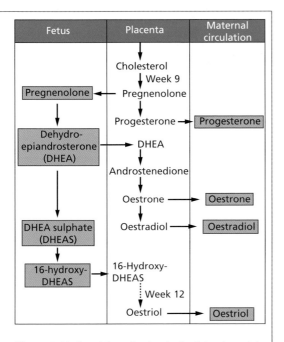

Fetus	Placenta	Maternal circulation

Figure 7.16 Steroid production in the feto-placental unit.

Box 7.17 Amenorrhoea

In the UK
- ~95% of girls have undergone menarche by 15 years
- ~50% have done so by 12½ years

Absence of periods is 'amenorrhoea'
- Primary amenorrhoea: menstruation not started by 16 years
- Secondary amenorrhoea: menstruation started but now absent for > 6 months

Defining the cause: first determine if oestrogen is present or absent

shoulder dystocia) and risk of neonatal hypoglycaemia (see Chapter 14).

Approaching term, cortisol stimulates synthesis of surfactant proteins, which decrease surface tension in the lungs (Box 7.16). This allows the fluid-filled alveoli to expand with air at birth and begin gas exchange. The mechanism is so important that dexamethasone, a synthetic glucocorticoid that crosses the placenta, is given to women in premature labour to decrease the incidence of neonatal respiratory distress syndrome.

The signal for birth (parturition) after ~9 months remains unclear. However, as progesterone levels fall, two factors, oxytocin and prostaglandins, are important [Box 7.16; the role of oxytocin in parturition and milk production (lactation) is described in Chapter 5]. Preparation for lactation begins with breast development (thelarche) ~2 years before menarche, under the influence of ovarian oestrogens, which initiate duct proliferation and accumulation of fat in the breast. During female adolescence, oestrogen, GH and adrenal steroids stimulate further growth of the duct system. Alveolar growth is promoted by oestrogen, progesterone,

glucocorticoids and prolactin with contributions from insulin and thyroid hormones [in boys, the process is inhibited by testosterone; however, some breast development (gynaecomastia) may occur (see Table 7.1)].

In early pregnancy, oestrogens cause further growth of the ducts and the breasts enlarge. Later on, glucocorticoids from the adrenal cortex, prolactin from the anterior pituitary and placental lactogen (a prolactin-like hormone from the placenta) induce enzymes needed for milk production (Box 7.16). So long as breast-feeding is continued, prolactin levels stay high and inhibit pituitary gonadotrophin release, tending to postpone cyclical ovulation. Even though this is unreliable for an individual unless the infant is exclusively breast-fed every few hours, globally this mechanism is an important contraceptive.

Clinical disorders

Amenorrhoea

Ovarian hormone disruption causes loss of ovulatory cycles and, consequently, absence of periods (amenorrhoea; Box 7.17). Amenorrhoea can be classified as either primary (periods never started) or secondary (periods started but now absent for >6 months); this distinction becomes arbitrary when the same pathology underlies both. Clinically, in determining the cause, the first task is to assess whether oestrogen is present or absent (Tables 7.3 and 7.4).

Amenorrhoea with absent oestrogen
Symptoms and signs

The commonest cause of amenorrhoea is secondary; temporary hypothalamic shutdown of pulsatile GnRH secretion during sub-optimal or challenging conditions (Table 7.3). This can be as subtle as major exercise or 'stress' (e.g. exams or bullying) and with its relief the menstrual cycle returns. Questioning such matters requires time and sensitivity. Broader questioning should address other pituitary pathology, including pregnancy, hypothyroidism, and potential galactorrhoea from excess prolactin (Case history 7.3, Table 7.3 and review Chapter 5).

Table 7.3 Approaching amenorrhoea with absent oestrogen	
History and examination	
Compassion and time are needed to elicit features of anorexia or bulimia nervosa, or bullying.	
Is there excessive physical exercise?	
Is there undiagnosed systemic illness, e.g. coeliac disease?	
Have the ovaries ever functioned?	
Question for a history of menopausal flushing (flashing) and look for evidence of breast development.	
Differential diagnosis	
Categories	*Examples*
Hypothalamic or anterior pituitary deficiency – indicated by low or 'normal' LH and FSH	Simple constitutional delay (i.e. not pathological)
	Transient, hypothalamic inhibition from 'higher' centres (e.g. extreme exercise, anorexia nervosa or stress)
	Head trauma
	Cranial irradiation
	Kallman syndrome (is there anosmia?)
	Congenital hypopituitarism
	Tumour affecting the pituitary gland (e.g. craniopharyngioma, non-functioning adenoma, or hormone-secreting tumour)
	Hyperprolactinaemia (e.g. dopamine antagonists, prolactinoma or stalk compression)
Ovarian (i.e. lack of follicles) – indicated by high LH and FSH	Absent or rudimentary ovaries, e.g. Turner syndrome (45,XO) or disorders of sex development
	Damage, e.g. chemotherapy, radiotherapy or autoimmune destruction
	Premature exhaustion of follicles, e.g. fragile X syndrome

LH, luteinizing hormone; FSH, follicle-stimulating hormone.

Assessment is needed of whether the ovaries ever functioned:

- Is there any breast development?
- Are there features of Turner syndrome?
  - Shield chest
  - Widely spaced nipples
  - Webbed neck
  - Increased carrying angle
- Have there been recent clear menopausal symptoms such as hot flushes (flashes) due to the acute withdrawal of oestrogen?

Investigation and diagnosis

Serum oestradiol is very low or undetectable.

If the aetiology is ovarian, loss of negative feedback causes a pronounced rise of serum gonadotrophins into the post-menopausal range (several-fold the upper limit of normal for the reproductive years; Table 7.3). Ultrasound can determine the presence and structure of the ovaries. A karyogram excludes gross chromosomal abnormality (e.g. Turner syndrome/45,XO) and screening is increasingly available for other genetic causes of premature ovarian failure (POF; menopause before 40 years of age), such as fragile X syndrome.

As for male hypogonadism (see earlier), low or inappropriately normal serum gonadotrophins indicate that the pathology is in the hypothalamus or anterior pituitary (Table 7.3; review Chapter 5). Although rarely performed, hypothalamic and anterior pituitary pathology can be distinguished by measuring LH and FSH 30 min after GnRH administration; if they rise adequately (more than twofold), this is indicative of hypothalamic pathology, while a poor response suggests a lesion in the anterior pituitary. In younger patients, craniopharyngioma or congenital deficiency needs to be excluded. The pituitary should be delineated by MRI (Figure 4.8).

Treatment

The primary issue is: '*if it is missing, replace it*'. Lack of oestrogen for prolonged spells leads to bone demineralization and risk of future osteoporosis. If persistent for longer than 6 months, oestrogen should be replaced, either by the combined oral contraceptive pill (COCP) or hormone replacement therapy (HRT) preparations of female sex hormones. Unopposed oestrogen increases the risk of endometrial carcinoma: if the uterus is present, treatment must include a progestogen. In permanent loss of ovarian function, HRT is advised until the normal age of the menopause at ~50 years, at which point DEXA can assess bone mineral density, allowing informed choices to be made on future fracture risk (see Chapter 9). Treatment relating to other pituitary hormone axes, if appropriate, is covered in Chapter 5.

Other treatment is more tailored, such as fertility management (see last section). In permanent secondary or tertiary hypogonadism (i.e. amenorrhoea due to pathology in the pituitary or the hypothalamus) the ovaries and uterus can potentially support pregnancy. Fertility can be restored by hCG and hMG injections to mimic the gonadotrophins. If GH-deficient, prior GH treatment may be needed to stimulate uterine growth prior to stimulating ovulation. Egg donation is required to achieve pregnancy in ovarian failure. These scenarios are emotionally charged, requiring specialist services, fertility experts and psychological support.

For Turner syndrome, there are additional considerations because of the X chromosome genes that play roles beyond the ovary. To collate these issues, dedicated clinics and care are indicated (Box 7.18).

Case history 7.3

A 25-year-old woman is referred because of spontaneous galactorrhoea. Her periods have stopped and she is sexually inactive. Serum prolactin is found to be 4500–6000 U/L (~212–283 ng/mL) on repeated investigation.

What other questions need to be asked?
What is the most likely diagnosis and would serum oestradiol be high or low?
What other investigations need to be considered?
What drug treatment will lower the prolactin and most likely stop the galactorrhoea?

Answers, see p. 163

Box 7.18 Caring for patients with Turner syndrome

During childhood and adolescence
- GH is used to maximize growth, compromised because of a missing copy of the *SHOX* gene
- Checks to ensure that hearing is satisfactory and thyroid function is normal
- Pubertal development is likely to need increasing doses of oestrogens, finally adding progestogens

During adulthood
- Oestrogen replacement (HRT or COCP) for bone mineral density
- Annual screening with thyroid function tests (increased incidence of primary hypothyroidism)

- Cardiology monitoring to detect abnormalities of the left outflow tract (ventricle, aortic value and aorta):
  - Increased risk of aortic dissection: rigorously treat hypertension and periodic imaging of aortic root (e.g. MRI)
  - Aortic valve may be bicuspid requiring prophylactic antibiotics during procedures to guard against endocarditis
  - Increased incidence of coarctation of aorta
- Remain mindful of increased risk of type 1 diabetes
- Assessment of bone mineral density by DEXA
- Psychological support may be necessary; interaction with patient support groups

---

Amenorrhoea with oestrogen present: polycystic ovarian syndrome and other causes

The commonest cause of decreased or irregular menstrual frequency with detectable oestrogen is PCOS. The pathological mechanism underlying PCOS is incompletely understood; however, it includes a polygenic predisposition to insulin resistance and altered insulin action in the ovary and in other sites (see Chapter 13).

PCOS is a diagnosis of exclusion. Other endocrine disorders can present similarly and must be ruled out before diagnosing PCOS.

Symptoms and signs

PCOS is encapsulated by amenorrhoea with relative clinical or biochemical androgen excess in the absence of other causes. Whether or not cysts contribute to making the diagnosis is contentious (see below). Symptoms and signs, and features of the history and examination are covered in Table 7.4. PCOS associates with an increased incidence of impaired glucose tolerance (IGT), gestational (GDM) and type 2 diabetes (T2DM), although the same is true of Cushing syndrome and other endocrinopathy. Maintaining a normal body mass index (BMI) is commonly difficult in PCOS. However,

weight gain *per se* increases resistance to insulin action and obesity associates with decreased menstrual frequency and subfertility. A key question to address this is whether, prior to weight gain, periods were regular. A persistent tendency to irregular periods soon after menarche is supportive of a true genetic predisposition to PCOS (Case history 7.4).

Investigation and diagnosis

PCOS is a diagnosis of exclusion, such that no test confirms PCOS and investigations must exclude other curable endocrinopathy. In PCOS, the ratio of LH to FSH tends to be increased and SHBG tends to be low. Low SHBG associates with hyperinsulinism (circulating insulin and C-peptide levels are increased), but this is also prevalent in simple obesity. The androgen excess of PCOS is both ovarian and adrenal in origin. A particularly high DHEA or DHEAS may suggest an adrenal tumour. The higher serum testosterone is greater than 4 nmol/L (~115 ng/mL), the more likely an ovarian or adrenocortical androgen-secreting tumour becomes, especially if supported by true virilization, which practically excludes PCOS (Table 7.4). Ultrasound can help to exclude ovarian tumours (the best views of the pelvic anatomy are

Table 7.4 Polycystic ovarian syndrome (PCOS)

The key principle: exclude other curable endocrinopathy with overlapping phenotype before diagnosing PCOS

This requires a full history, examination and investigations. Never miss pregnancy as a cause of amenorrhoea in the presence of circulating oestrogen.

Making the diagnosis and treatment

Were periods ever regular?

No	Supports the diagnosis of PCOS
Yes	Suspicion raised of:
	An androgen-secreting ovarian or adrenal tumour, especially if the patient is virilized, e.g. deepened voice and clitoromegaly
	Cushing syndrome (see Chapter 6), especially if physical stigmata, hypertension or glucose intolerance
	Hyperprolactinaemia
	Thyroid dysfunction

Other features to detect

Amenorrhoea/ oligomenorrhoea	Loss of ovulatory cycles decreases fertility
	Sub-optimal metabolic milieu increases spontaneous abortion even if pregnancy is achieved
Relative androgen excess	Acne
	Hirsuitism – commonly in distribution of male beard, chest and midline to umbilicus
	Frontal hair loss
Resistance to insulin action	Obesity or major difficulty restraining body mass index
	Positive family history for type 2 or gestational diabetes
	Acanthosis nigricans

Investigations

To exclude other causes	Pregnancy test
	Low-dose dexamethasone suppression test or equivalent (Cushing syndrome)
	Serum 17α-hydroxyprogesterone (late-onset congenital adrenal hyperplasia)
	Thyroid function test (hypothyroidism or hyperthyroidism)
	Serum prolactin (hyperprolactinaemia)
	Ovarian ultrasound (helps exclude an androgen-secreting tumour of the ovary)

(Continued)

Table 7.4 (*Continued*)		
Investigations (continued)		
To characterize biochemical hyperandrogenism	Serum testosterone, SHBG, androstenedione, DHEA(S)	
To characterize any wider metabolic disturbance	Fasting glucose or oral glucose tolerance test, glycated haemoglobin (IGT or T2DM)	
	Liver function tests – hepatitic markers (e.g. ALT)	
	Liver ultrasound may show fatty infiltration	
	Fasting lipid analysis – mixed dyslipidaemia common	
Treatment options and advice		
Common issues that precipitated the consultation		
Regular menstruation and contraception	Combined oral contraceptive pill	
To restore the normal cycle or improve fertility	Metformin (may also help weight loss)	
Hirsutism	See later section	
Simple reassurance	Exclusion of other endocrinopathies	
Promoted by the endocrinologist if not raised by the patient:		
Uterine health	Regular endometrial shedding every 3–4 months	
Health education/ information for the future	Plan pregnancy earlier rather than later as PCOS exacerbates decline in fertility with age	
	Maximal 'cardiovascular fitness' and weight control will improve symptoms and minimize risk of future IGT, GDM and T2DM	

SHBG, sex hormone-binding globulin; DHEA, dehydroepiandrosterone; IGT, impaired glucose tolerance; GDM, gestational diabetes mellitus; T2DM, type 2 diabetes.

transvaginal). Observing multiple, small cysts, as 'PCOS' implies, is not discriminatory. More than half of patients with Cushing syndrome have such cysts. Similarly, absence of cysts does not exclude PCOS. Once other conditions have been excluded, PCOS can be diagnosed (Table 7.4).

Treatment

Treatment is tailored according to what drove the initial consultation request (Table 7.4). However, two aspects are always important to the endocrinologist: uterine health, and minimizing future metabolic and cardiovascular risks.

Without menstruation, chronic low-level oestrogen stimulates endometrial growth that is not shed, increasing the risk of endometrial carcinoma ~six-fold. Withdrawal bleeds need to be induced by progesterone therapy (e.g. 5 mg norethisterone once daily for 7 days) every 3–4 months. The fall in progesterone after the last dose simulates the end of a menstrual cycle and provokes endometrial shedding.

Weight gain leading to obesity in patients with a polygenic tendency to insulin resistance massively increases risk of diabetes, either as GDM or T2DM. Encouragement, counselling and advice are important to maintain cardiovascular fitness and avoid obesity. These measures are also first-line fertility measures, followed by metformin (see Chapter 13), and, if this is insufficient, specialist referral (see later section). It is always useful to advise that female fertility declines progressively after the age of 30 years and if there are known potential problems, pregnancy should ideally be planned earlier rather than later. For women with a history of irregular periods presenting beyond 35 years, prompt referral is critical.

🔍 Case history 7.4

A 25-year-old woman is referred to the endocrinology clinic with irregular periods and hair growth affecting the chin and chest. On closer questioning, the menstrual cycle has never been shorter than 35 days in length since menarche. LMP was 7 months ago. Her mother has type 2 diabetes. Her BMI is 26.4 kg/m^2 and serum oestradiol is 340 pmol/L (~90 pg/mL). Pregnancy test is negative. She thinks she has PCOS.

Are any other tests necessary to make a diagnosis of PCOS?
In addition to the patient's issues, what two aspects of long-term healthcare should the clinician address?
What uterine treatment is indicated now?

Answers, see p. 163

Other female reproductive endocrinology referrals

Hirsuitism and male-pattern balding

Excess hair growth in women (hirsuitism) is a common endocrine referral. The first distinction to make is between androgen-dependent and independent growth. For the latter, hypothyroidism and causative drugs (e.g. phenytoin) should be excluded, after which effective treatment is difficult beyond standard cosmetic measures.

Androgen-dependent hair growth takes place in the region of the beard, chest and in the midline to the umbilicus (the male escutcheon). It may be accompanied by male-pattern scalp hair loss. Symptoms or signs of virilization imply major androgen excess. Consumption of performance enhancing drugs or supplements should be questioned. Some forms of the COCP possess androgenic activity.

Serum testosterone (ideally at 9 AM) greater than 4nmol/L (~115ng/mL) brings risk of androgen-secreting tumours when visualization by ultrasound, CT or MRI is indicated (Case history 7.5). If imaging is inconclusive (remembering the frequency of adrenal incidentalomas; see Chapter 6), venous sampling of adrenal and ovarian veins under radiological guidance may be helpful. Concomitant cortisol measurement can confirm cannulation of the adrenal veins. A clear androgen gradient between left or right adrenal or ovary and peripheral samples indicates the likely source of pathology. For a presumed ovarian source in post-menopausal women, both ovaries are usually removed (bilateral oophorectomy) laparoscopically. Removing both ovaries lowers risk of future ovarian cancer. Androgen-secreting tumours are most commonly benign and removal is curative, although frontal hair loss may not fully recover.

Clinical hyperandrogenism with normal serum testosterone is common. Individuals vary in their sensitivity to androgens. Serum total testosterone is a blunt measure of androgen action in target cells: free testosterone varies according to serum proteins; SRD5A2 is required to generate DHT (Figure 7.7); and AR activity differs between individuals through variability (polymorphism) in its first exon. Blocking DHT production (e.g. by SRD5A2 inhibitors such as finasteride) or androgen binding to AR (e.g. by antagonists such as spironolactone) can be effective. Waxing, plucking, laser therapy and the application of eflornithine cream that inhibits hair follicle cell division are also valid strategies that are free from systemic side-effects.

Galactorrhoea

Inappropriate milk production outside of breast-feeding is common in young women and results from excess prolactin (hyperprolactinaemia; see Chapter 5) or increased sensitivity to its action. Galactorrhoea with normal serum prolactin occurs with increased breast sensitivity (e.g. after cessation of breast-feeding), but still responds well to dopamine agonists, such as cabergoline.

Hormone-dependent gynaecological disorders

Endometriosis and uterine fibroids (leiomyomata) are hormone-dependent and prevalent in women during the reproductive lifespan. Both conditions are covered in greater depth in *Essential Reproduction*.

Endometriosis is the presence of endometrial tissue outside of the uterine cavity and may affect the ovaries, broad ligament, or other peritoneal surfaces. The cells contain oestrogen receptor that when bound by oestradiol mediates proliferation and hypertrophy. This can cause chronic pelvic pain or, if affecting the Fallopian tube, subfertility. In addition to surgery, decreasing the supply of oestrogen (e.g. by continuous GnRH agonist or the progesterone-only contraceptive pill) can help.

Fibroids are benign tumours of the muscle layer of the uterus (myometrium) and respond to oestrogen and, potentially, progesterone. Hormone modulation is most likely of short-term benefit, whereas surgery offers more definitive treatment. Total hysterectomy ends fertility. However, local laparoscopic resection can preserve the uterus, albeit with increased risk of rupture in future pregnancy.

Menopause and hormone replacement therapy

HRT in the menopausal period can overcome the acute symptoms of oestrogen withdrawal, typified by hot flushes (flashes). The duration and relative benefit of HRT therapy is contentious. Historically, it has been given to maintain bone mineral density, but this effect is rapidly lost upon cessation (see Chapter 9). It has also been used to protect against cardiovascular disease until trials showed the opposite effect. One approach is to prioritize HRT for symptoms of oestrogen withdrawal during the 5 years around and following the menopause. This largely avoids any increased risk, potential or otherwise, of cardiovascular disease and breast cancer from longer term use. In the presence of a uterus, oestrogen needs to be combined with progesterone, which reduces oestrogen receptor number in target cells and increases inactivation of oestradiol to oestrone. Given intermittently, withdrawal bleeding can continue with this combined therapy. Progesterone can also be administered by an intrauterine coil, in which case vaginal bleeding may be erratic or cease completely.

🔍 Case history 7.5

A 72-year-old woman presents with frontal hair loss over the last 5 years. Serum total testosterone was 7.4 nmol/L (~213 ng/mL). She is otherwise very fit.

Name two clinical features that might characterize this androgen level in a woman?
What is the diagnosis until proven otherwise and in which two organs might it be located?
What investigations need to be considered and what is the most likely eventual treatment they may lead to?

Answers, see p. 163

Pubertal disorders

Children with endocrine abnormalities causing pubertal precocity or delay must be distinguished from those who simply represent the extremes of the normal range (Case history 7.6). Even where observation may be feasible in the latter group, there are major psychosocial consequences of puberty occurring out of synchrony with the individual's peer group. Early puberty, subject to ethnic differences, also induces the growth spurt, which ultimately causes earlier epiphyseal fusion and shorter adult height.

Precocious puberty

Precocity may result from either the normal process, driven by GnRH pulses, occurring abnormally early (central or true), or aetiology extrinsic to the hypothalamic–anterior pituitary–gonadal axis that results in premature sex steroid biosynthesis (Table 7.5). Precocity may be caused by oestrogen in boys and androgen in girls, leading to inappropriate feminization or virilization respectively (contra-sexual precocity). The goal is to treat the underlying cause and avoid significant disruption of psychosocial development or the attainment of predicted final height. It needs to focus on the individual cause. For true precocity, continuous GnRH can be used to suppress the pituitary gonadotrophins. For isolated premature breast development ('thelarche'), reassurance is appropriate.

Delayed puberty

As well as slow entry into puberty, delay may also occur within pubertal stages (Box 7.19). The commonest cause is constitutional or chronic illness when bone age is also appropriately delayed. Delayed puberty may also reflect gonadal failure when serum gonadotrophins are raised and sex steroids are low. In females, ultrasound may show streak gonads and a karyotype might indicate Turner syndrome (45,XO). Secretion of pituitary gonadotrophins can be assessed in response to GnRH (see earlier section on amenorrhoea with absent oestrogen). In boys, a rise in testosterone after hCG injection indicates normal testicular potential. If necessary, treatment is with increasing doses of sex steroids to induce pubertal changes with close monitoring of pubertal progression and growth.

In females, progesterone is added once uterine bleeding starts (Case history 7.6).

Case history 7.6

A 15-year-old girl was referred because of a failure to commence periods. Her mother frequently interrupted the consultation and strongly wished for 'something to be done'. The patient declined examination but was noted to look healthy if rather short for predicted family height. She agreed to some blood tests, which revealed LH and FSH below the normal range and undetectable oestradiol. Thyroid function, karyotype and serum prolactin were normal.

Does anything need to be done urgently? What other questioning might be insightful?

Answers, see p. 164

Box 7.19 Delayed puberty: defined as >2 standard deviations above mean age

- Boys ≥ 16 years of age
- Girls ≥ 14 years

Subfertility

Subfertility is defined as the failure of a woman to become pregnant despite a year of unprotected regular intercourse with her male partner (Case history 7.7). Both partners must be assessed (Table 7.6).

Male factor treatment

Review earlier sections on semen analysis (Box 7.7) and hypogonadism. Treatment depends on cause. In secondary hypogonadism, testicular function can be restored with injections of hCG and, if needed, hMG to mimic endogenous LH and FSH. In the

Table 7.5 Precocious puberty

Definition	>2 standard deviations below the mean age
	Boys ≤ 9 years of age
	Girls ≤ 7 years
Types	'True' or 'central'
	Idiopathic
	Disruption to the central nervous system (e.g. tumour/infection/trauma)
	Gonadotrophin-independent isosexual
	hCG-secreting tumour
	Androgen excess in males, e.g. CAH or tumour of the adrenal cortex or testis
	Genetic, e.g. McCune–Albright syndrome
	Gonadotrophin-independent contrasexual
	Male, e.g. tumour with aromatase activity generating oestrogens
	Female, e.g. androgen excess from CAH or tumour of the adrenal cortex or ovary
History	Age and order of onset, e.g. breast growth/body odour/genital enlargement/menstruation
	Are there other medical conditions?
	Is it familial?
	Has there been a recent growth spurt or weight gain?
Examination	Are there signs of secondary sexual development, e.g. breast or pubic hair growth?
	Are the changes out of keeping with the child's sex?
	Full neurological examination
	'Café-au-lait' spots (patches of brown skin pigment) may indicate McCune–Albright syndrome (review Figure 3.14)
Investigation	Serum testosterone, oestradiol, androstenedione and DHEA or DHEAS
	17α-hydroxyprogesterone (to exclude CAH due to 21-hydroxylase deficiency)
	GnRH test – LH and FSH at 0 min and 30 min after GnRH
	Tumour markers, e.g. AFP and hCG
	X-ray to estimate bone age

hCG, human chorionic gonadotrophin; CAH, congenital adrenal hyperplasia; DHEA, dehydroepiandrosterone; AFP, α-fetoprotein; GnRH, gonadotrophin-releasing hormone; LH, luteinizing hormone; FSH, follicle-stimulating hormone.

Table 7.6 An approach to subfertility

Female factor subfertility	Male factor subfertility
Was there normal development at birth?	
Was childhood normal?	
Did the individual enter puberty at the appropriate time?	
Consider PCOS, pituitary, thyroid or adrenal disease	All the potential causes of primary or secondary hypogonadism need consideration
Pelvic inflammatory disease (PID) can block the Fallopian tubes – symptoms include discharge and pain	Examination
	Is testicular size normal (20–25 mL)?
What is the cycle length and regularity?	Is there a varicocoele?
A regular 28-day cycle is likely to be ovulatory	Are the external genitalia structurally normal?
Biochemical profile and investigation	
Day 2–5: serum LH, FSH, oestradiol, prolactin and thyroid function tests	Serum LH, FSH, testosterone, SHBG, prolactin and thyroid function tests
Consider investigations related to PCOS (Table 7.4)	Consider testing for other anterior pituitary disorders
Day 21: serum progesterone to assess ovulation	Consider analyzing karyotype (Klinefelter syndrome/46,XXY)
BMI – fertility declines with obesity	Semen analysis – volume, concentration, motility and morphology
Swab for PID, e.g. chlamydia	
Consider laparoscopy (or hysterosalpingogram) to assess tubal patency	

PCOS, polycystic ovarian syndrome; LH, luteinizing hormone; FSH, follicule-stimulating hormone; SHBG, sex hormone-binding globulin; BMI, body mass index.

event of spermatozoa being deemed inadequate for spontaneous fertilization *in vivo* or *in vitro*, they can be assessed for suitability for intra-cytoplasmic sperm injection (ICSI).

Female factor treatment

The initial goal is to regularize the ovulatory cycle to no longer than ~28 days in length to maximize the frequency of egg release by the ovary (i.e. the number of opportunities for pregnancy).

Cycles of longer than 30 days are increasingly likely to be anovulatory. In overweight individuals or those with PCOS, increased cardiovascular fitness and weight reduction may be sufficient to generate this regular pattern. Metformin, an insulin sensitizer, can be useful, prescribed as for type 2 diabetes (see Chapter 13). The importance of fitness and weight control prior to pregnancy cannot be over-emphasized: patients with PCOS are already at higher risk of first trimester miscarriage; PCOS (with its resistance to insulin action) and obesity link to GDM; and obesity and GDM can cause difficulties at term and in labour.

Other methods of ovulation induction increase risk of multiple pregnancies, which, in turn, increases risk of maternal and fetal morbidity. Blocking oestrogen feedback at the gonadotroph (most commonly with clomiphene) is the simplest approach. Ovulation induction using a cycle of hCG and hMG injections is used for women with secondary or tertiary hypogonadism whose ovaries are healthy and/or to recover ova for *in vitro* fertilization (IVF) or ICSI (e.g. if there was co-existing tubal damage or male factor concerns). For women with primary ovarian failure, egg donation can be considered. Other aspects of fertility management are described in *Essential Reproduction*.

🔍 Case history 7.7

A couple attends the subfertility clinic. Semen analysis was satisfactory. The female partner had a regular 28-day cycle and normal BMI. However, 5 years previously, she had had a 6-month history of pelvic pain and some green coloured vaginal discharge that resolved on treatment with antibiotics.

What investigations are warranted?
What treatments can be offered?

Answers, see p. 164

🔑 Key points

- In the relative absence of androgens and AMH, the default in utero is female development
- Disorders of sexual development present to the paediatric endocrinologist and are highly emotive
- The critical aspects of male and female reproductive endocrinology are sex hormone biosynthesis and gamete production

- Disorders of male and female reproductive endocrinology are investigated by interrogating negative feedback within the hypothalamic–anterior pituitary–gonadal axis
- The reproductive axis in both sexes is vulnerable to disruption from other endocrine disorders
- Subfertility requires assessment of both partners

🔍 Answers to case histories

Case history 7.1

The ambiguous genitalia and potential signs of hypoadrenalism made the endocrinologist consider CAH, most likely caused by deficiency of CYP21. Raised urea would be consistent with dehydration; hyponatraemia and hyperkalaemia may be present; ACTH would be raised, with cortisol very low [e.g. <100 nmol/L (~3.6 µg/dL)]; 17α-hydroxyprogesterone would be expected to be raised. Renin might be raised and aldosterone low if this is salt-wasting CAH.

Intravenous hydrocortisone is indicated in potential hypoadrenal crisis. This could be given after the first blood sample was taken. Although ACTH stimulation test with measurement of cortisol and 17α-hydroxy-progesterone would be desirable, emergency treatment with cortisol outweighs this wish.

The baby actually has 46,XX DSD caused by CAH, i.e. a virilized female, who in all likelihood will be raised as a girl. This is incredibly emotive to parents. Sexual identity in the presence of ambiguous genitalia should not have been ascribed without investigation.

Case history 7.2

The pathology lies in the testes. Serum testosterone is very low. LH and FSH are high. The diagnosis is primary hypogonadism.

Karyotype analysis is important given suspicion of Klinefelter syndrome (47,XXY).

The patient should be commenced on testosterone, initially at low dose (gel administration would be a good option) given the likely long-standing deficiency. Sudden full replacement in Klinefelter syndrome can impact adversely on mood and other psychosocial issues. If confirmed, information should be offered about the Klinefelter support group. The patient can anticipate increased beard growth, improved energy levels and sexual drive. The gynaecomastia might persist, at least in part, at which point cosmetic correction should be offered.

A DEXA scan would probably demonstrate bone demineralization and quite possibly osteoporosis due to the hypogonadism (see Chapter 9). Performing this investigation at diagnosis offers a 'benchmark' against which replacement therapy can be judged.

Case history 7.3

A drug history should be obtained. Chronic medical illnesses should be excluded. Pregnancy should not be an issue. Thyroid function tests should be performed, although

the prolactin level is atypically high for primary hypothyroidism.

At this level, a microprolactinoma is the most likely diagnosis. Oestradiol would be low and may well be undetectable.

MRI of the pituitary gland is indicated, which may appear normal as some lactotroph tumours are tiny and below resolution of the imaging.

Once a microprolactinoma has been diagnosed, the patient should be reassured that these tumours are benign and offered treatment with a dopamine agonist, such as cabergoline. She should be warned that periods and fertility are likely to return with treatment. The galactorrhoea should stop within a matter of weeks. After 5 years, ~60% of patients with microprolactinomas can stop treatment and serum prolactin remains normal. Further details relevant to this case are provided in Chapter 5.

Case history 7.4

PCOS is a diagnosis of exclusion; therefore, other investigations are very important (see Table 7.4).

Advice should be given on (1) future cardiovascular and diabetes risk with encouragement to stay fit, active and of ideal body weight; and (2) endometrial shedding during reproductive years at least every ~4 months to normalize the risk of endometrial carcinoma.

It is 7 months since LMP. A week-long course of progesterone is indicated (e.g. norethisterone 5 mg daily for 7 days) to stimulate endometrial shedding on withdrawal.

Case history 7.5

The woman might be virilized with clitoromegaly and deepened voice.

This level of serum testosterone in a woman is indicative of an androgen-secreting tumour until proven otherwise, most likely located in the ovary or adrenal gland.

Imaging is needed; ultrasound (useful for the ovaries), CT or MRI. Venous sampling might be useful. The tumour needs removal, most likely laparoscopically as unilateral adrenalectomy or bilateral oophorectomy.

Case history 7.6

In the absence of major signs of pituitary disease (e.g. no visual disturbance, normal prolactin), nothing needs to be done instantly. The features are consistent with simple constitutional delay.

It would be helpful to know whether menarche had been delayed in other family members. Delicate questioning might reveal stresses (e.g. bullying) as a cause of hypothalamic amenorrhoea. Commonly, in constitutional delay, growth and sexual development will occur during follow-up and periods will commence spontaneously.

Case history 7.7

Although most women with signs of pelvic inflammatory disease are asymptomatic at the time of infection, this woman has a clear history raising the possibility of tubal scarring and blockage. It is important to confirm ovulation with day 21 progesterone measurements. However, the major question is to assess patency of the Fallopian tubes by laparoscopy and dye infusion. The dye, inserted via the vagina, should be seen spilling bilaterally from the fimbriated ends of the oviducts by the laparoscope. An alternative is hysterosalpingogram, which employs X-ray and radio-opaque dye. Evidence of current infection should be sought with serology, swabs and culture.

Evidence of current infection should be treated with antibiotics. For restoring fertility, Fallopian tube microsurgery has poor success rates; however, IVF has among its best chances of pregnancy (rates are published for individual UK fertility clinics on a government website) because the female and male endocrinology is normal, meaning quality of the ova and spermatozoa should be excellent.

CHAPTER 8
The thyroid gland

Key topics

- Embryology   166
- Anatomy and vasculature   168
- Thyroid hormone biosynthesis   168
- Circulating thyroid hormones   172
- Metabolism of thyroid hormones   172
- Function of thyroid hormones   173
- Clinical disorders   175
- Key points   187
- Answers to case histories   187

Learning objectives

- To appreciate the development of the thyroid gland and its clinical consequences
- To understand the regulation, biosynthesis, function and metabolism of thyroid hormones
- To recognize the clinical consequences of thyroid underactivity and overactivity
- To understand the clinical management of thyroid nodules and cancer

This chapter integrates the basic biology of the thyroid gland with the clinical conditions that affect it

Essential Endocrinology and Diabetes, Sixth Edition. Richard IG Holt, Neil A Hanley.
© 2012 Richard IG Holt and Neil A Hanley. Publlished 2012 by Blackwell Publishing Ltd.

To recap

- Regulation of the thyroid gland occurs as part of a negative feedback loop, the principle of which is introduced in Chapter 1
- Thyroid hormones are synthesized from tyrosine; review the biosynthesis of hormones derived from amino acids (Chapter 2)
- Like steroid hormones, thyroid hormones act in the nucleus; review the principles of nuclear hormone action covered in Chapter 3

Cross-reference

- The thyroid is regulated by the hypothalamus and anterior pituitary thyrotroph, which are covered in Chapter 5
- Medullary carcinoma of the thyroid is part of multiple endocrine neoplasia type 2, covered in Chapter 10
- Other autoimmune endocrinopathies can co-exist with autoimmune thyroid disease, especially Addison disease (see Chapter 6) and type 1 diabetes (see Chapter 12)

The thyroid gland is responsible for making thyroid hormones by concentrating iodine and utilizing the amino acid tyrosine (review Chapter 2). The hormones play major metabolic roles, affecting many different cell types in the body. Clinical conditions affecting the thyroid gland are common. Therefore, a thorough understanding is important.

Embryology

Understanding development of the thyroid and its anatomical associations underpins the gland's examination and surgical removal to treat overactivity or enlargement. In the fourth week of human embryogenesis, the thyroid begins as a midline thickening at the back of the tongue that subsequently invaginates and stretches downward (Figure 8.1). This creates a mass of progenitor cells that migrates in front of the larynx and comes into close proximity with the developing parathyroid glands (see Chapter 9). In adulthood, the pea-sized parathyroids located on the back of the thyroid as pairs of upper and lower glands regulate calcium by secreting parathyroid hormone (PTH). The lower parathyroids originate higher in the neck than the upper glands and only achieve their final position by migrating downwards. The migrating thyroid also comes into

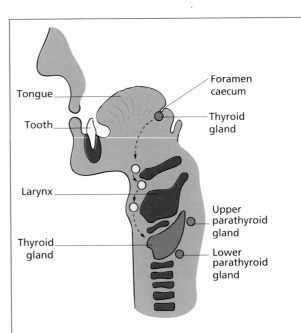

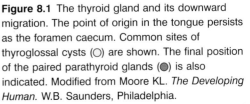

Figure 8.1 The thyroid gland and its downward migration. The point of origin in the tongue persists as the foramen caecum. Common sites of thyroglossal cysts (○) are shown. The final position of the paired parathyroid glands (●) is also indicated. Modified from Moore KL. *The Developing Human.* W.B. Saunders, Philadelphia.

contact with cells from the lower part of the pharynx. These latter cells eventually comprise ~10% of the gland as future C-cells, which will secrete calcitonin (see Chapter 9).

Towards the end of the second month, the thyroid comprises two lobes joined at an isthmus in front of the trachea. It lies just below the larynx, which forms a convenient landmark for locating the bowtie-shaped gland during clinical examination (see Box 8.12). The thyroglossal duct atrophies and loses contact with the thyroid in all but ~15% of the population, in whom a finger-like pyramidal lobe of thyroid projects upward. By ~11 weeks, primitive follicles are visible as simple epithelium surrounding a central lumen (Figure 8.2). This signals the gland's first ability to trap iodide and synthesize thyroid hormone, although it only responds to thyroid-stimulating hormone (TSH) from the anterior pituitary towards the end of the second trimester.

Abnormal embryology can be clinically important (Box 8.1). Thyroid agenesis or hypoplasia caused by loss-of-function mutation in genes, such as *PAX8*, requires immediate detection and treatment with thyroid hormone in order to minimize severe and largely irreversible neurological damage

---

Box 8.1 Embryological abnormalities with clinical consequences

- Failure of the gland to develop causes congenital hypothyroidism
- Under- or over-migration of the thyroid can cause a lingual or retrosternal thyroid respectively
- Failure of thyroglossal duct to atrophy can lead to a thyroglossal cyst

---

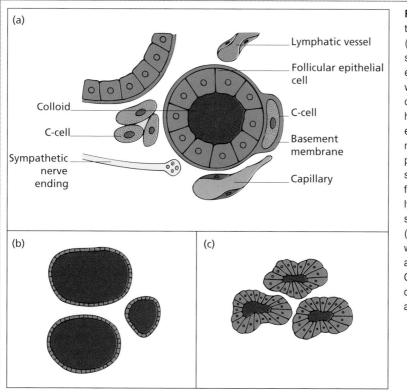

Figure 8.2 Histology of the human thyroid gland. (a) Euthyroid follicles are shown lined with cuboidal epithelium and lumens filled with gelatinous colloid that contains stored thyroid hormone. Surrounding each follicle is a basement membrane enclosing parafollicular C-cells within stroma containing fenestrated capillaries, lymphatic vessels and sympathetic nerve endings. (b) Underactive follicles with flattened epithelial cells and increased colloid. (c) Overactive follicles with tall, columnar epithelial cells and reduced colloid.

in the infant. Less critically, thyroglossal cysts can occur in the midline and move upwards on tongue protrusion (a clinical test).

Anatomy and vasculature

The adult thyroid weighs 10–20 g, is bigger in women than men and is also larger in areas of the world with iodine deficiency. It enlarges during puberty, pregnancy and lactation. The right lobe is usually slightly larger than the left. Its outer capsule is not well-defined, but attaches the thyroid posteriorly to the trachea. The parathyroid glands are situated between this and the inner capsule, from which trabeculae of collagen pervade the gland carrying nerves and a rich vascular supply (Figure 8.2). The thyroid receives ~1% of cardiac output from superior and inferior thyroid arteries, which are branches of the external carotid and subclavian arteries respectively. Per gram of tissue, this blood supply is almost twice that of the kidney and is increased during autoimmune overactivity when it may cause a bruit on auscultation (Box 8.2; and see Box 8.12). Blood flow through fenestrated capillaries is controlled by post-ganglionic sympathetic nerves from the middle and superior cervical ganglia.

The functional unit of the thyroid is the follicle, comprised of cuboidal epithelial ('follicular') cells around a central lumen of colloid. Colloid is composed almost entirely of the iodinated glycoprotein, thyroglobulin (pink on periodic acid-Schiff (PAS) staining). There are many thousands of follicles 20–900 μm in diameter, interspersed with blood vessels, an extensive network of lymphatic vessels, connective tissue and the parafollicular calcitonin-secreting C-cells. When the gland is quiescent (e.g. in hypothyroidism from iodine deficiency), follicles

are distended with colloid and the epithelial cells are flattened with little cytoplasm. Conversely, in an overactive gland, follicular cells are columnar and there is less stored colloid (Figure 8.2).

Thyroid hormone biosynthesis

There are two active thyroid hormones: thyroxine (3,3′,5,5′-tetra-iodothyronine; abbreviated to T_4) and 3,5,3′-tri-iodothyronine (T_3); the subscripts 4 and 3 represent the number of iodine atoms incorporated on each thyronine residue (Figure 8.3). These hormones are generated from the sequential iodination and coupling of the amino acid tyrosine and inactivated by de-iodination and modification to 3,3′,5′-tri-iodothyronine [reverse T_3 (rT_3)] and di-iodothyronine (T_2). The equilibrium between these different molecules determines overall thyroid hormone activity. Synthesis of thyroid hormone can be broken down into several key steps (Figure 8.4).

Uptake of iodide from the blood

Synthesis of thyroid hormone relies on a constant supply of dietary iodine as the monovalent anion iodide (I^-). When the element is scarce the thyroid enlarges to form a goitre (Figure 8.5 and Box 8.3). Circulating iodide enters the follicular cell by active transport through the basal cell membrane. The sodium (Na^+)/I^- pump is linked to an adenosine triphosphate (ATP)-driven Na^+/potassium (K^+) pump. This process concentrates I^- within the thyroid gland to 20–100-fold that of the remainder of the body. This selectivity allows use of radioiodine both diagnostically and therapeutically (see later). Several structurally related anions can competitively inhibit the I^- pump. For instance, large doses of perchlorate (ClO_4^-) can block I^- uptake in the short term (e.g. to treat accidental ingestion of radioiodine). The pertechnetate ion incorporating a γ-emitting radioisotope of technetium is also taken up by the I^- pump, allowing the thyroid to be imaged diagnostically.

The synthesis of thyroglobulin

Thyroglobulin (Tg) is the tyrosine-rich protein that is iodinated within the colloid to yield stored

---

Box 8.2 The thyroid gland

- Thyroid enlargement is called goitre
- The gland is encapsulated:
  - Breaching the capsule is a measure of invasion in thyroid cancer
- The thyroid receives a large arterial blood supply:
  - May cause a bruit in Graves disease

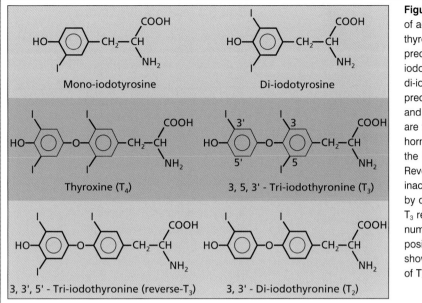

Figure 8.3 The structures of active and inactive thyroid hormones and their precursors. Mono-iodotyrosine and di-iodotyrosine are precursors. Thyroxine (T_4) and tri-iodothyronine (T_3) are the two thyroid hormones, of which T_3 is the biologically more active. Reverse T_3 and T_2 are inactive metabolites formed by de-iodination of T_4 and T_3 respectively. The numbering of critical positions for iodination is shown on the structure of T_3.

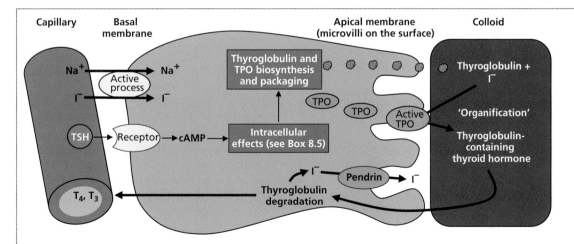

Figure 8.4 Thyroid hormone biosynthesis within the follicular cell. Active iodide (I^-) import is linked to the Na^+/K^+-ATPase pump. Thyroglobulin is synthesized on the rough endoplasmic reticulum, packaged in the Golgi complex and released from small, Golgi-derived vesicles into the follicular lumen. Its iodination is also known as 'organification'. Cytoplasmic microfilaments and microtubules organize the return of iodinated thyroglobulin into the cell as endocytotic vesicles of colloid, which is broken down to release thyroid hormone. TSH, thyroid-stimulating hormone; TPO, thyroid peroxidase; T_4, thyroxine; T_3, tri-iodothyronine. Modified from *Williams' Textbook of Endocrinology*, 10th edn. Saunders, 2003, p. 332.

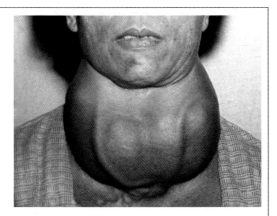

Figure 8.5 A large goitre caused by iodine deficiency in rural Africa. Note the engorged veins overlying the gland, implying venous obstruction. Image kindly provided by Professor David Phillips, University of Southampton.

thyroid hormone. It is synthesized exclusively by the follicular cell, such that the small amount in the circulation can serve as a tumour marker for thyroid cancer. Tg contains ~10% carbohydrate, including sialic acid responsible for the pink PAS staining of colloid. Tg is transcribed, translated, modified in the Golgi apparatus and then packaged into vesicles that undergo exocytosis at the apical membrane to release Tg into the follicular lumen (Figure 8.4; and review Figures 2.3 and 2.4).

Iodination of thyroglobulin

Thyroid peroxidase (TPO) catalyzes the iodination of Tg (mature Tg is ~1% iodine by weight). The enzyme is synthesized and packaged alongside Tg into vesicles at the Golgi apparatus (Figure 8.4). TPO becomes activated at the apical membrane where it binds I^- and Tg (at different sites), oxidizes I^-, and transfers it to an exposed Tg tyrosine residue. The enzyme is particularly efficient at iodinating fresh Tg; as the reaction proceeds, the efficiency of adding further I^- decreases. Drugs inhibiting TPO and iodination are used to treat hyperthyroidism (Box 8.4). Some naturally-occurring chemicals [e.g. milk from cows fed on certain green fodder or from

Box 8.3 Iodine deficiency

Some areas of the developing world remain iodine-deficient, which can cause particularly large goitres (Figure 8.5) and hypothyroidism. Thyroglobulin in the normal thyroid stores enough thyroid hormone to supply the body for ~2 months. When dietary I^- is limited (<50 μg/day), less is incorporated into thyroglobulin, providing a higher proportion of the more active T3 compared to T4. However, eventually thyroid hormone synthesis fails. Diminished negative feedback increases TSH secretion, which induces thyroid enlargement (a compensatory mechanism to increase capacity for I^- uptake). This may restore sufficient thyroid hormone biosynthesis for normal circumstances; however, during pregnancy, the supply of iodine and thyroid hormones is insufficient for the fetus, which becomes at risk of severe neurological damage and may also develop a goitre. Post-natally, the syndrome of intellectual impairment, deafness and diplegia (bilateral paralysis) has been termed cretinism and affects many millions of infants worldwide. Decreased iodine intake with a marginal but chronic elevation of TSH may also increase the incidence of thyroid cancer, especially if irradiation is involved, as with the Chernobyl disaster. Prophylaxis with iodine supplements has reduced the incidence of cretinism, although tends not to shrink adult goitres effectively. Many countries supplement common dietary constituents such as salt or bread. In extremely isolated communities, depot injections of iodized oils can supply the thyroid for years.

brassicae vegetables (cabbages, sprouts)] may also inhibit Tg iodination. This leads to diminished negative feedback at the anterior pituitary causing TSH secretion to rise (Figure 8.6), which chronically can stimulate a goitre; hence the chemicals are known as 'goitrogens'.

Box 8.4 Antithyroid drugs – effective at suppressing the synthesis and secretion of thyroid hormones

- Carbimazole
- Methimazole (active metabolite of carbimazole; used in the USA)
- Propylthiouracil (PTU)

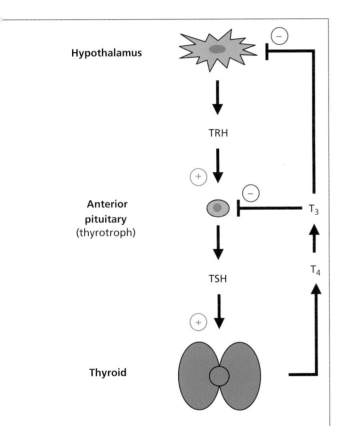

Figure 8.6 The hypothalamic–anterior pituitary–thyroid axis. The more active hormone, T_3, provides the majority of negative feedback. TRH, thyrotrophin-releasing hormone; TSH, thyroid–stimulating hormone.

The production of thyroid hormone

Iodination of Tg initiates thyroid hormone formation (Figures 8.3 and 8.4). Within the Tg structure, di-iodotyrosine couples to either mono-iodotyrosine or another di-iodotyrosine to generate T_3 or T_4 respectively. This coupling occurs during the TPO-mediated iodination, yielding thyroid hormone stored as colloid in the lumen of the thyroid follicle.

The secretion of thyroid hormone

To secrete thyroid hormone, colloid is first enveloped by microvilli on the cell surface (endocytosis) to form colloid vesicles within the cells that fuse with lysosomes (Figure 8.4). The enzymes from the lysosomes break down the iodinated Tg, releasing thyroid hormones. Other degradation products are recycled; for instance, the transporter, Pendrin, moves I$^-$ back into the follicular lumen. Loss-of-function mutations in the *PENDRIN* gene cause a congenital form of hypothyroidism (Pendred syndrome).

The thyroid hormones move across the basal cell membrane and enter the circulation, ~80% as T_4 and 20% as T_3.

Regulation

The thyroid is controlled by TSH from the anterior pituitary, which in turn is regulated by thyrotrophin-releasing hormone (TRH) from the hypothalamus (review Chapter 5). Thyroid hormone, predominantly T_3 (the more active), completes the negative feedback loop by suppressing the production of TRH and TSH (Figure 8.6). TSH binds to its specific G-protein–coupled receptor on the surface of the thyroid follicular cell and activates both adenylate cyclase and phospholipase C (review Chapter 3). The former predominates and cAMP mediates most of the actions of TSH (Box 8.5). This increases fresh thyroid hormone stores and, within ~1 h, increases hormone release. The most recently synthesized Tg is the first to be resorbed as it is nearest to the microvilli. This Tg has also had less time to be iodinated than the mature, central colloid, such that

---

Box 8.5 Thyroid-stimulating hormone action on the follicular cell

Increases
- Intracellular cAMP concentration
- Tg iodination
- Apical microvilli number and length
- Endocytosis of colloid droplets
- Thyroid hormone release
- I⁻ influx into the cell (relatively late effect as activation of the I⁻ pump requires protein synthesis)
- Cellular metabolism
- Protein synthesis (including Tg)
- DNA synthesis

Box 8.6 Circulating thyroid hormones

- Thyroid hormones are almost entirely bound to serum proteins (in order of decreasing affinity):
  - Thyroxine-binding globulin (TBG)
  - Thyroxine-binding pre-albumin (TBPA)
  - Albumin
- The unbound fraction is tiny, yet critical – *only free thyroid hormone enters cells and is biologically active*:
  - Free T_4 (fT_4) ~0.015% of total T_4
  - Free T_3 (fT_3) ~0.33% of total T_3
  - Circulating half-life of T_3, ~1–3 days – needs to be prescribed several times a day if used to achieve steady levels
  - Circulating half-life of T_4, ~5–7 days – can be prescribed as single daily dose
  - Both fT_4 and fT_3 are measured by immunoassay
- T_3 is more potent than T_4 (~2–10-fold depending on response monitored)

---

it releases thyroid hormone with a relatively higher T_3:T_4 ratio and, consequently, greater activity.

Circulating thyroid hormones

From ~3 days after birth serum levels of free thyroid hormones remain relatively constant in normal individuals throughout life. Thyroid hormones are strongly bound to serum proteins, with only a tiny amount free to enter and function in cells (Box 8.6). The free (f)T_3 concentration is ~30% that of fT_4. T_3 is bound slightly less strongly than T_4 to each of the three principal serum-binding proteins. The interaction with albumin is relatively non-specific.

Total thyroid hormone levels can alter. For instance, some drugs, such as salicylates, phenytoin or diclofenac, which structurally resemble iodothyronine isoforms, can compete for protein binding; starvation or liver disease lowers the concentration of binding proteins. However, free thyroid hormone concentrations remain essentially unaltered.

Metabolism of thyroid hormones: conversion of T_4 to T_3 and rT_3

T_3 is the more active hormone, yet only 20% of thyroid hormone output. Most T_3 is generated by removing one iodine atom from the outer ring of T_4 (de-iodination) (Figures 8.3 and 8.7). This step is catalyzed by selenodeiodinase enzymes, which contain selenium that accepts the iodine from the thyroid hormone. Selenium deficiency in parts of western China or Zaire can be a rare contributory factor to hypothyroidism. Type 1 selenodeiodinase (D1) predominates in the liver, kidney and muscle, and is responsible for producing most of the circulating T_3. It is inhibited by PTU (Box 8.4 and Figure 8.7). The type 2 enzyme (D2) is predominantly localized in the brain and pituitary, key sites for regulating T_3 production for negative feedback at the hypothalamus and thyrotroph. The third selenodeiodinase, D3, de-iodinates the inner ring and converts T_4 to rT_3 (Figures 8.3 and 8.7). rT_3 is biologically inactive and cleared very rapidly from the circulation (half-life ~5 h). D3 action on T_3 is one method by which inactive T_2 is generated. These combined steps are important: at least in part, T_4 can be thought of as a 'prohormone'; when a given cell has sufficient T_3, it can limit its exposure

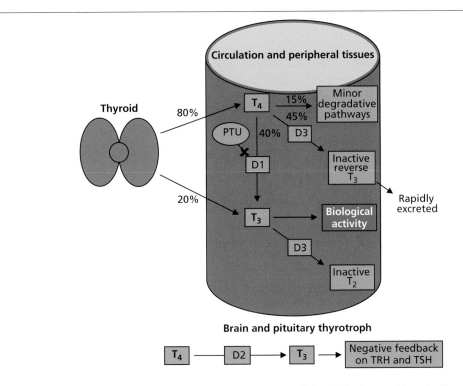

Figure 8.7 Metabolism of thyroid hormones in the circulation. Four times more T_4 is produced by the thyroid gland than T_3. Under normal 'euthyroid' physiology, ~40% of circulating T_4 is converted to active T_3 by type 1 selenodeiodinase (D1; inhibited by propylthiouracil – see Box 8.4) and ~45% of T_4 is converted to rT_3 by the type 3 selenodeiodinase (D3). The remaining 15% of T_4 is degraded by minor pathways, such as deamination. The conversion of T_3 to T_2 by D3 is shown, although other pathways also exist for this reaction. The type 2 selenodeiodinase (D2) is predominantly located in the brain and pituitary gland where it catalyzes the production of T_3 for negative feedback at the hypothalamus and anterior pituitary. TRH, thyrotrophin-releasing hormone; TSH, thyroid-stimulating hormone.

to further thyroid hormone action by switching to rT_3 generation (review Table 3.2).

Function of thyroid hormones

Thyroid hormones affects a vast array of tissue and cellular processes, most obviously increasing metabolic rate, but also influencing the actions of other hormones. For instance, they synergize with catecholamines to increase heart rate, causing palpitations in thyrotoxicosis. In amphibians, thyroid hormones cause metamorphosis, a highly complex reprogramming of several internal organs and the growth of limbs.

T_3 acts in the target cell nucleus as a ligand for the thyroid hormone receptor (TR), which itself functions as a transcription factor altering gene expression (review Chapter 3 and Figure 3.20). It binds TR with a 15-fold greater affinity than T_4, which is the main reason why T_3 is the more potent hormone. The predominantly genomic action explains why most effects of thyroid hormones occur slowly, in days rather than minutes or hours.

TR is not identical in all tissues. There are two predominant isoforms, TRα and TRβ, each encoded by different genes and each subject to alternative promoter use and/or mRNA splicing (review Figure 2.2). This creates a number of receptor sub-types, all of which perform the basic activities of binding thyroid hormone, binding DNA and influencing target genes, but with subtly different efficacy. Clinically, this can be evidenced in the rare condition of thyroid hormone resistance caused by mutations mostly located in the $TR\beta$ gene. Some tissues show thyroid hormone overactivity (e.g. tachycardia), while the pituitary thyrotroph responds as if thyroid hormone is inadequate (i.e. TSH secretion is maintained or slightly raised).

Thyroid function tests

Clinical investigation of thyroid activity hinges upon immunoassay of circulating free thyroid hormones and TSH, in combination termed thyroid function tests (TFTs). They indicate whether the thyroid gland is overactive ('hyperthyroid'), underactive ('hypothyroid') or normal ('euthyroid') (Table 8.1). Interpretation is based on understanding negative feedback (Figure 8.6 and review Chapter 1). Serum TSH is the critical measurement as, in the absence of pituitary disease, it illustrates the body's response to its own thyroid hormone levels. Low TSH indicates hyperthyroidism; raised TSH indicates hypothyroidism. The normal range for serum TSH is wide (~0.3–5.0 mU/L) but for the large majority of the population, TSH is less than 2.0 mU/L.

Pituitary underactivity can reduce TSH levels and cause secondary hypothyroidism, in which case it is very important to consider the other pituitary hormone axes, which might also be underactive. Similar TFT results may be seen in patients suffering from physical (or in some instances psychiatric) illnesses that do not directly involve the thyroid gland. Severe illness in a patient is usually obvious, when fT_4, and especially fT_3, may fall below normal without a compensatory increase in TSH. The body's type 1 selenodeiodinase activity is low. This condition is referred to as the 'sick euthyroid' syndrome. Although contentious, treatment is not normally undertaken. If recovery occurs, T_3 and T_4 spontaneously return to normal. In pregnancy, TSH is low in the first trimester, as human chorionic gonadotrophin (hCG) from the placenta mimics TSH action (see Chapter 7).

Table 8.1 Interpretation of thyroid function tests

Test results			Interpretation
TSH	**fT_4**	**fT_3**	
Normal	Normal	Normal	Euthyroidism
Low	High	High	Primary hyperthyroidism
Low	(High) normal	(High) normal	Sub-clinical primary hyperthyroidism or early pregnancy
Low	Normal	High	T_3-toxicosis
High/normal	High	High	Pituitary (secondary) hyperthyroidism or thyroid hormone receptor mutation; both are very rare
High	Low	Low	Primary hypothyroidism
High	(Low) normal	(Low) normal	Sub-clinical primary hypothyroidism
Low	Low	Low	Consider secondary hypothyroidism (assess other pituitary hormone axes)
Normal/low	Low	Low	'Sick euthyroid' syndrome

For simplicity, higher axis disorders have been listed as secondary, i.e. pituitary, although tertiary hypothalamic disease is possible.

Clinical disorders

The major clinical disorders affecting the thyroid gland arise from over- or under-activity, goitre or cancer.

Hypothyroidism

Thyroid hormone deficiency is most commonly a primary disease of the thyroid (primary hypothyroidism) and less frequently caused by deficiency of TSH (secondary hypothyroidism) (Box 8.7). Tertiary hypothyroidism, which results from loss of hypothalamic TRH, is rare.

Primary hypothyroidism

In the western world, thyroid underactivity from autoimmune attack on the gland is very common. It is six-fold more frequent in women than men and incidence increases with age (up to 2% of adult women). This autoimmune thyroiditis can be classified by the presence (Hashimoto thyroiditis) or absence (atrophic thyroiditis or primary myxoedema) of goitre. However, the disease process is essentially the same for both and even overlaps with that of hyperthyroidism secondary to Graves disease (see

later). This common genetic predisposition leaves the patient at increased risk of other autoimmune endocrinopathies as part of type 2 autoimmune polyglandular syndrome (APS-2, see Chapter 9 for APS-1) (Box 8.8). In autoimmune hypothyroidism, an extensive lymphocytic infiltration is accompanied by autoantibodies blocking the TSH receptor and also directed against Tg and TPO. Progressive destruction of thyroid follicular tissue results in hypothyroidism.

Riedel thyroiditis is rare and results from progressive fibrosis that causes a hard goitre. Congenital failure of thyroid gland formation, migration or hormone biosynthesis (~1/4000 births) usually presents early to the paediatric endocrinologist; the biosynthetic defects, collectively called 'thyroid dyshormonogenesis', usually present with goitre. Along with testing for phenylketonuria (the eponymously named Guthrie test) and other conditions, using a dried blood spot to measure TSH in the neonatal period is aimed at early postnatal detection of congenital hypothyroidism (see Table 8.1).

Some exogenous factors can lead to thyroid underactivity. Excessive iodine intake, such as from radiocontrast dyes, can transiently block synthesis and hormone release. Lithium, used in the treatment of bipolar disorder, can do the same. Indeed, lithium and iodine (either as potassium iodide or Lugol's iodine) can be used to control hyperthyroidism temporarily (see next section).

Box 8.7 Causes of hypothyroidism

Primary
- Goitre
  - Autoimmune Hashimoto thyroiditis
  - Iodine deficiency (Box 8.3 and Figure 8.5)
  - Drugs (e.g. lithium)
  - Riedel thyroiditis
  - Congenital hypothyroidism
    – dyshormonogenesis
- No goitre:
  - Autoimmune atrophic thyroiditis
  - Post-radioiodine ablation or surgery (see treatment of hyperthyroidism)
  - Post-thyroiditis (hypothyroidism is transient)
  - Congenital hypothyroidism – hypoplasia or aplasia

Secondary/tertiary
- Pituitary or hypothalamic disease (assess other hormone axes)

Box 8.8 Organ-specific autoimmune diseases with shared genetic predisposition (type 2 autoimmune polyglandular syndrome)

- Autoimmune hyperthyroidism (Graves disease)
- Autoimmune hypothyroidism
- Addison disease (see Chapter 6)
- Type 1 diabetes mellitus (see Chapter 12)
- Premature ovarian failure (see Chapter 7)
- Pernicious anaemia:
  - Destruction of the parietal cells with loss of intrinsic factor secretion causing vitamin B_{12} deficiency
- Autoimmune atrophic gastritis
- Coeliac disease

Viral infection, e.g. Echo or Coxsackie virus, can cause painful inflammation of the thyroid and release of stored hormone. A brief thyrotoxicosis is followed by transient hypothyroidism and is known as 'De Quervain's subacute thyroiditis'.

Symptoms and signs

Hypothyroidism in adults lowers metabolic rate. Common symptoms and signs are listed in Box 8.9 (Case history 8.1). The facial appearance and the potential for carpal tunnel syndrome are caused by the deposition of glycosaminoglycans in the skin. Children tend to present with obesity and short stature. Distinguishing between hypothyroidism that is permanent (treatment mandatory) and transient (treatment usually not needed) is important. Short-lived symptoms (less than a few months) preceded by sore throat or upper respiratory tract infection may indicate the latter. Permanent hypothyroidism is more likely if other family members have thyroid disease. A drug history should be taken and questions should address the chance of other coincident endocrinopathies (Box 8.8).

Box 8.9 Symptoms, signs and features of hypothyroidism

- Weight gain
- Cold intolerance, particularly at extremities
- Fatigue, lethargy
- Depression
- Coarse skin and puffy appearance
- Dry hair
- Hoarse voice
- Constipation
- Menstrual irregularities (altered luteinizing hormone/follicle-stimulating hormone secretion)
- Possible goitre
- 'Slow' reflexes, muscles contract normally, but relax slowly
- Generalized muscle weakness and paraesthesia
- Bradycardia (with reduced cardiac output)
- Cardiomegaly (with possible pericardial effusion)
- Possible carpal tunnel syndrome
- Loss of outer third of eyebrows (reason unclear)

Case history 8.1

A 45-year-old woman attended her doctor having felt 'not quite right' for the last 6 months. She was tired and her hair had been falling out. She had noticed her periods being heavy and rather erratic and wondered whether she was entering the menopause. She had put on 5 kg during the last 6 months. The doctor did some blood tests: Na^+ 134 mmol/L (134 mEq/L), K^+ 3.8 mmol/L (3.8 mEq/L), urea 4.2 mmol/L (~11.8 mg/dL), creatinine 95 μmol/L (~1.1 mg/dL), TSH 23.4 mU/L, fT_4 6.7 pmol/L (~0.5 ng/dL), Hb 112 g/L, gonadotrophins were normal.

What is the endocrine diagnosis and why?
What is the treatment?
What is the potential significance of the haemoglobin level?

Answers, see p. 187

Investigation and diagnosis

TFTs are mandatory as thyroid disease can be insidious, especially primary hypothyroidism in the elderly (see Table 8.1). Four scenarios are commonly encountered.

• Raised TSH at least twice the normal upper limit (can be >10-fold increased) plus thyroid hormone levels clearly below the normal range. This diagnosis of primary hypothyroidism is clear-cut. When accompanied by long-standing symptoms, underactivity will be permanent.

• Raised TSH at least twice the normal upper limit with normal thyroid hormone levels. The biochemistry implies compensation to try and retain normal thyroid hormone levels. With significant symptoms, treatment is worthwhile. Even as sub-clinical hypothyroidism, treatment can be justified, as ultimately the gland is likely to fail and produce frank hypothyroidism, especially if auto-antibodies are detected or if there is a family history of thyroid disease.

• TSH is only moderately raised and thyroid hormone levels are normal. These patients have an increased progression to frank hypothyroidism and, in the presence of significant symptoms, a therapeutic trial of thyroxine is one option. If the results are an incidental finding, repeat testing over the following months is an alternative, especially if there is concern over a transient viral hypothyroidism.

• All aspects of the TFTs are unequivocally normal. Do not treat with thyroxine, regardless of symptoms, as the patient is not hypothyroid.

Other investigations are commonly not needed; however, if measured, a raised titre of thyroid auto-antibodies may be detected. Creatinine kinase may be elevated. Dyslipidaemia is common with raised low-density lipoprotein (LDL)–cholesterol. Serum prolactin may be elevated (stimulated by increased TRH secretion; see Chapter 5).

Treatment

Clear-cut hypothyroidism requires life-long replacement with oral thyroxine (T_4, 100 μg/day is the starting point for standard adult replacement; ~100 μg/m^2/day in children). The goal of replacement is to normalize TSH, ideally in the range 0.5–2.0 mU/L,

assessed by repeat TFTs 6 weeks later (the pituitary thyrotroph responds sluggishly to acute changes in thyroid hormones). Thyroxine may need slight increases or decreases until the correct replacement dose is reached. In patients with long-standing hypothyroidism and co-existing ischaemic heart disease, graded introduction of replacement therapy over several weeks is frequently used (e.g. escalate from a starting dose of 25 μg/day). A final caveat to initiating treatment is to be confident of excluding Addison disease (see Chapter 6), a clue to which might be hyperkalaemia or postural hypotension. Increasing basal metabolic rate with thyroxine increases the body's demand for an already vulnerable cortisol supply and can send a patient into Addisonian crisis. The rare, yet high, mortality clinical scenario of myxoedema coma is summarized in Box 8.10.

Box 8.10 Myxoedema coma: very severe hypothyroidism

Features
• Diminished mental function → confusion → coma
• Usually in the elderly
• Hypothermia
• Low cardiac output/cardiac failure
• Pericardial effusion
• Hyponatraemia and hypoglycaemia
• Hypoventilation

Management
• Identify any precipitating cause (e.g. infection)
• Gradual re-warming
• Supportive ITU management (protect airway in coma, oxygen, broad-spectrum antibiotics, cardiovascular monitoring, glucose, monitor urine output)
• Take blood for TFTs
• Treat with hydrocortisone until hypoadrenalism excluded
• Thyroid hormone replacement – both oral and intravenous T_4 and T_3 have been advocated with no clear consensus
• Recognize and counsel that even with treatment, mortality is high

Monitoring

Once stable, TFTs can be measured annually, although replacement rarely changes. Compliance issues can be encountered where fT$_4$ is normal (the patient took a tablet prior to clinic) but TSH is raised (chronically, the patient is missing tablets). Despite large trials, there is no convincing evidence that treatment with T$_3$ is better than with thyroxine. T$_3$ needs to be taken three times daily and usually only worsens adherence. All other forms of thyroid hormone replacement (e.g. 'natural' gland extracts sold over the internet) are unregulated and are to be avoided.

Secondary hypothyroidism

If the anterior pituitary thyrotrophs are underactive, TSH-dependent thyroid hormone production fails (see Chapter 5). The principle of thyroxine treatment is similar to that in primary hypothyroidism, although TSH is no longer a reliable marker of adequate replacement. The easiest approach is to treat with sufficient thyroxine for fT$_4$ to lie in the upper half of the normal range and for fT$_3$ also to lie within the normal range.

Hyperthyroidism

Hyperthyroidism is thyroid overactivity causing increased circulating thyroid hormones (thyrotoxicosis). Note that release of stored hormone during a viral infection or overdose of oral thyroxine will cause transient thyrotoxicosis, but this is not hyperthyroidism. Most commonly, hyperthyroidism has an autoimmune origin, is 10-fold more common in women than men, and is named after its discoverer, Thomas Graves. Other causes are associated with the antiarrhythmic drug amiodarone and overproduction of hormone from an autonomous thyroid nodule, either single or part of a multinodular goitre. Occasionally, thyroid overactivity can be a feature of the first few months of pregnancy associated with hyperemesis. The pathology involves high human chorionic gonadotrophin (hCG) levels capable of signalling via the TSH receptor (see pregnancy in Chapter 7). Overactivity from excess TSH is incredibly rare.

Graves disease

Autoimmune hyperthyroidism affects ~2% of women in the UK. Its immune pathogenesis includes thyroid-stimulating IgG antibodies that activate the TSH receptor on the follicular cell surface (Box 8.5), leading to hyperthyroidism and, in many cases, goitre (Figure 8.8).

Symptoms and signs

The natural history of Graves disease is waxing and waning. However, the diagnosis is important as symptoms are unpleasant, potentially serious, yet

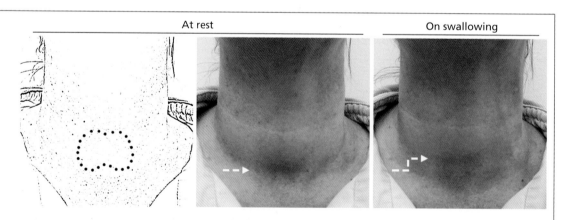

At rest	On swallowing

Figure 8.8 Hyperthyroidism caused by Graves disease in a young woman. The dotted outline in the line drawing illustrates the position of the goitre visible at rest in the central image. The broken line and arrowhead illustrate the goitre's lower margin. Upon swallowing (right image), the goitre rises in the neck; its lower margin is demarcated by the stepped arrow.

Box 8.11 Symptoms and signs of thyrotoxicosis plus features associated with Graves disease

- Weight loss despite full, possibly increased, appetite
- Tremor
- Heat intolerance and sweating
- Agitation and nervousness
- Palpitations, shortness of breath/ tachycardia ± atrial fibrillation
- Amenorrhoea/oligomenorrhoea and consequent subfertility
- Diarrhoea
- Hair loss
- Easy fatigability, muscle weakness and loss of muscle mass
- Rapid growth rate and accelerated bone maturation (children)
- Goitre, diffuse and reasonably firm ± bruit in Graves disease (Figure 8.8)

Extra-thyroidal features associated with Graves disease
- Thyroid eye disease, also called Graves orbitopathy (Figure 8.9)
- Pretibial myxoedema – rare, thickened skin over the lower tibia (Figure 8.9d)
- Thyroid acropachy (clubbing of the fingers)
- Other autoimmune features, e.g. vitiligo

Box 8.12 3-min clinical assessment of the thyroid and thyroid hormone status

- General inspection:
  - Is there obvious goitre (Figure 8.8) or thyroid eye disease (Figure 8.9)?
  - Is the patient appropriately dressed for the temperature?
  - Is the patient underweight, normal weight or overweight?
  - Note nearby pill containers or medicines (e.g. lithium or throat lozenges)
- Start with the hands:
  - Are they warm and sweaty? Is there onycholysis (detachment of the nail from the nail bed) or palmar erythema?
  - Is there thyroid acropachy (similar to clubbing)?
  - Place sheet of paper on outstretched hands to assess tremor
  - Assess rate and rhythm of the radial pulse
  - Briefly assess character of pulse at the brachial artery
- Inspect front of neck, ask patient to swallow with the aid of a sip of water; is the neck tender?
- Move behind patient to palpate neck – is there a goitre? If so:
  - Assess size and movement on swallowing (Figure 8.8)
  - Can the lower edge be felt (if not, it may extend retrosternally)?
  - Assess quality (e.g. firm, soft or hard)
  - Is it symmetrical?
  - Palpate for lymphadenopathy, especially if there is a goitre in a euthyroid patient
- Percuss for retrosternal extension
- Auscultate for a bruit
- Examine for other features of Graves disease (thyroid eye disease, pre-tibial myxoedema)

amenable to treatment. The commonest symptoms are attributable to an increased basal metabolic rate and enhanced β-adrenergic activity (Box 8.11and Case history 8.2). Additional features specific to Graves disease are caused by the autoimmune disease process affecting other sites in the body. Thyroid acropachy and pre-tibial myxoedema are caused by cytokines that stimulate the deposition of glycosaminoglycans. (Figure 8.9d)

Efficient clinical assessment of thyroid status is required (Box 8.12).

Investigation and diagnosis

Thyrotoxicosis requires biochemical proof of suppressed TSH and raised free thyroid hormone levels

(Table 8.1). In the absence of extra-thyroidal features (e.g. Graves orbitopathy or pre-tibial myxoedema), additional tests may help to distinguish between Graves disease and other forms of hyperthyroidism. There may be elevation of the titre of anti-Tg and anti-TPO antibodies, which are more commonly assayed than anti-TSH receptor antibodies (the disease-relevant auto-antibody); thyroid ultrasound should show generalized increased vascularity in Graves disease (features that correlate to a bruit on auscultation); and radionuclide scans [commonly using iodine-123 (I^{123}) which has a short half-life] may show diffuse (Graves disease), patchy (toxic multinodular goitre) or localized uptake (a single toxic nodule). Transient hyperthyroidism will appear normal on ultrasound and have normal isotope uptake.

Treatment
There are three options for treatment.

Antithyroid drugs
Since Graves disease waxes and wanes, a valid approach is to block hyperthyroidism until remission. It is common to maintain patients on antithyroid drugs (Box 8.4) for 12–18 months and then to withdraw treatment to test for spontaneous remission. During this period, TFTs are needed to ensure biochemical euthyroidism (i.e. thyroid hormones in the normal range). A high dose of drug can be started (e.g. carbimazole 40 mg/day) and titrated down according to falling fT_4 levels on TFTs. Alternatively, antithyroid drugs can be maintained at high dose in combination with thyroxine (100 μg/day) as a 'block and replace' regimen. Very rarely, antithyroid drugs can cause agranulocytosis and the patient must be warned to attend for a blood neutrophil count in the event of sore throat or fever. Rash is a common side-effect and may settle with hydrocortisone cream.

The success of antithyroid drug treatment can be broken down into three categories: approximately one-third of patients remits and remains well; one-third remits but relapses at some future time; and one-third relapses soon after stopping the

drug and requires further treatment. The risk of falling into the last group is increased for men, or those presenting with a particularly high fT_4 [e.g. >60 pmol/L (4.7 ng/dL)] or large goitre, and for those in whom TSH remains suppressed despite antithyroid drug treatment that normalizes serum fT_4.

Surgery
If drugs fail or if a prompt definitive outcome is required (e.g. in pregnancy), sub-total or increasingly commonly total thyroidectomy can be used so long as the patient is adequately blocked pre-operatively. Operating on an acutely overactive gland risks 'thyroid storm' when physical handling releases huge stores of hormone, causing raging, life-threatening thyrotoxicosis. Over weeks pre-operatively, carbimazole can be used to achieve biochemical euthyroidism; more acutely, Lugol's iodine or potassium iodide temporarily blocks thyroid hormone release. Sub-total thyroidectomy leaves a small amount of tissue to try and minimize the risk of post-operative hypothyroidism (Box 8.7). Complications include: bleeding; damage to the recurrent laryngeal nerve controlling the laryngeal muscles and voice; and transient or permanent hypoparathyroidism from damage or removal of the parathyroids (see Chapter 9). The scar, parallel to natural skin creases, usually becomes barely noticeable over time.

Radioiodine
Iodine-131 (I^{131}) can be used to treat thyroid overactivity. It requires the same preparation as surgery to avoid thyroid storm. In the UK, I^{131} has tended to be reserved for women who have completed their family, although there is little evidence to suggest that the radiation increases tumour risk or diminishes fertility. It is used more liberally in Europe. It is taken orally and absorbed by the stomach. Compared to surgery it carries no risk to surrounding structures but it is more likely to induce permanent hypothyroidism than sub-total thyroidectomy; the patient needs pre-operative counselling, postoperative monitoring and, in all likelihood, life-long thyroxine replacement. I^{131} is contraindicated in

pregnancy, children, thyroid eye disease (it can make this worse) and incontinence. It is also inappropriate where small children or babies need close contact with the patient in the immediate post-administration period.

For all three treatment approaches, β-blockers, most commonly propranolol, can be used to control the symptoms of adrenergic excess, especially as antithyroid drugs take two weeks to have much effect. As a minor effect, propranolol also inhibits selenodeiodinase, thus tending to prevent the conversion of T4 to T3.

Graves disease in pregnancy

Autoimmune disorders, including Graves disease, tend to ameliorate during pregnancy. A common scenario is one of relative subfertility while hyperthyroidism is undiagnosed, followed by pregnancy once treatment becomes effective. If surgery to the mother's thyroid is required during pregnancy, it is best planned for the second trimester. Post-partum, the relative immunosuppression of pregnancy abates and Graves disease may relapse. Monitoring TFTs is warranted.

Two scenarios can arise in the fetus during pregnancy:

• If blocking the mother's thyroid, the minimum dose should be used and 'block and replace' avoided as antithyroid drugs cross the placenta more efficiently than thyroxine, risking fetal hypothyroidism. As carbimazole increases the risk of aplasia cutis (a rare scalp defect), propylthiouracil (PTU) has been preferred in the past. However, PTU has recently acquired a US Food & Drug Administration alert for idiosyncratic liver toxicity. Monitoring LFTs in each trimester should be considered.

• In ~1% of mothers with Graves disease, past or present, high levels of thyroid-stimulating antibodies cross the placenta. Fetal hyperthyroidism is easy to miss if the mother has had previous definitive treatment (surgery or I[131]) and is euthyroid. Fetal heart rate is a useful guide to fetal thyroid status and goitre may be visible on fetal ultrasound. If needed, antithyroid drugs can be used. After delivery, symptoms recede as maternal antibodies are cleared.

Case history 8.2

A 32-year-old man attended his doctor having lost 10 kg in weight and with poor sleep. He felt on edge and had had difficulty concentrating at work. He smokes five cigarettes/day. Colleagues had commented on his staring appearance. The doctor completes the history and examination and takes a blood test. He knew the likely diagnosis beforehand, however, the results provided proof: TSH less than 0.01 mU/L, fT$_4$ 82.7 pmol/L (~6.5 ng/dL), fT$_3$ 14.2 pmol/L (~0.9 ng/dL).

What is the biochemical diagnosis and why?
What features of the examination could have implied the diagnosis without the blood test?
Describe a suitable management plan?
Once the thyrotoxicosis has settled, what definitive treatment of hyperthyroidism might be ill-advised at present?

Answers, see p. 188

Thyroid eye disease (Graves orbitopathy)

The same autoimmune inflammation that affects the thyroid can also affect the extra-ocular muscles of the orbit, causing Graves orbitopathy, also known as ophthalmopathy (Table 8.2 and Figure 8.9). It is most commonly synchronous with hyperthyroidism when it confirms Graves disease as the cause of thyrotoxicosis. However, it is possible for thyroid eye disease to occur separately. For reasons that are unclear, it is much worse in smokers.

Symptoms of grittiness are common, for which liquid teardrops are effective. All but minor thyroid eye disease warrants referral to ophthalmology (Case history 8.3). Patients who can no longer close their eyes because of proptosis (forward displacement of the orbit; Figure 8.9) are at risk of ulcerated cornea; taping the eyelids closed may be necessary at night.

Table 8.2 Symptoms, signs and examination of thyroid eye disease	
Symptoms and signs	Gritty, weepy, painful eyes
	Retro-orbital pain
	Difficulty reading
	Diplopia
	Loss of vision
	'Staring' appearance (Figure 8.9a)
	Proptosis (Figure 8.9b)
	Periorbital oedema and chemosis (redness; Figure 8.9c) of the conjunctiva
	Injection (redness) over the insertion point of lateral rectus (Figure 8.9c)
	Lid retraction
Examination	Inspect from the front for signs of inflammation and lid retraction
	Is the sclera visible around the entire eye (this is not normal) (Figure 8.9a)?
	Inspect from the side for proptosis
	Assess eye movements from the front asking the patient to report double vision
	Assess visual fields
	Ask the patient to look away while retracting the lateral portion of each eyelid in turn. The insertion point of lateral rectus is visible
	Is it inflamed?
	Assess whether the patient can close the eyelids completely

Although cosmetically undesirable, proptosis acts as a safeguard, relieving the retro-orbital pressure from swollen muscles. A relatively normal external appearance associated with retro-orbital pain or visual disturbance is worrying as pressure on the optic nerve risks loss of vision.

The degree of retro-orbital inflammation and compression can be assessed by magnetic resonance imaging (MRI). Treatment begins with advice to stop smoking. Carbimazole possibly possesses some immunosuppressive qualities, so 'block and replace' (see earlier) may be useful if there is co-existing thyroid disease. Radioiodine is contraindicated during active orbitopathy. Anti-inflammatory or immunosuppressive agents such as glucocorticoid or azathioprine can be used. The efficacy of orbital radiotherapy is contentious. Surgery can relieve sight-threatening compression. The natural disease history is for regression, leaving fibrosed muscles such that diplopia may remain; however, at this late stage, corrective surgery is highly effective.

Amiodarone-associated thyroid disease

Amiodarone is frequently used in cardiology to treat arrhythmias. It contains a lot of iodine and has a half-life longer than 1 month. In addition to potential pulmonary fibrosis, it causes disordered TFTs in as many as 50% of patients as well as frank hyperthyroidism or hypothyroidism in up to 20% (Box 8.13 and Case history 8.4).

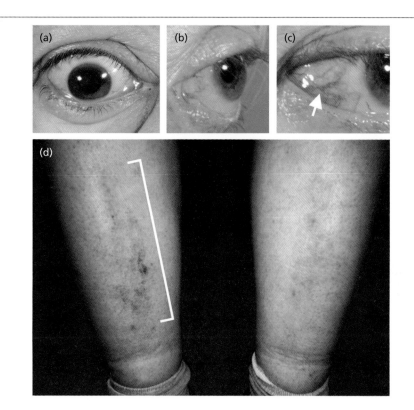

Figure 8.9 Complications of Graves disease. (a–c) Examples of thyroid eye disease. Images courtesy of Dr Anne E Cook, Consultant Oculoplastic & Orbital Surgeon, Central Manchester University Hospitals NHS Foundation Trust. (a) Note the sclera clearly visible above the iris consistent with a degree of lid retraction and proptosis in a right eye. There is also the suggestion of some periorbital puffiness. Fluorescein drops have been added to examine under fluorescent light the cornea for injury or dryness (because propotosis may have inhibited eyelid closure). (b) Propotosis of the left eye. (c) Lateral inflammation (arrow) of the right eye. (d) Pretibial myxoedema, particularly marked with slight discolouring on the tibial surface of the right leg (white line) with some excoriation of the skin. Note the bilateral oedematous appearance (indentations from socks).

Case history 8.3

A 45-year-old woman attends her family doctor because of pain in her right eye, which has been weepy, sore, red and protuberant for the last 2 weeks. She also has pain behind her left eye which otherwise appears normal. She smokes 10 cigarettes/day. The doctor notices a scar on her neck.

Why is the scar of interest?
What is significant about the pain behind the left eye?
What investigations and management should be considered?

Answers, see p. 188

> ### Case history 8.4
>
> An 81-year-old man was referred by the cardiologist with TSH less than 0.14 mU/L, fT$_4$ 32.4 pmol/L (~2.5 ng/dL), and fT$_3$ 6.2 pmol/L (0.4 ng/dL). He has been taking amiodarone for the last 6 months for supraventricular arrhythmia. On questioning he has shortness of breath.
>
> Give three possible causes of the mild thyrotoxicosis.
> If considered to be hyperthyroidism, what treatment would restore euthyroidism?
> Give one drug-related reason why the patient might be short of breath.
>
> *Answers, see p. 189*

Box 8.13 Amiodarone affects the thyroid gland and thyroid function tests

Effects on peripheral hormone metabolism and TFTs

- fT$_3$ slightly decreased ⎫ inhibition of D1
- fT$_4$ slightly increased ⎬ and D2 activity
- rT$_3$ formation increased ⎭ (Figure 8.7)
- Transient TSH increase

Amiodarone-associated hypothyroidism

- Iodine content may inhibit hormone synthesis and release

Amiodarone-associated hyperthyroidism

- Iodine content may stimulate overactivity in susceptible individuals (type 1 amiodarone-induced thyrotoxicosis)

- Potential thyroid toxicity by causing thyroiditis (type 2 amiodarone-induced thyrotoxicosis), possibly followed by hypothyroidism

Treatment

- Hypothyroidism: thyroxine
- Hyperthyroidism:
  - Consider withdrawal of amiodarone (but treatment may be needed during long washout period)
  - Try carbimazole
  - I^{131} uptake may be limited as thyroid already loaded with iodine
  - If drugs fail, surgery can be considered

Toxic adenoma

Hyperthyroidism other than Graves disease is usually secondary to autonomous function of a benign adenoma (a single 'toxic nodule') or dominant nodule(s) within a multinodular goitre (see below). Occasionally, nodules secrete an excess of T$_3$ to cause 'T$_3$-toxicosis' with normal fT$_4$ levels (a specific request to the laboratory may be needed to measure serum fT$_3$).

Such patients will not have the diffuse and symmetrical goitre of Graves disease, nor will they have signs of Graves eye disease. Ultrasound and I^{123} uptake scans will demonstrate the lesion. Unlike Graves disease, spontaneous remission does not occur and definitive treatment with surgery or I^{131} radioiodine is indicated. With thyroid lobectomy or with radioiodine (when the remainder of the gland is quiescent and will not take up the I^{131}), the risk of post-treatment hypothyroidism is low.

Single thyroid nodules and multinodular goitre

For nodules that are not functional (i.e. 'cold' nodules that lack I^{123} uptake in a euthyroid patient), the critical diagnosis to exclude is thyroid malignancy (see Box 8.14):

- Single cold nodules must always be regarded with suspicion
- Multinodular goitres contain many colloid-filled follicular nodules. Frequency is increased in women, with age and with iodine deficiency. The pathogenesis is unclear, although clinically, they almost always behave benignly.

Absence of lymphadenopathy, no family history of thyroid cancer, no rapid growth, no alteration of voice, and a goitre that moves freely on swallowing (as shown in Figure 8.8) are all reassuring features.

Fine needle aspiration cytology (FNAC) under ultrasound guidance is an excellent modality to investigate nodules greater than 0.5 cm diameter. Whether and when nodules require FNAC is debatable. The American Thyroid Association has comprehensive recommendations governed by ultrasound characteristics and clinical suspicion. FNAC tends to produce four results: normal, suspicious, malignant and 'non-diagnostic'. Pragmatically, if history (Box 8.14) and ultrasound are encouraging, and histology is normal, FNAC should be repeated once after a few months for reassurance. In part, this caution has been precipitated by histology showing atypical cells even in clinically benign goitres. For suspicious, malignant and non-diagnostic FNAC, see the next section.

Having addressed malignancy risk, most commonly no treatment is needed for multinodular goitres (Case history 8.5). If local compressive symptoms occur (e.g. on the trachea, assessed by spirometry) or if there is cosmetic dissatisfaction from a large goitre, surgery is the best treatment. Autonomous function can develop in the largest ('dominant') nodule(s) and cause thyrotoxicosis. Long-term, even sub-clinical thyrotoxicosis (suppressed serum TSH and normal fT_4 and fT_3; see Table 8.1) increases mortality from cardiovascular disease. I^{131} is effective with a relatively low risk of post-treatment hypothyroidism compared to Graves disease. If no treatment is needed or if treatment is decided against, annual TFTs are useful as progression to frank thyrotoxicosis occurs in ~1%, particularly with nodule(s) greater than 2 cm in diameter.

Case history 8.5

A 55-year-old woman who had lived in the UK all her life attended her family doctor because of a sense of fullness in her neck. It had been present for at least 5 years and had not changed in nature but was perhaps minimally larger. The patient was worried. The doctor examined her and discovered a non-symmetrical firm mass either side of and close to the midline at the base of her neck that moved on swallowing. There was no palpable lymphadenopathy. There was no family history of cancer. TSH 1.34 mU/L, fT_4 21.4 pmol/L (~1.7 ng/dL), fT_3 4.7 pmol/L (~0.3 ng/dL).

What is the likely diagnosis?
What further investigation would help provide complete reassurance?
What follow-up might be suggested?

Answers, see p. 189

Thyroid cancer

The various types of thyroid cancer have quite different prognoses (Table 8.3). There is a female predominance, but as all thyroid disease has much higher incidence in women, goitre in a man increases the relative risk of malignancy (Box 8.14 and Case history 8.6). In any patient with goitre, hyperthyroidism greatly reduces the likelihood of thyroid malignancy. Overall, ~12% of 'cold' nodules prove to be malignant.

Clear malignancy on FNAC requires total thyroidectomy. Suspicious FNAC in high-risk individuals is probably best managed by local resection to provide a clear tissue diagnosis followed by total thyroidectomy if malignancy is confirmed. Repeated non-diagnostic aspirations and biopsies are relatively common and, if clinical suspicion is high, local surgery is probably the best option (as for suspicious biopsies).

Papillary cell cancer carries a good prognosis. Spread is characteristically via the lymphatic system. Following thyroidectomy, slightly high doses of

Table 8.3 Thyroid malignancy			
Type	**% of thyroid malignancies**	**Groups affected**	**Outcome**
Follicular cell origin			
Papillary carcinoma	70–75	Young women	Good
Follicular carcinoma	15–20	Middle-aged women	Good
Anaplastic	5	Older people	Very poor
C-cell origin			
Medullary carcinoma	<10	Can be part of MEN	Poor
Others			
E.g. lymphoma, sarcoma	<10	Variable	
MEN, multiple endocrine neoplasia.			

Box 8.14 Approach to diagnosing thyroid malignancy

Suspicious features in the history
- Rapid growth of goitre, especially in a man
- Alteration of the voice or dysphagia
- Previous irradiation of the neck
- Familial tumour predisposition syndrome (e.g. multiple endocrine neoplasia; see Chapter 10)

Suspicious features on examination
- Firm, irregularly shaped goitre with euthyroidism

- Tethering to other structures
- Local lymphadenopathy

Investigation
- Radioiodine scanning looking for a 'cold' nodule (decreased uptake in comparison to normal tissue)
- Ultrasound-guided fine needle aspiration or biopsy followed by cytology
- Histological diagnosis

---

replacement thyroxine are given to suppress TSH, thus removing trophic drive to any remaining thyroid cells. This allows Tg to serve as a very sensitive marker of persisting or recurrent disease, for which ablative doses of I^{131} can be administered. Follicular carcinoma also carries a good prognosis. It consists of a mixture of neoplastic colloid-containing follicles, empty acini and alveoli of neoplastic cells. Follicular carcinomas predominate in geographical areas with low dietary iodine. Treatment and postoperative follow-up are similar to papillary carcinoma. In contrast, anaplastic carcinoma is a fast-growing, poorly differentiated tumour that is almost always fatal. Mean survival from diagnosis is only 6 months. Despite the link to familial syndromes (Table 8.3), most medullary carcinoma is sporadic. Calcitonin serves as a circulatory marker (see Chapter 10).

Case history 8.6

A 48-year-old man presented to his family doctor with a swelling at the base of the neck that had come on over the last 3 months. He had had a hoarse voice for the last 2 weeks. TFTs were normal.

Is this presentation concerning?
What additional features might be present on examination of the neck?

Answers, see p. 189

Key points

- T_3 and T_4 are produced by the thyroid gland in response to TSH stimulation
- The thyroid stores significant amounts of hormone compared to other endocrine organs
- T_3 is the major, active thyroid hormone
- The effects of thyroid hormone happen rather slowly by virtue of its action on gene expression

- Overactive and underactive thyroid disease are common, especially in women
- TSH levels are the main diagnostic biochemical measure of hypothyroidism and hyperthyroidism
- Most goitres are benign
- The majority of thyroid malignancy has a good outcome

Answers to case histories

Case history 8.1

The woman has primary hypothyroidism, which probably accounts for the tiredness and the hair loss. TSH is markedly elevated and fT_4 levels are below the normal range. fT_3 measurement is not needed. The slightly low serum sodium is probably associated with the hypothyroidism. Treatment is life-long oral thyroxine to normalize serum TSH on repeat TFTs, which should be performed 6 weeks to 2 months after starting treatment. Commonly, replacement is a single daily tablet of 100 µg, which in the UK does not currently attract a prescription charge. She could start on this dose straight away.

She has mild anaemia, possibly secondary to iron deficiency from menorrhagia, which might also contribute to the hair loss. Alternatively, hypothyroidism can cause anaemia, usually normochromic normocytic, but possibly associated with mild macrocytosis. Macrocytosis would also raise concern over pernicious anaemia, of which this patient is at increased risk. The mean cell volume should be measured and the anaemia should be investigated further by examining iron stores. If low, then a course of ferrous sulphate would be appropriate, but this can affect absorption of thyroxine so should be taken separately from the thyroxine.

Finally, the patient should be advised that euthyroidism by itself will not necessarily promote weight loss. However, alongside careful diet and exercise, this may be attainable.

Case history 8.2

The TFTs reveal thyrotoxicosis. TSH is undetectable and both free thyroid hormones are ~three-fold the normal upper limit.

The scale of these blood results is very unlikely to be caused by transient thyrotoxicosis and the history contains no clues of recent viral infection. The diagnosis is clinched by the thyroid eye disease. The staring appearance is explained by the entire sclera being visible because of lid retraction and possible proptosis. In combination with the thyrotoxicosis, this diagnoses primary hyperthyroidism caused by Graves disease. The other relevant feature of the examination could have been the detection of a thyroid bruit on auscultation over each lobe of the gland. A characteristic goitre is strongly suggestive of Graves disease; however, the bruit, indicative of diffusely increased vascularity, confirms the diagnosis. Although rare, pre-tibial myxoedema would also indicate thyrotoxicosis from Graves disease. A family history of autoimmune thyroid disease would also be supportive.

The patient should be referred to an endocrinologist. However, treatment could be initiated with antithyroid drugs to attain biochemical euthyroidism. The most likely treatment plan is their use for 12–18 months, followed by withdrawal. In the UK, the most common agent is carbimazole at a starting dose of ~40 mg daily for this level of thyroid hormone excess. The prescription should be issued with a warning over the rare side-effect, agranulocytosis, and the need for urgent consultation in the event of sore throat or fever. Rash is a more common side-effect and may settle after a few days. Propranolol 40 mg three times daily could be prescribed to control symptoms, certainly

during the 2 weeks or so while the carbimazole begins to take effect. Endocrinologists vary in their follow-up strategy; either titrating the dose of carbimazole or using 'block-and-replace'. By either approach, TSH would most likely remain undetectable at first; however, in time, it should rise back towards the normal range. Biochemical hypothyroidism should be avoided. As a man with high levels of free thyroid hormones at diagnosis, the patient should be advised of the increased risk of future relapse and the need for definitive treatment. Persistently undetectable TSH during treatment and a large goitre would increase this risk further. Further assessment of thyroid eye disease is needed. The patient should be advised to stop smoking. If symptoms are limited to minor 'grittiness', the patient can close his eyes completely, and the remainder of the eye examination is largely unremarkable (e.g. vision normal, no retro-orbital pain), then observation would suffice. However, if the disease is any more significant, he should be referred to an ophthalmologist.

Radioiodine would be ill-advised as definitive treatment, especially in an active smoker, as it would risk exacerbating the eye disease.

Case history 8.3

The scar is a clue to diagnosing thyroid eye disease because it suggests previous thyroidectomy for Graves disease, which should be the topic of specific questions.

The left retro-orbital pain is very significant for a number of reasons. It makes a unilateral retro-orbital mass (e.g. lymphoma) less likely to explain the more obvious right-sided symptoms and signs. Bilateral symptoms make the diagnosis of thyroid eye disease far more probable. It is easy to be distracted by the more obvious signs on the right; however, the normal appearance of the left eye plus retro-orbital pain may indicate significant retro-orbital pressure and potential damage to the optic nerve and vision. Urgent referral to ophthalmology is warranted.

Vision should be assessed and imaging (e.g. MRI) of the orbits undertaken. It should be ensured that the right eye can close properly. Liquid tears may be useful. TFTs should be done and treatment for hypothyroidism or hyperthyroidism started, if necessary. The patient should be advised and helped to stop smoking. If specific treatment of thyroid eye disease is needed, this requires specialist input and may involve anti-inflammatory glucocorticoids, immunosuppression and/or decompression surgery.

Case history 8.4

The patient may have a transient thyroiditis (e.g. has he had a recent sore throat or fever?). Graves disease is relatively unlikely *de novo* at 81 years, but possible. An alternative is a toxic adenoma, either as a solitary nodule or as part of a multinodular goitre. However, in this history, the most likely cause is hyperthyroidism secondary to amiodarone therapy.

Low-dose carbimazole (or equivalent antithyroid medication) would most likely be effective at restoring euthyroidism, which is important as thyrotoxicosis risks destabilizing the patient's well being, especially given the supraventricular arrhythmia and risk of cardiac failure, which would exacerbate the shortness of breath.

There are several reasons why the man might be short of breath (e.g. cardiac failure); however, amiodarone can cause pulmonary fibrosis. It has been advocated that baseline pulmonary function tests should be done before treatment to allow monitoring for this.

Case history 8.5

The patient most likely has a multinodular goitre. She is euthyroid.

This is highly unlikely to be malignancy as the mass has not changed, particularly over 5 years, and there is no lymphadenopathy, tethering, symptoms such as hoarseness (implies local invasion), or family history. Ultrasound of the neck would confirm a multi-nodular goitre with FNAC possible for any of the larger nodules.

For any nodules that were aspirated and unremarkable, repeat FNAC a few months later accords with the British Thyroid Association guidelines. There is a risk of future hyperthyroidism in multi-nodular goitre such that annual TFTs could be suggested even though there is no current suspicion of TSH suppression.

Case history 8.6

Yes. The presentation is suspicious of thyroid malignancy. There is a rapidly growing mass in the region of the thyroid in a euthyroid patient. There is alteration of the voice. This warrants urgent specialist referral as suspected cancer.

The goitre may be hard, tethered to the skin and underlying structures and not move with swallowing. There may be associated lymphadenopathy.

CHAPTER 9

Calcium and metabolic bone disorders

Key topics

- Calcium   191
- Hormones that regulate calcium   192
- Clinical disorders of calcium homeostasis   198
- Bone health and metabolic bone disorders   203
- Clinical conditions of bone metabolism   205
- Key points   211
- Answers to case histories   211

Learning objectives

- To understand normal calcium homeostasis and its principal regulators
- To recognize the causes, clinical features and treatment of hypocalcaemia and hypercalcaemia
- To understand normal bone formation and turnover
- To recognize the causes, clinical features and treatment of osteoporosis
- To understand the causes, clinical features and treatment of osteomalacia and rickets

This chapter is divided into sections on calcium and associated clinical conditions, and bone health and associated metabolic disorders

To recap

- Regulation of calcium by parathyroid hormone occurs as part of a negative feedback loop, the principle of which is introduced in Chapter 1
- Calcium is regulated by parathyroid hormone and vitamin D, making it timely to review the biosynthesis of peptide hormones and those derived from cholesterol, covered in Chapter 2
- Understanding how parathyroid hormone and vitamin D act requires an understanding of hormone action at the cell surface and in the nucleus, covered in Chapter 3

Essential Endocrinology and Diabetes, Sixth Edition. Richard IG Holt, Neil A Hanley.
© 2012 Richard IG Holt and Neil A Hanley. Publlished 2012 by Blackwell Publishing Ltd.

Cross-reference

■ The development of the parathyroid and parafollicular C-cells is described alongside the thyroid in Chapter 8

■ Tumours of the parathyroid glands are an important component of multiple endocrine neoplasia, covered in Chapter 10

■ Other hormones such as cortisol (see Chapter 6) and sex hormones (see Chapter 7) affect mineralization of the bones

Calcium

Calcium (Ca^{2+}) performs vital functions (Box 9.1) and its concentration at all locations requires tight control [serum, 2.20–2.60 mmol/L (8.8–10.4 mg/dL); interstitium, ~1.5 mmol/L (6.0 mg/dL); and inside the cell, 0.1–1.0 mmol/L (0.4–4.0 mg/dL)]. In the circulation, Ca^{2+} is bound to plasma proteins, mainly albumin, with ~10% complexed with citrate. The important fraction is the ~50% that is unbound (free) and biologically active. Thus, serum Ca^{2+} always requires correction for albumin concentration. An approximation is to increase or decrease Ca^{2+} by 0.02 mmol/L for every gram that albumin is below or above 40 g/L (or by 0.08 mg/dL for 0.1 g that albumin is below or above 4.0 g/dL) (Case history 9.3). Otherwise, hypocalcaemia or hypercalcaemia may be erroneously diagnosed if albumin concentrations are respectively low or high.

Under normal circumstances Ca^{2+} is in equilibrium across different 'pools' in the body (i.e. bones, circulation, tissues and organs) (Figure 9.1). During

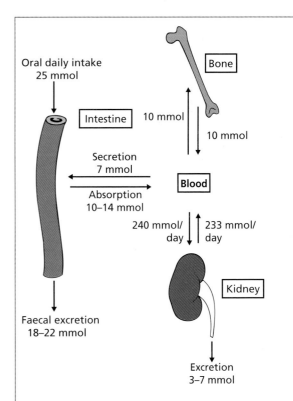

Figure 9.1 Calcium homeostasis. In an adult, daily net absorption from the gut equals urinary loss. For a child in positive Ca^{2+} balance, net absorption exceeds renal excretion with retention of Ca^{2+} in the growing skeleton.

Box 9.1 Key facts about calcium

Ca^{2+} is critical for:
• Bone mineralization
• Blood clotting
• Muscle contraction
• Enzyme action
• Exocytosis of hormones and neurotransmitters
• Nerve function
• Intracellular signaling (review Figure 3.16)

childhood, overall Ca^{2+} balance is positive as new bone is laid down. During young adulthood, the daily uptake of Ca^{2+} from the gut matches losses, mainly from urine (but some from sweat and the bowels). In older age, particularly in post-menopausal women, output (from bone) is greater than input, putting Ca^{2+} into negative balance. Ca^{2+} is in part regulated alongside phosphate [PO_4^{3-}; normal range in serum, 0.8–1.45 mmol/L (2.5–4.5 mg/dL), higher in children]. However, a higher proportion of PO_4^{3-} than Ca^{2+} is absorbed from the diet and so correspondingly more PO_4^{3-} is excreted in the urine. PO_4^{3-} absorption and excretion is also increased with high meat intake. A gene on the short arm of the X chromosome, *PHEX*, is important in regulating renal PO_4^{3-} excretion. Mutations in this gene cause X-linked hypophosphataemic rickets (see last section of the chapter).

Ca^{2+} is a major constituent of all cell types and acts as an intracellular signalling mechanism (review Figure 3.16) linking external stimulation of a cell to function. For instance, in myocytes, Ca^{2+} mediates contraction.

Dietary intake of calcium

The recommended daily allowance for Ca^{2+} is ~1 g. Ca^{2+} is abundant in many foods, especially dairy products such as cheese, yoghurt and milk. Absorption from the gut is inefficient; only ~30% of ingested Ca^{2+} is absorbed. However, gut absorption is highly regulated as one method of controlling serum Ca^{2+}. Absorption increases in childhood and during pregnancy and lactation, but decreases with age and if Ca^{2+} intake is high.

A number of dietary factors also affect Ca^{2+} absorption. Basic amino acids and lactose enhance absorption, making milk supplementation particularly effective at increasing Ca^{2+} in children. In contrast, phytic acid, present in unleavened or brown bread, inhibits Ca^{2+} absorption by chelating it in the gut. During the Second World War, bread was fortified with Ca^{2+} in the UK and this practice continues to this day.

Hormones that regulate calcium

Vitamin D and parathyroid hormone (PTH) are the two major hormones that regulate Ca^{2+} through a complex interaction (Box 9.2). Both hormones increase serum Ca^{2+} levels. Calcitonin and parathyroid hormone-related peptide (PTHrP) can affect Ca^{2+}, but they play limited roles in human physiology.

Box 9.2 Major hormones that regulate serum calcium

Serum Ca^{2+} concentration is increased by two hormones:
- PTH
- Vitamin D

Box 9.3 Why vitamin D is a hormone

- By definition, a vitamin must be provided in the diet; 90% of vitamin D is synthesized in the skin
- Active vitamin D mainly circulates via the bloodstream to act on a distant tissue (a feature of a hormone)
- The receptor for vitamin D is a member of the nuclear hormone receptor superfamily

---

Vitamin D

Vitamin D functions more like a hormone than a vitamin (Box 9.3). It is derived from cholesterol and has a similar structure to steroid hormones (review Chapter 2). There are a number of different forms of vitamin D. At least 10% is acquired from dietary sources like fish and eggs as vitamin D_2 (ergocalciferol; Figure 9.2), which places vegans at increased risk of vitamin D deficiency (see Box 9.18). Several foodstuffs, including margarine and milk, are fortified with vitamin D_2. Vitamin D_3 (cholecalciferol) accounts for 90% of total vitamin D and is synthesized in the skin by photoisomerization induced by ultraviolet (UV) light (see below and Figure 9.2). The last section of the chapter provides details on vitamin D deficiency.

Synthesis of active vitamin D

Vitamin D_2 and vitamin D_3 serve as precursors for active hormone synthesis and are structurally identical except for the double bond in vitamin D_2 between carbon (C) 22 and C23 of the side chain. In the inner layers of the sun-exposed epidermis, vitamin D_3 is synthesized from 7-dehydrocholesterol. The B ring opens to form pre-vitamin D followed

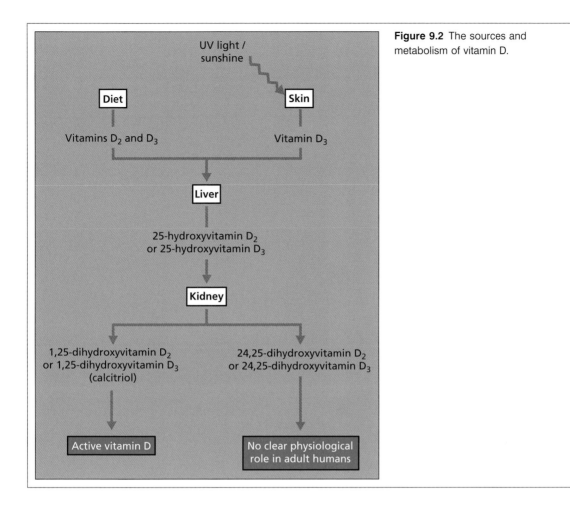

Figure 9.2 The sources and metabolism of vitamin D.

by rotation of the A ring (Figure 9.3). Activation occurs by two hydroxylation steps. The first occurs predominantly in the liver at C25 to form 25-hydroxyvitamin D, which circulates at quite high concentrations [20–40 nmol/L (8–16 ng/mL)] and is then converted in the kidney to fully active 1,25-dihydroxyvitamin D (calcitriol; Figure 9.3), the serum concentration of which is very low [48–110 pmol/L (20–46 pg/mL)]. As for steroid hormones (review Chapter 2), there is a circulating vitamin D-binding protein with high affinity for 25-hydroxyvitamin D but low affinity for calcitriol. This means calcitriol circulates largely free and has a short half-life of ~15 h, compared to 15 days for 25-hydroxyvitamin D. The longer half-life of 25-hydroxyvitamin D makes it a more reliable measure of overall vitamin D status in patients.

Regulation of vitamin D synthesis

Prevailing Ca^{2+} levels control production of active or inactive vitamin D by negative feedback (review Chapter 1). Inactivation of vitamin D occurs in the kidney by 24-hydroxylation to 1,24,25-trihydroxyvitamin D. 24-hydroxlyase also acts on 25-hydroxyvitamin D to form 24,25-dihydroxyvitamin D. This metabolite may play a role in bone development; however, no clear function is apparent in adulthood, other than to limit formation of calcitriol. For instance, high Ca^{2+} increases activity of 24-hydroxylase, thereby restricting levels of active vitamin D in circumstances where it would be detrimental to increase serum Ca^{2+} (Figure 9.4). Conversely, low Ca^{2+} or PO_4^{3-} levels stimulate 1α-hydroxylase (a cytochrome P450 enzyme officially known as CYP27B1) to

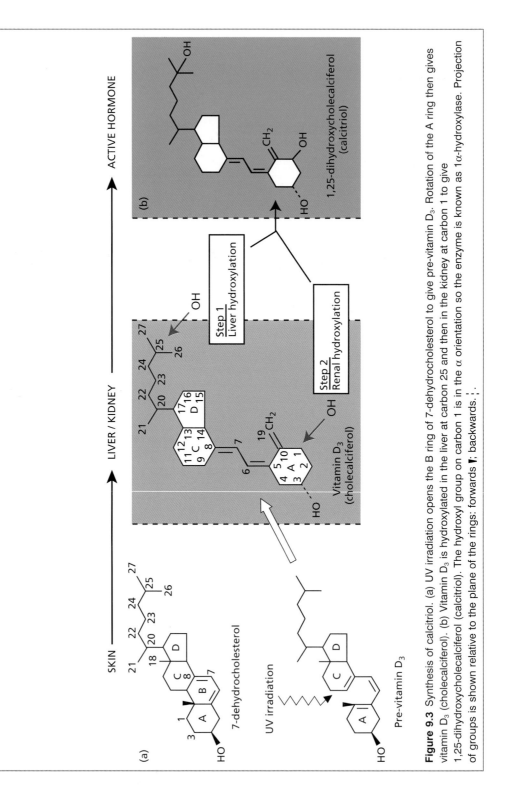

Figure 9.3 Synthesis of calcitriol. (a) UV irradiation opens the B ring of 7-dehydrocholesterol to give pre-vitamin D₃. Rotation of the A ring then gives vitamin D₃ (cholecalciferol). (b) Vitamin D₃ is hydroxylated in the liver at carbon 25 and then in the kidney at carbon 1 to give 1,25-dihydroxycholecalciferol (calcitriol). The hydroxyl group on carbon 1 is in the α orientation so the enzyme is known as 1α-hydroxylase. Projection of groups is shown relative to the plane of the rings: forwards ▼; backwards ┆.

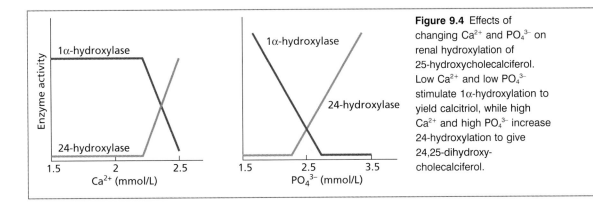

Figure 9.4 Effects of changing Ca^{2+} and PO_4^{3-} on renal hydroxylation of 25-hydroxycholecalciferol. Low Ca^{2+} and low PO_4^{3-} stimulate 1α-hydroxylation to yield calcitriol, while high Ca^{2+} and high PO_4^{3-} increase 24-hydroxylation to give 24,25-dihydroxy-cholecalciferol.

Table 9.1 Comparative actions of vitamin D, parathyroid hormone (PTH) and calcitonin

	Vitamin D	PTH	Calcitonin
Bone	↑ Osteoclast activity ↑ Bone resorption (but note that vitamin D deficiency causes demineralization)	↓ Osteoblast activity (if constant) ↑ Bone resorption (if constant) ↑ Osteoblast activity (if intermittent) ↓ Bone resorption (if intermittent)	↓ Osteoclast activity ↓ Bone resorption
Kidney	↑ Calcium re-absorption ↑ Phosphate re-absorption	↑ 1α-hydroxylase synthesis ↑ Calcium re-absorption ↓ Phosphate re-absorption	↓ Calcium re-absorption ↓ Phosphate re-absorption
Gut	↑ Calcium absorption ↑ Phosphate absorption	(Indirect action only) ↑ Calcium absorption ↑ Phosphate absorption	
Blood	↑ Calcium ↑ Phosphate	↑ Calcium ↓ Phosphate	↓ Calcium ↓ Phosphate

encourage active vitamin D synthesis. The expression of 1α-hydroxylase requires and is increased by PTH. As a consequence, calcitriol rather than cholecalciferol or ergocalciferol needs to be given to treat hypocalcaemia secondary to hypoparathyroidism (see later). 1α-hydroxylase expression is also increased by growth hormone (GH), cortisol, oestrogen and prolactin.

Function of vitamin D

Like steroid and thyroid hormones, calcitriol binds a specific nuclear receptor, the vitamin D receptor (VDR), which functions as a ligand-activated transcription factor in the nucleus by heterodimerizing with the retinoid X receptor (RXR) [RXR also interacts with thyroid hormone receptor (review Figure 3.20) and PPARγ (see Chapter 13)]. The VDR–RXR heterodimer orchestrates the expression of genes involved in Ca^{2+} absorption and homeostasis, mainly in the intestine, bone and kidney (Table 9.1). In the gut, vitamin D increases the absorption of dietary Ca^{2+} and PO_4^{3-}. Vitamin D's effects on bone are complex and in part mediated via complex interactions with PTH. On the whole, if vitamin D is deficient, bones can become demineralized, leading to osteomalacia. However, direct vitamin D action in bone tends to increase the release of Ca^{2+} and PO_4^{3-} by some activation of osteoclast activity (see section on metabolic bone

disease for detailed roles of the osteoblast and osteoclast in bone turnover). In the kidney, vitamin D
increases Ca^{2+} and PO_4^{3-} re-absorption.

Vitamin D is implicated outside of Ca^{2+} metabolism in direct effects on the vasculature, insulin
secretion and immune function.

Parathyroid glands and parathyroid hormone

PTH is secreted by four parathyroids, located as
upper and lower glands behind each lobe of the
thyroid. They are small, lentil-sized glands, each
weighing 40–60 mg. They develop from the third
and fourth pharyngeal pouches, which emerge at
the upper end of the foregut during the third week
of development (Figures 9.5 and 8.1). During
embryogenesis, the two uppermost glands on each
side descend to become the lower parathyroids; this
complex migration can go wrong leaving ectopic
tissue in the neck or mediastinum. If overactive, this
can present a challenge to the endocrine surgeon.

There are two parathyroid cell types: chief cells
secreting PTH and oxyphil cells, the function of
which is unknown. There is a rich vascular supply
mainly from the inferior thyroid arteries. Blood
drains into the thyroid veins.

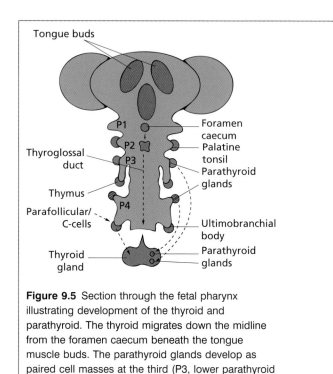

Figure 9.5 Section through the fetal pharynx
illustrating development of the thyroid and
parathyroid. The thyroid migrates down the midline
from the foramen caecum beneath the tongue
muscle buds. The parathyroid glands develop as
paired cell masses at the third (P3, lower parathyroid
gland) and fourth (P4, upper parathyroid gland)
pharyngeal pouches and migrate to the posterior
surface of the thyroid. The origins of the thymus and
palatine tonsils are also shown.

Synthesis of parathyroid hormone

PTH is produced from a single gene as a precursor
peptide that is cleaved to a mature single-chain 84-
amino acid hormone stored in vesicles in the chief
cells (review Figures 2.2 and 2.4). The potential for
rapid changes in PTH secretion indicates that it is
not dependent on *de novo* synthesis. Full biological
activity resides within the first 34 amino acids,
which are now synthetically available as a treatment
for osteoporosis (teriparatide, see later).

Regulation of parathyroid hormone production

PTH release is controlled by negative feedback
according to serum Ca^{2+} concentration via the
G-protein–coupled Ca^{2+}-sensing receptor (CaSR)
(Figure 9.6). This 'calciostat' regulates serum Ca^{2+}
around a set point. If serum Ca^{2+} falls below this
threshold, signalling downstream of the CaSR

increases PTH production; at levels above the set
point, PTH secretion is shut off. Alterations to this
mechanism explain biochemical findings in primary
hyperparathyroidism and rare individuals with inactivating mutations in the CaSR (see later).

Function of parathyroid hormone

In general, PTH acts to increase serum Ca^{2+}. The
hormone acts via a specific G-protein–coupled
receptor on the surface of renal tubule, osteoblast
and gut epithelial cells (review Chapter 3). In the
kidney, PTH increases 1α-hydroxylase expression,
thereby activating vitamin D. PTH also increases
Ca^{2+} and hydrogen absorption at the distal tubule.
Unlike vitamin D, PTH decreases PO_4^{3-} and bicarbonate re-absorption. Collectively, this promotes a
metabolic acidosis. In the bone, constant PTH
inhibits bone-forming osteoblast activity but signals
via this cell type to stimulate osteoclasts, leading to

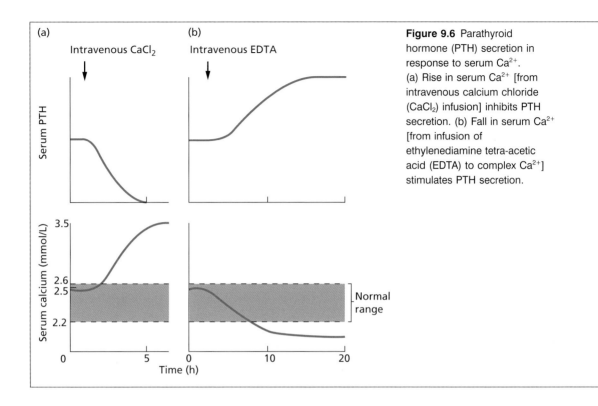

Figure 9.6 Parathyroid hormone (PTH) secretion in response to serum Ca^{2+}. (a) Rise in serum Ca^{2+} [from intravenous calcium chloride ($CaCl_2$) infusion] inhibits PTH secretion. (b) Fall in serum Ca^{2+} [from infusion of ethylenediamine tetra-acetic acid (EDTA) to complex Ca^{2+}] stimulates PTH secretion.

net release of Ca^{2+} and PO_4^{3-} into the circulation (see Box 9.15). Of these opposing effects on PO_4^{3-}, the renal action is larger such that the net effect of PTH is to lower serum PO_4^{3-}. Intermittent PTH can stimulate osteoblasts (injection regimens now exploit this clinically; see later section on osteoporosis). PTH also acts via osteoblasts to increase the number of haematopoietic stem cells in adjacent bone marrow. There appears to be no direct effect of PTH in the gut but there is an indirect increase in Ca^{2+} uptake by enhanced formation of active vitamin D.

Parathyroid hormone-related peptide

During evolution, duplication has given rise to a second gene very closely related to *PTH* that encodes PTH-related peptide (PTHrP). PTHrP is larger but acts via the same cell surface receptor to raise cAMP levels. PTHrP was discovered as the hormonal cause of hypercalaemia of malignancy (see later). Ordinarily, it does not regulate serum Ca^{2+} levels but is synthesized by the placenta and

lactating breast, when it can contribute to 1α-hydroxylase activation. PTHrP is very important in the fetus for bone development.

Calcitonin

Calcitonin is secreted from the parafollicular or C-cells of the thyroid gland (see Figure 8.2) in response to a rise in extracellular Ca^{2+}. It acts to reduce Ca^{2+} levels via binding to its specific G-protein–coupled receptor on the surface of renal tubule cells, where it inhibits Ca^{2+} and PO_4^{3-} reabsorption, and osteoclasts, where it suppresses the release of Ca^{2+} and PO_4^{3-}.

The physiological relevance of calcitonin is unknown because no clinical syndrome arises from its deficiency, e.g. after total thyroidectomy, or excess, as in medullary thyroid cancer (see Chapters 8 and 10). It may be important in growing children and pregnant women, contributing to growth or preservation of the skeleton, and it may have a role in the treatment of several metabolic bone diseases. In birds, it regulates eggshell formation.

Clinical disorders of calcium homeostasis

Most clinical problems reflect either too much (hypercalcaemia) or too little (hypocalcaemia) circulating Ca^{2+}.

Hypocalcaemia

The commonest cause of hypocalcaemia (Box 9.4) is lack of PTH due to hypoparathyroidism (Box 9.5).

Box 9.4 Causes of hypocalcaemia

- Hypoparathyroidism
- Hypomagnesaemia
- Renal failure
- Neonatal hypocalcaemia (temporary suppression of PTH following maternal hypercalcaemia during gestation; see hyperparathyroidism)
- Pancreatitis
- Pseudohypoparathyroidism

Box 9.5 Causes of hypoparathyroidism

In approximate order of descending frequency:
- Surgical – damage or unintended removal during thyroid surgery
- Autoimmune – isolated or part of type 1 autoimmune polyglandular syndrome (APS-1)
- Congenital – may be part of DiGeorge syndrome

Approximately 1–2% of patients undergoing thyroid surgery experience damage to the parathyroids (Case history 9.1). Autoimmune damage to the parathyroids can be isolated or occur as part of type 1 autoimmune polyglandular syndrome (APS-1), an autosomal recessive disorder caused by mutations in the *AIRE* gene (Case history 9.2). Along with a tendency to mucosal candidiasis, adrenocortical, thyroid and gonadal failure can occur (see Chapters 6–8; see Box 8.8 for APS-2). Parathyroid under-development (hypoplasia) or absence (agenesis) occurs in DiGeorge syndrome when the third and fourth pharyngeal pouches fail to develop properly. The thymus may also be missing and there may be variable congenital heart disease (see Figure 4.4).

When hypocalcaemia is not caused by hypoparathyroidism, it is most commonly a result of ineffective PTH action, e.g. due to lack of magnesium (Mg^{2+}) (hypomagnesaemia; Box 9.4). Mg^{2+} is required as a co-factor for PTH action. In renal failure, PTH can no longer increase 1α-hydroxylase activity, leading to a lack of active vitamin D and potential hypocalcaemia.

Neonatal hypocalcaemia can occur *per se* in premature babies. It can also reflect maternal hypercalcaemia (see later) that suppressed fetal PTH *in utero* and continued to cause transient low Ca^{2+} in the neonate.

Inactivating mutations in the PTH signalling pathway cause hypocalcaemia due to PTH resistance. Collectively, these conditions are termed pseudohypoparathyroidism. In addition to the hypocalcaemia and hyperphosphataemia, patients are short with a round face and characteristically short fourth metacarpals (Figure 9.7). There may be

---

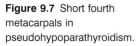

Figure 9.7 Short fourth metacarpals in pseudohypoparathyroidism.

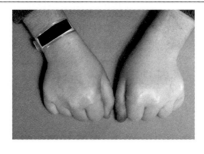
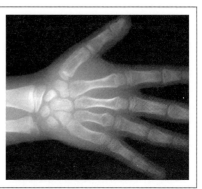

Box 9.6 Symptoms and signs of hypocalcaemia

- Muscle cramps and carpopedal spasm – when induced by applying a blood pressure cuff to the arm, it is called Trousseau's sign
- Numbness and paraesthesiae
- Mood swings and depression
- Tetany and neuromuscular excitability – tapping over the facial nerve causes the facial muscles to twitch (Chvostek's sign)
- Convulsions
- Cardiac arrythmias (long QT interval on ECG)
- Cataract

paradoxical ectopic calcification in muscle and brain and some degree of intellectual impairment. Mutations in the $G_s\alpha$ subunit downstream of the PTH receptor cause autosomal dominant Albright hereditary osteodystrophy (review Box 3.8).

Symptoms and signs

Other than when caused by surgical hypoparathyroidism, hypocalcaemia is usually insidious in onset (Box 9.6). However, once corrected serum Ca^{2+} falls below 1.5 mmol/L (6.0 mg/dL), the condition becomes increasingly dangerous.

Investigation and diagnosis

Low serum Ca^{2+} makes the diagnosis. Concomitant assessment of serum PO_4^{3-}, renal function and PTH levels are helpful. Serum Mg^{2+} rarely needs checking.

Treatment

The broad aim is Ca^{2+} restoration to prevent symptoms and signs. In hypoparathyroidism, treatment with PTH, although possible (see later section on osteoporosis), is expensive and would need to be given by injection. Therefore, treatment is commonly with oral Ca^{2+} and calcitriol tablets (because in the absence of PTH, renal 1α-hydroxylation of ergocalciferol or cholecalciferol would be lacking). The goal is to restore serum Ca^{2+} to the lower end of the normal range. Complete normalization of

Ca^{2+}, in the absence of PTH, leads to excessive Ca^{2+} flux through the urine, risking renal calcification and stone formation, especially if the renal anatomy is abnormal.

Case history 9.1

A 30-year-old woman underwent a difficult thyroidectomy for the treatment of Graves disease. She is anxious about the outcome of her operation and 2 days postoperatively, she complains of tingling in her fingers and mouth.

What are the possible explanations for her symptoms?
What would be your management?

Answers, see p. 211

Case history 9.2

A 26-year-old woman was referred by her family doctor because of hypocalcaemia [corrected serum Ca^{2+} 1.94 mmol/L (7.76 mg/dL)]. The doctor had measured serum PTH, which was also low. On close questioning, her parents were cousins, and a cousin and a grandparent of the patient took long-term Ca^{2+} replacement. The cousin also took thyroxine. The patient had always suffered from recurrent sore throats; on examination, white plaques were visible.

What diagnosis is consistent with all aspects of the history and examination? What is the differential diagnosis?
Assuming the unifying diagnosis is correct, what endocrine management would you consider beyond the hypocalcaemia and sore throat?

Answers, see p. 211

Box 9.7 Causes of hypercalcaemia

Common
- Primary hyperparathyroidism
- Malignancy
- Drugs and dietary causes

Rare
- Familial benign hypercalcaemia
- Thyrotoxicosis
- Hypoadrenalism
- Acromegaly
- Sarcoidosis
- Tertiary hyperparathyroidism

Box 9.8 Primary tumours that commonly metastasize to bone

- Lung
- Breast
- Prostate
- Kidney
- Thyroid

Hypercalcaemia

Primary hyperparathyroidism and malignancy are the commonest causes of raised serum Ca^{2+} levels. However, several other conditions need consideration (Box 9.7) (Case history 9.3). Hypercalcaemia can be severe [serum $Ca^{2+} > 3.0$ mmol/L (12.0 mg/dL)] and can be exacerbated by dehydration.

Primary hyperparathyroidism

Primary hyperparathyroidism is common after middle age with a female predominance of ~2:1 and an incidence of 1 in 1000. It reflects elevation of the set-point at which serum Ca^{2+} signals via the CaSR to shut off PTH production (review Figure 9.6). Around 80% of cases are caused by a single parathyroid adenoma with the remainder resulting from hyperplasia of all glands. Parathyroid cancer is extremely rare; however, primary hyperparathyroidism in someone younger than 45 years should raise suspicion of multiple endocrine neoplasia (MEN) type 1 (see Chapter 10).

Secondary and tertiary hyperparathyroidism usually occur in renal failure, although they can occasionally result from Ca^{2+} malabsorption. Failure of 1α-hydroxylation of vitamin D in renal impairment causes a compensatory increase in PTH to maintain normal serum Ca^{2+} (secondary hyperparathyroidism). This is at the expense of normal bone health and a typical osteodystrophy occurs. With prolonged high secretion of PTH, there is a risk that the parathyroid glands then become autonomous and over-secrete PTH even after Ca^{2+} concentrations are normalized. This leads to hypercalcaemia and tertiary hyperparathyroidism.

Malignancy

Hypercalcaemia is frequently seen in later stage malignancy either because of eroding local bony metastases, secretion of paracrine factors, such as prostaglandins, that activate osteoclasts (Box 9.8) or because of humoral hypercalcaemia of malignancy from PTHrP secretion (see earlier).

Drugs and dietary causes

It is important to take a drug history as thiazide diuretics cause hypercalcaemia by increasing Ca^{2+} resorption at the distal tubule. Overdose of vitamin D may also cause hypercalcaemia, sometimes from non-prescription multivitamins. Rarely, ingestion of large amounts of milk or Ca^{2+}-containing antacids can cause hypercalcaemia, although this is much less common now that H_2 antagonists and proton pump inhibitors exist to treat peptic ulceration.

Familial benign hypercalcaemia

Also known as familial hypocalciuric hypercalcaemia, this autosomal dominant condition of inactivating mutations in CaSR can masquerade as primary hyperparathyroidism (Case history 9.4). The main difference is that 24-h urine Ca^{2+} excretion tends to be diminished, not raised. The distinction is important as falsely diagnosing primary hyperparathyroidism in the paediatric clinic would raise concern of MEN1. CaSR inactivation reduces negative feedback from Ca^{2+} and consequently leads to increased PTH and mild hypercalcaemia; however, familial benign hypercalcaemia requires no treatment.

Other causes

Hypercalcaemia may occur in thyrotoxicosis because of increased osteoclast activity. In 1–2% of patients with sarcoidosis, serum Ca^{2+} rises because of 1α-hydroxylase activity in the non-caseating granulomata. Somewhat similarly, excessive GH in acromegaly can stimulate renal 1α-hydroxylase.

Symptoms and signs

Automated biochemistry laboratories have meant that most patients are identified with asymptomatic mild hypercalcaemia [e.g. 2.5–2.8 mmol/L (10.0–11.2 mg/dL)] (Box 9.9). Common symptoms are non-specific. Others associated with more severely elevated serum Ca^{2+} [>3.0 mmol/L (>12.0 mg/dL)] led to the clinical adage 'bones, stones, abdominal groans and psychic moans'. Persistent hypercalcaemia can lead to ectopic calcification visible on plain radiographs of the heart, joints and kidney, and more rarely seen in the liver and pancreas. Hypercalcaemia resulting from PTHrP tends to be a late feature of malignancy.

Investigation and diagnosis

Commonly, raised serum Ca^{2+} is a serendipitous finding. If there is any doubt, a fasting sample taken without use of a tourniquet in a well-hydrated patient minimizes spurious minor rises in Ca^{2+}.

Investigations for primary hyperparathyroidism are shown in Box 9.10. Serum PTH is either inappropriately 'normal' (in the presence of raised serum Ca^{2+}, PTH should be suppressed) or raised. Serum PO_4^{3-} is likely to be low. Note that PTH is increased in vitamin D deficiency (very common in the UK), making it important to be clear that serum Ca^{2+} is truly raised. 24 hour urinary Ca^{2+} is always expected to be increased in primary hyperparathyroidism (note this assay requires an acidified container, see Box 4.1).

Box 9.9 Symptoms and signs of hypercalcaemia

- Asymptomatic serendipitous finding
- Tiredness and fatigue
- Anorexia and nausea
- Thirst and polyuria
- Muscle weakness
- Headache
- Hypertension
- Bony pain
- Renal stones
- Abdominal pain from constipation, peptic ulceration or, rarely, acute pancreatitis
- Confusion and mood disturbance
- Palpitations through cardiac arrhythmias
- Bone fractures
- Convulsions and coma if severe
- Corneal calcification

Box 9.10 Investigating hypercalcaemia

- Serum Ca^{2+}
- Investigating primary hyperparathyroidism:
  - Serum PO_4^{3-} (decreased)
  - 24-h urinary Ca^{2+} (increased)
  - Serum PTH (normal or raised)
  - DEXA (to assess bone mineralization)
  - Plain X-ray of kidneys (potential calcification)
  - Neck ultrasound (if surgery is considered)
  - Isotope scan using technicium 99m-sestamibi
  - CT or MRI
  - Venous sampling (if surgery if necessary and adenoma unlocalized)
- Serum angiotensin-converting enzyme (ACE) and chest X-ray (can be helpful if considering sarcoidosis)
- Serum cholecalciferol (25-hydroxycalciferol) (if vitamin D toxicity is possible)
- Investigating malignancy (see Box 9.8):
  - Chest X-ray (carcinoma of the bronchus)
  - Prostate examination and serum prostate-specific antigen (PSA)
  - Mammogram
  - Thyroid ultrasound (see Chapter 8)
  - Bone scintigraphy using technicium 99m-methylene diphosphate (bone scan)
  - Serum electrophoresis and urinary Bence-Jones proteins (for multiple myeloma)
  - PTHrP (rarely assayed but distinguishable from PTH which is low)

Prior to automated biochemical analyses, hyper-calcaemia as a result of primary hyperparathyroidism tended to present more severely (Box 9.9), when hand X-rays would show characteristic features of bone resorption. This is uncommon now but dual X-ray absorptiometry (DEXA) should still be done to assess bone mineralization and fracture risk.

Having made the diagnosis of primary hyper-parathyroidism and if surgery is desired, locating the causative gland(s) may be difficult because of variation in embryological migration. Ultrasound scanning may indicate a single adenoma. Selective venous sampling can occasionally be undertaken (Figure 9.8). Isotope uptake scans and computed tomography (CT) or magnetic resonance imaging (MRI) may be useful (Box 9.10).

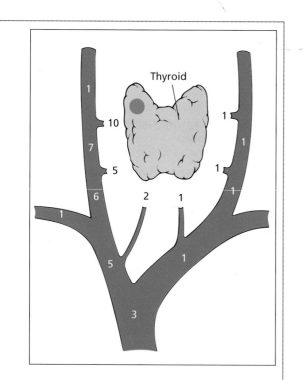

Figure 9.8 Venous sampling for parathyroid hormone (PTH) prior to surgery to localize a tumour in the upper right parathyroid gland (blue circle). The numbers indicate relative PTH levels (arbitrary scale). Values are higher in the right superior thyroid and right internal jugular veins than in other places such as the inferior thyroid veins and superior vena cava.

Treatment

Severe hypercalcaemia [> 3.0 mmol/L (12.0 mg/dL)] may present as a medical emergency (e.g. with arrhythmias) (Box 9.11). Most patients are dehydrated and simple rehydration can significantly reduce serum Ca^{2+}. Intravenous bisphosphonates (see section later on osteoporosis), such as pamidronate, inhibit bone resorption and rapidly reduce Ca^{2+} in the emergency setting. Glucocorticoids are effective in cases of haematological malignancy or sarcoidosis (see Chapter 6). Calcitonin also lowers serum Ca^{2+}. Dietary Ca^{2+} intake should be restricted.

Primary hyperparathyroidism with mildly increased serum Ca^{2+} in asymptomatic individuals can commonly be monitored as it rarely worsens. However, some argue that even mild hypercalcaemia is associated with excess morbidity, including depression, malaise and hypertension. Features other than very high Ca^{2+} levels that warrant definitive surgical treatment are clearly associated symptoms, renal impairment, stones or structural abnormality (increasing the risk of calcification or stone formation), and bone demineralization (see later section on osteoporosis) (Box 9.12). Although guidelines for when to intervene are relatively flexible, primary hyperparathyroidism associated with raised Ca^{2+} excretion and evidence of bone demineralization in a younger and otherwise fit patient should prompt serious thought of surgery, even when there are no symptoms, as long-term fracture risk is a concern. Even asymptomatic individuals may feel better once their Ca^{2+} has fallen to normal.

For a discrete adenoma, single parathyroidectomy with visualization of the normal glands is usually curative. Intraoperative dyes taken up by parathyroid tissue and histology of snap-frozen samples can improve the likelihood of curative removal.

Box 9.11 Emergency management of hypercalcaemia

- Intravenous rehydration
- Bisphosphonates
- Steroids if vitamin D toxicity or haematological malignancy
- Loop diuretics may be of limited value

Box 9.12 Indications for parathyroidectomy in primary hyperparathyroidism

- Renal stones, structural abnormality or impairment
- Bone disease (history of fractures, osteopaenia or osteoporosis)
- Clearly associated symptoms
- Age < 50 years irrespective of symptoms if otherwise fit
- More severe hypercalcaemia [>3.0 mmol/L (12.0 mg/dL)]

Other possible indications should be considered carefully and may include:
- Hypertension
- Psychiatric morbidity

Case history 9.3

An overweight, 50-year-old woman with a history of hypertension was found to have a serum Ca^{2+} of 2.58 mmol/L (10.32 mg/dL) and albumin of 36 g/L (3.6 g/dL). She consumed multiple supplements from health food shops. Her mother died aged 35 years from breast cancer and our patient is concerned that she may have breast cancer too.

What is her corrected calcium?
What are the possible explanations for the hypercalcaemia?

Answers, see p. 211

Removing all four glands would be necessary to treat parathyroid hyperplasia and is less readily undertaken; in the past, fragments of one gland have been re-implanted in the forearm to avoid hypoparathyroidism. Repeat neck surgery is technically difficult and it was considered easier to re-operate on the forearm if the patient redeveloped hypercalcaemia post-operatively.

For decision making in MEN1, see Chapter 10. For any parathyroid surgery, monitoring for hypoc-

Case history 9.4

At a routine occupational health check a 30-year-old man was found to have mild hypercalcaemia. He is anxious because the problem failed to resolve in his father, despite neck surgery. His uncle also has high Ca^{2+} levels. Both men are well into their late 50s.

What are the possible familial causes of hypercalcaemia?

Answers, see p. 212

alcaemia in the immediate postoperative period is mandatory, although most patients can be discharged with outpatient follow-up the following day if serum Ca^{2+} is normal.

Cinacalcet is a new drug that activates the CaSR. It can be used in secondary hyperparathyroidism and is licensed to treat hypercalcaemia in the very rare setting of parathyroid carcinoma.

For most other causes of hypercalcaemia (e.g. thyrotoxicosis; see Box 9.7), normalization occurs with treatment of the underlying condition.

Bone health and metabolic bone disease

Bone and its composition

The skeleton comprises two types of bone (Box 9.13). Even in adulthood, bone remodelling is perpetual and involves two matrices: ~35% of bone mass is organic matrix (osteoid), of which 90–95% is collagen (mainly type 1) (Box 9.14), with the remainder being proteoglycans, glycoproteins, sialoproteins and a small amount of lipid. Osteoid is subsequently mineralized into a hard, calcified extracellular matrix of hydroxyapatite [$3Ca_3(PO_4)_2$.$Ca(OH)_2$]. This inorganic component accounts for ~65% of bone mass and contains the vast majority of the adult body's ~1.2 kg of Ca^{2+}, 90% of its PO_4^{3-}, 50% of its Mg^{2+} and 33% of its Na^+.

Box 9.13 The two types of bone

Lamellar or compact bone
- In the shaft of adult long bones
- Consists of concentric lamellae around a central blood vessel
- Relatively inert metabolically

Cancellous or spongy bone
- In young subjects, at fracture sites and at the end of long bones
- Collagen fibres in loosely woven bundles
- Proportion increased in hyperparathyroidism
- High rate of turnover
- Large numbers of osteocytes present

Box 9.14 What is collagen?

- Many different types, bone contains mainly type 1 collagen
- Each type composed of different sub-units
- Large protein (MW ~300,000 kDa) rich in amino acids glycine, proline and hydroxyproline
- General formula is (glycine–proline.X)$_{333}$ (i.e. 333 repeating units) where X is another amino acid
- Semi-rigid, rod-like molecule of ~300 × 1.5 nm
- Molecules readily polymerize to form microfibrils and fibrils
- Secreted in immature form and cleaved into mature collagen in extracellular space
- Major component of osteoid
- Framework for initiating hydroxyapatite crystallization

Box 9.15 Osteoblasts and osteoclasts

Osteoblasts
- Synthesize new bone
- Stimulated by intermittent PTH, GH/IGF-I, androgens
- Differentiate from osteoprogenitors
- Differentiate into osteocytes

Osteoclasts
- Differentiate from haematopoietic stem cells
- Break down bone
- Stimulated by constant PTH, glucocorticoids and oestrogen withdrawal
- Inhibited by anti-resorptive agents (see Table 9.2)

Cell types in bone

Although several cell types lie in the bony matrix, it is the balance of action between two that determines bone formation versus resorption (Box 9.15 and Figure 9.9).

The bone-forming osteoblasts arise from immature fibroblast-like precursor cells called osteoprogenitors. Osteoblasts stimulate new bone formation by synthesizing osteoid and then help its mineralization. Although osteoid formation is relatively rapid (<1 day), its secondary mineralization takes much longer (1–2 months). Once bone formation is complete, the osteoblasts, embedded in new inorganic matrix, differentiate into relatively inactive cells called osteocytes.

Osteoclasts are responsible for resorption of bone at its surfaces through the action of lysosomal enzymes. They are large, multinucleated cells that differentiate as part of the myeloid lineage from haematopoietic stem cells in response to a range of growth factors and cytokines, some of which are secreted by osteoblasts, such as the ligand for the receptor activator of nuclear factor-kappa B (RANK ligand) (Figure 9.9).

Bone growth and remodelling during life

During childhood new bone formation matches requirements for linear growth, with both length and diameter of long bones increasing. Bone mass peaks in early adulthood (Figure 9.10). Thereafter, turnover of bone probably reflects the need to repair microtrauma and contribute to Ca^{2+} and PO_4^{3-} metabolism. It is tightly regulated by paracrine and endocrine factors. Although the mechanisms are

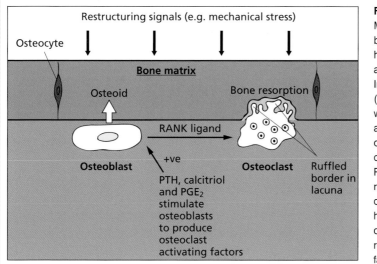

Figure 9.9 Bone remodelling. Mechanical stress influences bone remodelling while hormones control osteoblast and osteoclast activity. Intermittent parathyroid hormone (PTH) stimulates bone formation, while constant PTH, calcitriol and prostaglandin E_2 (PGE_2) act on the osteoblast to produce osteoclast-activating factors (e.g. RANK ligand) that result in bone resorption. Calcitonin inhibits osteoclast activity. Thyroid hormones can increase osteoclast activity. RANK, receptor activator of nuclear factor-kappa B.

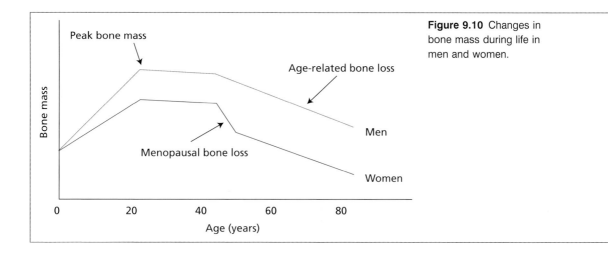

Figure 9.10 Changes in bone mass during life in men and women.

complex and frequently both direct and indirect (e.g. oestrogen action on resident immune cells), resorption is accurately coupled to formation (Box 9.15 and Figure 9.9). However, particularly in post-menopausal women lacking oestrogen, a small mismatch develops whereby resorption exceeds new bone formation. Consequently, as an individual ages, bone mass falls (Figure 9.10). Bone mass is also proportional to stature and weight. Larger gravitational forces are reflected by increased bone mass. At an extreme, astronauts experiencing weightlessness lose bone mass.

Clinical conditions of bone metabolism

Osteoporosis

Osteoporosis is characterized by low bone mass and micro-architectural deterioration. By WHO criteria (the data actually originate only from women), low bone mass is defined by its investigation using DEXA. DEXA measures bone mineral density (BMD) to generate a T-score, which represents the number of standard deviations above or below the

---

Box 9.16 Diagnostic criteria for osteoporosis on DEXA

Mean reference value:	T score of 0
Normal:	T score above −1.0
Osteopaenia:	T score −1.0 to −2.5
Osteoporosis:	T score below −2.5
Severe osteoporosis:	T score below −2.5 plus one or more fractures

---

Box 9.17 Risk factors for osteoporosis

Non-modifiable
- Age
- Female sex
- Polygenic inheritance; Caucasian or Asian race and family history
- Low body mass index

Modifiable
- Hypogonadism (see Chapter 7)
- Cushing syndrome or glucocorticoid therapy (e.g. for asthma) (see Chapter 6)
- Thyrotoxicosis (see Chapter 8)
- Hyperparathyroidism
- Type 1 diabetes (see Chapter 12)
- Drugs (alcohol, heparin, tobacco smoking, some antipsychotics)
- Chronic disease:
  - Liver
  - Renal
  - Malabsorption/bowel
  - Post-transplantation
  - Rheumatoid arthritis
  - Malignancy
  - Connective tissue disorders

---

mean reference value for healthy young individuals with peak bone mass. Osteoporosis is defined when the T-score is −2.5 or lower (Box 9.16).

Osteoporosis increases the risk of fracture, mainly at the hip, spine and wrist. The scale of the problem is massive. The lifetime risk of a fracture related to osteoporosis is 1 in 2 for US women compared to 1 in 8 for US men. In the UK, it is estimated that 1.2 million women have osteoporosis; ~60,000 hip fractures, 50,000 distal radial fractures and 40,000 vertebral fractures occur annually. This may be an underestimate as many vertebral fractures may not come to clinical attention. Hip fractures occupy 20% of all orthopaedic hospital beds. Up to 20% of patients with osteoporotic hip fracture die within 1 year and up to 50% lose their independence. The estimated total NHS cost of acute management of osteoporotic fractures is ~£2 billion in 2011.

Age is the major risk factor for osteoporosis as bone mass gradually declines after the mid-20s (Box 9.17). Elderly women are at the greatest risk because bone loss is accelerated to varying degrees after the menopause secondary to the loss of oestrogen. This makes women with premature ovarian failure and no oestrogen replacement at particular risk (review hormone replacement therapy in Chapter 7). Polygenic factors and race are other non-modifiable risk factors. Lighter, slight individuals are also at greater risk as BMD is lower throughout life. Osteoporosis may also be secondary to a number of other more modifiable causes (Box 9.17). This can be so predictable that anti-resorptive agents should be started routinely when patients commence long-term glucocorticoids (Table 9.2).

Table 9.2 Drugs used to prevent bone demineralization and to treat osteoporosis

Inhibitors of resorption	Stimulators of bone formation
Calcium and vitamin D	Parathyroid hormone (intermittent)
Bisphosphonates	Strontium ranelate
Sex hormone replacement therapy*	Sodium fluoride
Selective oestrogen receptor modulators (SERMS)	
Calcitonin (rarely used)	
Denosumab	

*In men and pre-menopausal women.

Symptoms and signs

The most common presentation of osteoporosis is fracture (or bone pain); particularly suspicious is fracture following trivial impact (Case history 9.5). Many patients will also be diagnosed by DEXA performed routinely in high-risk individuals, such as those with hypogonadism.

Investigation and diagnosis

Osteoporosis is diagnosed on the basis of T-score measured by DEXA (see Box 9.16). DEXA values are obtained bilaterally at the hip, spine and sometimes the wrist. T-scores that are abnormally low (below −1.0) but not osteoporotic are termed osteopaenic (T-score of −1.0 to −2.5).

Where osteoporosis has been detected unexpectedly, history, examination and investigations should seek to exclude modifiable factors (Box 9.17).

Treatment

Management can be divided into treating osteoporosis with drugs and supplements, and addressing wider issues. As immobilization causes bone loss, weight-bearing activity is important. This should not be so excessive as to cause oestrogen deficiency through hypothalamic amenorrhoea, as occurs in elite female runners and ballet dancers (see Chapter 7). Patients should moderate alcohol consumption and be encouraged to stop smoking. Other modifiable risk factors should be minimized (Box 9.17). As the major outcome measure is morbidity and mortality, not T-score, risk of falls should be addressed, especially in the elderly and infirm. Sometimes, very simple interventions are possible such as avoiding ill-fitting slippers and removing rugs. Additional risk factors for falls include dehydration, postural hypotension and untreated Parkinson disease.

In the UK 10–20% of women receive drug treatment for bone mineralization. The choice of anti-resorptive or anabolic agent is influenced by age, BMD, stage of disease, whether there has been a fracture (and if so, where and what type), co-morbidities and side-effects (Table 9.2). Anti-resorptive drugs preserve existing bone mass, while anabolic agents increase *de novo* cancellous bone mass.

Anti-resorptive drugs

The two first-line therapies for osteoporosis are both primarily anti-resorptive. Combined dietary Ca^{2+} and vitamin D supplementation reduces fracture rates in the elderly. Bisphosphonates, such as alendronate, zoledronic acid and risedronate, robustly reduce fracture risk; 40–50% reduction for vertebrae, 40–60% for hip and 30–40% at other non-vertebral sites. Bisphosphonates are synthetic analogues of pyrophosphate that become incorporated into bone where they have a very long half-life. They inhibit osteoclast activation and function and promote their apoptosis. Many are now available as long-acting preparations (e.g. once yearly zoledronate infusion). All bisphosphonates raise concern that while profound suppression of bone turnover enhances BMD on DEXA, it may also compromise the bone's capacity to repair minor trauma. Alendronate can cause significant upper gastrointestinal symptoms and lower oesophageal erosions.

In women with premature ovarian failure, sex steroid hormone replacement therapy (HRT) should be given to maintain bone mineralization until the normal time of the menopause (~50 years; review Chapter 7). Similarly, the need for sex steroid action on bone is why it is important to treat hyperprolactinaemia that results in secondary hypogonadism. HRT was used previously to treat post-menopausal osteoporosis. It is effective at reducing fracture rates while it is taken. However, bone mass rapidly declines after cessation of treatment such that 5 years of peri-menopausal therapy fails to protect against fracture two to three decades later (when it matters). Long-term HRT is reported to increase the risk of cardiovascular disease and stroke, and some forms of cancer. Selective oestrogen receptor modulators (SERMs, e.g. raloxifene) act as weak oestrogen receptor (ER) agonists in some tissues, including bone, and as ER antagonists in others. As such, they significantly reduce vertebral fracture risk while minimizing side-effects of HRT. In male hypogonadism, androgen should be replaced long term when it has beneficial effects on bone mass (review Chapter 7).

Calcitonin nasal spray is associated with reduced fracture risk but is not routinely used.

Denosumab is a human monoclonal antibody that binds RANK ligand and prevents its activation of osteoclasts (review Figure 9.9). Its use is approved in women with post-menopausal osteoporosis and high fracture risk.

Anabolic drugs

Intermittent PTH stimulates new bone formation. Synthetic PTH(1-34) (teriparatide; the first 34 amino acids of PTH, see earlier) can be given by daily injection in osteoporosis with high fracture risk refractory to first-line approaches. There is some concern that it increases risk of osteosarcoma.

Strontium ranelate (registered in the UK and much of Europe but not in the USA) is the only agent that both activates osteoblasts and inhibits osteoclasts. It has been shown to reduce vertebral and non-vertebral fracture risk.

Monitoring

Treatment can be monitored by serial DEXA every 2 years or so. More frequent investigation is unhelpful. Although some serum biomarkers of bone turnover have been identified, large inter- and intra-individual variability restricts their value in clinical practice; serial measurements may be useful in monitoring short-term responses to therapy.

🔍 Case history 9.5

A 57-year-old woman with long-standing, severe asthma tripped on the carpet. She now complains of a pain in her back and a radiograph suggests demineralized bone and a wedge fracture of her L3 vertebra.

Why has this woman had a fracture?
What are the possible treatments?

Answers, see p. 212

Vitamin D deficiency, osteomalacia and rickets

Although vitamin D intimately regulates Ca^{2+} metabolism, its deficiency tends not to cause hypocalcaemia, but does cause failure of osteoid mineralization (Figure 9.11). In growing children this presents more severely as rickets with bowing deformity of long bones, which are described as rachitic. The normal columnar arrangement of chondrocytes in the hypertrophic zone of cartilaginous growth is elongated and distorted, and calcification is delayed or absent (Figure 9.11). There are vascular abnormalities. In adulthood, once bones have stopped growing, presentation is that of milder osteomalacia with bone pain and fragility.

Vitamin D deficiency in children was a major public health problem in industrialized nations in the northern hemisphere (i.e. poor sunlight exposure) until the 1920s when it was discovered that cod liver oil could cure rickets. This led to widespread vitamin D fortification of milk, which was effective in virtually eliminating rickets. More recently, ceasing free milk programmes in UK schools, coupled to very effective total sun block marketing, has led to a resurgence of vitamin D deficiency. A number of groups are at particularly high risk (Box 9.18) (Case history 9.6).

Symptoms and signs

Bone pain is now the predominant clinical feature, which may occur because of mineralization defects leading to the X-ray appearance of pseudofractures (also called Looser zones). In addition, there may be a proximal myopathy causing profound weakness of the hip and shoulder girdle. Hypocalcaemia may occur (see Box 9.6).

Specifically in rickets, physical and radiological signs tend to be found where bone growth is most active; usually the metaphyseal region of long bones. At birth, the skull is growing most rapidly and therefore neonatal rickets may show craniotabes, where the cranial vaults have the consistency of a ping-pong ball. From the age of 1 year, rickets manifests as swollen epiphyses of the wrist and swelling of the costochondral junction, so-called 'rickety rosary'.

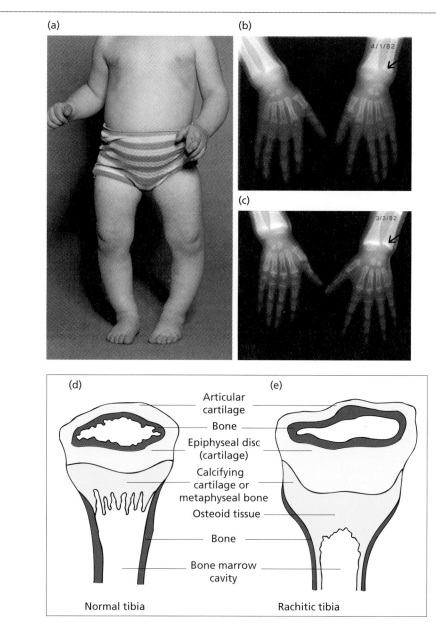

Figure 9.11 Rickets. (a) Bowing of the tibiae in a 3-year-old. (b) Radiological features showing expansion, irregularity and 'cupping' of the metaphyses (arrow). (c) Radiological features of healing rickets: note the increased density and definition of the metaphysis (arrow). Note also the reduced thickness of the radiolucent radial epiphyseal cartilage from (b) to (c). (d) During normal growth, epiphyseal disc with the underlying zone of calcifying cartilage. (e) In rickets, the epiphyseal disc is greatly enlarged [as in (b)] with a thick underlying zone of osteoid tissue, i.e. uncalcified matrix.

Box 9.18 Groups at risk of vitamin D deficiency

- The elderly, particularly those in residential care
- Babies of vitamin D-deficient mothers
- Those with skin conditions where avoidance of sunlight is advised
- Dark skinned people, particularly if fully veiled for cultural or religious beliefs
- Vegans
- Patients with malabsorption

Box 9.19 Secondary causes of rickets and osteomalacia

- Chronic renal failure – lack of 1α-hydroxylase activity
- Drugs – barbiturate and phenytoin interfere with vitamin D metabolism
- Congenital deficiency of 1α-hydroxylase activity
- PO_4^{3-} depletion
- Renal tubular disorders – these may be congenital, e.g. inactivating *PHEX* mutations in X-linked dominant hypophosphataemic rickets

Investigation and diagnosis

Vitamin D measurement is usually done as cholecalciferol (25-hydroxyvitamin D) rather than calcitriol (1,25-hydroxyvitamin D) because of the former's longer half-life. Serum alkaline phosphatase is raised and Ca^{2+} and PO_4^{3-} may be low. Plain X-rays of painful sites may show pseudofractures. Conditions causing osteomalacia and rickets other than dietary vitamin D deficiency should be considered (Box 9.19).

Treatment

The normal treatment of vitamin D deficiency is oral cholecalciferol, either as a daily dose, e.g. 25 µg (1000 IU) in adults or as a single large dose, e.g. 5 mg (225,000 IU). Improvement occurs within weeks, but it may take as long as a year before the skeleton returns to normal. Although vitamin D replacement leads to rapid normalization of 25-hydroxycholecalciferol concentrations, calcitriol levels become and remain elevated for many months because of increased 1α-hydroxylase activity; a consequence of secondary hyperparathyroidism.

Other causes of rickets and osteomalacia will respond to vitamin D replacement, although much higher doses may be required in hypophosphataemic rickets. As in primary hypoparathyroidism leading to lack of 1α-hydroxylase activity active vitamin D (calcitriol) should be given.

Long-term, it is important not to over-treat to avoid hypercalcaemia (see Box 9.9).

Case history 9.6

A 73-year-old South Asian woman taking bendrofluazide for hypertension attended her local practitioner because of tiredness. She was vegan and wore a veil. The doctor identified a corrected serum Ca^{2+} of 2.60 mmol/L (10.4 mg/dL) and went on to measure PTH, which was increased several fold above the upper limit of normal. Primary hyperparathyroidism was diagnosed.

Is the diagnosis necessarily correct? What other hormone measurement might demonstrate an alternative diagnosis?

Answers, see p. 212

🔑 Key points

- Hormonal Ca^{2+} homeostasis is via PTH and vitamin D
- Hypocalcaemia in the western world is commonly from surgical trauma/removal or autoimmune destruction of the parathyroids
- Hypocalcaemia may be asymptomatic, but can present with muscle cramps, numbness and paraesthesia
- Hypocalcaemia is treated with Ca^{2+} and vitamin D
- Common causes of hypercalcaemia include primary hyperparathyroidism and malignancy
- Hypercalcaemia may be asymptomatic, but remember 'bones, stones, moans and groans'
- Osteoporosis, defined by DEXA T-score, is low bone mass and micro-architectural deterioration leading to increased fracture risk
- Osteomalacia (adults) and rickets (children) result from vitamin D deficiency causing a failure to calcify osteoid

🔍 Answers to case histories

Case history 9.1

The most likely explanation of the paraesthesia is hypocalcaemia because of inadvertent removal of or damage to the parathyroid glands (i.e. hypoparathyroidism). Alternatively, she may be hyperventilating because of her anxiety. The symptoms are the same because over-breathing may induce a fall in serum ionized Ca^{2+} concentration. This results from the disturbance of the following equilibria:

$$CO_2 + H_2O \rightleftharpoons H_2CO_3^-$$

$$H_2CO_3^- \rightleftharpoons H^+ + HCO_3^-$$

$$Albumin\text{-}H \rightleftharpoons Albumin^- + H^+$$

$$Albumin^- + Ca^{2+} \rightleftharpoons Albumin\text{-}Ca$$

As the woman over-breathes, the partial pressure of carbon dioxide falls, leading to respiratory alkalosis from decreased production of hydrogen ions (H^+) from $H_2CO_3^-$. To compensate H^+ ions dissociate from albumin allowing increased binding of Ca^{2+} to the protein. Thus, ionized Ca^{2+} concentration falls and can be sufficient to induce tetany or paraesthesia. The two causes can be easily distinguished because total serum Ca^{2+} would not change in hyperventilation, while it would fall if there were parathyroid dysfunction.

Hypoparathyroidism is treated by supplementation with Ca^{2+} and vitamin D, usually α-calcidol (because 1α-hydroxylase activity is lacking), to maintain serum Ca^{2+} values at the lower end of normal (to avoid excessive Ca^{2+} flux through the kidney). The hypoparathyroidism may be temporary from reversible operative trauma. Withdrawal of treatment could be trialled at out-patient follow-up. Hyperventilation can be treated by re-breathing into a paper bag.

Case history 9.2

Type 1 autoimmune polyglandular syndrome (APS-1) is consistent with all aspects of the history and examination. The patient has primary hypoparathyroidism with a family history suggesting an inherited cause. The white plaques are suggestive of candidiasis ('thrush'), more commonly found in the genital tract, but in APS-1 this manifests in the throat. The syndrome is very rare; therefore, it is important to consider more common diagnoses, e.g. by taking a history and examining for previous neck surgery. The sore throat and family history could also be chance findings in a patient with isolated autoimmune hypoparathyroidism.

If the family has APS-1, gaining a molecular genetic diagnosis is important as a mutation would allow straightforward identification or exclusion of the syndrome in other family members. The *AIRE* gene should be amplified and sequenced from genomic DNA (review Chapter 4). To facilitate this investigation and family assessment, referral to clinical genetics should be considered. The patient and affected family members are at risk of other autoimmune endocrinopathies; e.g. hypoadrenalism, which can be life-threatening. Therefore, potential underactivity of the thyroid, adrenal cortex and reproductive axis should be assessed by history, examination and investigation (see Chapters 6–8). Follow-up should ideally be in a specialist endocrinology clinic. Finally, a young woman at risk of premature ovarian failure should be counselled on future fertility and family planning to allow her to make informed choices.

Case history 9.3

Albumin is 4 units below 40 g/L; therefore 4×0.02 (i.e. 0.08) needs to be added to the uncorrected serum Ca^{2+} of 2.58 mmol/L, making the corrected serum Ca^{2+} 2.66 mmol/L (10.64 mg/dL).

There are several potential reasons for her hypercalcaemia: vitamin D excess from her non-prescribed supplements; venesection may have been difficult with prolonged tourniquet application; she may be taking a thiazide diuretic for hypertension; she may have a familial form of breast cancer with hypercalcaemia of malignancy. These possibilities need addressing alongside potential primary hyperparathyroidism.

Case history 9.4

There are several causes of familial hypercalcaemia. The most serious one is MEN1 (primary hyperparathyroidism is commonly the first manifestation; see Chapter 10). However, the fact that both men are well and neck surgery was unsuccessful suggests familial benign hypercalcaemia. It is benign in most situations but is important to recognize so that parathyroidectomy for mis-diagnosed primary hyperparathyroidism is avoided.

Case history 9.5

Although we do not know the force with which she fell, the impact seems rather trivial, suggesting a pathological fracture. Given the X-ray, the most likely cause is osteoporosis, although other pathology like tumour metastasis needs consideration. Likely contributing factors to osteoporosis here are post-menopausal age and severe asthma, most likely treated with glucocorticoids (possibly systemic). Other factors need interrogation (e.g. smoking and alcohol intake).

Having made a diagnosis of osteoporosis by DEXA, calcium and vitamin D supplementation, and bisphosphonate therapy (especially if on long-term oral glucocorticoid therapy) would be first-line treatments.

Case history 9.6

The diagnosis is not necessarily correct. Bendrofluazide could cause mildly increased serum Ca^{2+}. Raised serum PTH could reflect vitamin D deficiency. She most likely has poor UV light exposure and a diet quite possibly deficient in vitamin D. Serum vitamin D should be measured, most likely as cholecalciferol. If low, vitamin D should be replaced. Once replete, PTH is likely to have fallen to normal. It would also be worth re-checking the serum Ca^{2+} as the first very subtly raised value might have been spurious.

CHAPTER 10

Pancreatic and gastrointestinal endocrinology and endocrine neoplasia

Key topics

- Pancreatic and gastrointestinal endocrinology — 214
- Familial endocrine neoplasia — 223
- Ectopic hormone syndromes — 227
- Hormone-sensitive solid tumours — 228
- Key points — 230
- Answers to case histories — 231

Learning objectives

- To appreciate and understand the roles of gastrointestinal and pancreatic hormones
- To recognize the clinical consequences of gut hormone tumours
- To understand how hormone-secreting tumours can be inherited
- To appreciate ways in which endocrinology may interact with oncology:
  - ☐ The clinical manifestations of ectopic hormone production
  - ☐ How hormones can affect other solid tissue tumours

This chapter discusses pancreatic and gastrointestinal endocrinology and endocrine tumours

Essential Endocrinology and Diabetes, Sixth Edition. Richard IG Holt, Neil A Hanley.
© 2012 Richard IG Holt and Neil A Hanley. Publlished 2012 by Blackwell Publishing Ltd.

To recap

- Gastrointestinal and pancreatic hormones are peptides, the biosynthesis of which is covered in Chapter 2
- Some solid tumours in the breast and prostate are sensitive to steroid hormones, providing therapeutic strategies and making it timely to review nuclear hormone action (see Chapter 3)

Cross-reference

- Function of the pancreatic islet β-cell and α-cell is also covered in Chapter 11 on diabetes mellitus
- Tumours secreting adrenomedullary hormones are an important component of familial neoplasia syndromes and are also covered in Chapter 6
- Tumours of the thyroid present with goitre, the examination and investigation of which is described in Chapter 8
- Tumours and hyperplasia of the parathyroid glands, part of multiple endocrine neoplasia syndromes, cause primary hyperparathyroidism (see Chapter 9)
- Incretin hormones, an important area of gastrointestinal endocrinology, are now exploited therapeutically in diabetes (see Chapter 13)

This chapter is arranged into three sections: pancreatic and gastrointestinal endocrinology as a forerunner to understanding hormone-secreting tumours from these sites; familial endocrine neoplasia syndromes; and other tumours and hormone-sensitive cancers. While the latter are the mainstay of other specialties, antagonizing hormone action can be an important component of therapy.

Pancreatic and gastrointestinal endocrinology

Endocrine cells secreting a multitude of hormones are present throughout the gastrointestinal tract and in the pancreas (Table 10.1). Their development is similar and regulated by critical transcription factors, foremost amongst which is neurogenin-3 (Neurog3 or Ngn3). If Neurog3 fails to act, no endocrine cell types are formed either in the pancreas or in the gastrointestinal tract.

Pancreatic and gastrointestinal hormones regulate digestion and broad aspects of metabolism. Therefore, tumours secreting inappropriate or excessive amounts of these hormones can cause syndromes with distinctive symptoms and signs. Some of the tumours arise as part of multiple endocrine neoplasia (MEN) type 1 (see later section).

Pancreatic islet endocrinology

In the pancreas, endocrine cell types aggregate as islets of Langerhans and comprise ~1% of the organ embedded within the surrounding exocrine tissue that secretes digestive enzymes (Table 10.1 and Chapter 11).

Insulin

The predominant islet cell type is the insulin-secreting β-cell (Table 10.1 and Figure 10.1). Insulin acts to lower blood glucose. Its release is proportional to the ambient glucose concentration. Its inadequacy leads to diabetes (Chapters 11–14). The hormone is synthesized initially as pre-proinsulin and stored in intracellular granules complexed with zinc. Enzymatic cleavage by prohormone convertase 1/3 (PC1/3) during hormone secretion yields mature insulin and equimolar amounts of

Table 10.1 Pancreatic and gastrointestinal hormones

Hormone	Amino acids (active form)	Cell type	Location	Major stimulus	Major action	Receptor-signalling (review Chapter 3)
Pancreas						
Insulin	51	β-cell	Islet	High glucose	Lowers serum glucose (see Chapter. 11)	IR-TK
Glucagon	29	α-cell	Islet	Low glucose	Raises serum glucose (see Chapter 11)	GPCR
Somatostatin (SS)	28, 14	δ-cell	Islet		Inhibits secretion of insulin, glucagon, VIP, GIP, secretin, motilin, CCK and GH (SS also in brain – see Chapter 5)	GPCR
Pancreatic polypeptide (PP)	36	PP-cell	Islet	Fasting, hypoglycaemia	Poorly understood; seems to coordinate islet function	GPCR
Ghrelin	28 (+ modification by fatty acid)	ε-cell D1-cell	Islet Stomach	Fasting	Stimulates hunger (see Chapter 15)/stimulates GH (see Chapter 5)	GPCR
Gastrointestinal						
Gastrin	34 (big), 17 (little), 14 (mini)	G-cell	Stomach, duodenum and pancreas	Stomach distension, vagal input, Ca^{2+}, amino acids	Stimulates gastric acid secretion from parietal cells; stimulates pepsinogen secretion	GPCR
Vasoactive intestinal peptide (VIP)	28	Enteric neurones	Nerves in islet and throughout intestine	Cholinergic nerve activity	A range of effects that in combination stimulate intestinal motility	GPCR

(Continued)

Table 10.1 (Continued)

Hormone	Amino acids (active form)	Cell type	Location	Major stimulus	Major action	Receptor-signalling (review Chapter 3)
Glucagon-like peptide 1 (GLP-1)	37	L-cell	Small intestine, especially the terminal ileum*	High intestinal glucose/nutrients	Incretin; enhances glucose-sensitive insulin secretion (GSIS) by pancreatic β-cell	GPCR
Glucose-dependent insulinotropic peptide (GIP)	42	K-cell	Duodenum and jejunum	High intestinal glucose/nutrients	Incretin; enhances GSIS by pancreatic β-cell	GPCR
Cholecystokinin (CCK)	58, 33, 8	I-cell	Duodenum	Fat/protein in duodenum	Stimulates bile and pancreatic secretion to allow fat digestion	GPCR
Secretin	27	S-cell	Duodenum	Low pH	Stimulates pancreatic bicarbonate secretion to buffer stomach acid in small intestine; stimulates bile secretion	GPCR
Motilin	22	M-cell	Duodenum and jejenum	High pH	Stimulates intestinal motility	GPCR
Serotonin	Synthesized from tryptophan	Enteroendocrine cells and enteric neurones	Throughout intestine	Food in intestine causing enteric nerve activity	Regulates intestinal motility	GPCR

*Some GLP-1 is most likely produced by the α-cell in the pancreatic islet and also from the large bowel.
IR, insulin receptor; TK, tyrosine kinase; GH, growth hormone; GPCR, G-protein–coupled receptor.

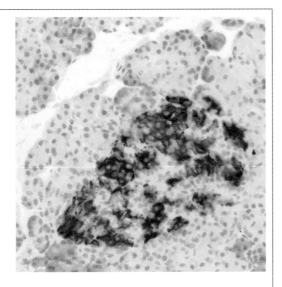

Figure 10.1 A pancreatic islet surrounded by exocrine tissue. β-cells are demonstrated by immunohistochemistry for stored insulin (brown staining). Image courtesy of Rachel Salisbury, University of Manchester.

C-peptide [PC1/3 also cleaves adrenocorticotrophic hormone (ACTH) from pro-opiomelanocortin (POMC); review Figure 2.4 and Chapter 5].

Insulinoma (and the differential diagnosis of hypoglycaemia)

Insulinomas are rare β-cell tumours that secrete insulin excessively and inappropriately (i.e. when blood glucose is already low; Table 10.1). They are usually benign with a median age of presentation of ~50 years. However, they may present earlier and be malignant, especially when part of MEN-1.

Symptoms and signs

The major clinical feature is a tendency to hypoglycaemia. Symptoms include light-headedness and hunger, precipitated by fasting or exercise and relieved temporarily by eating. More profound hypoglycaemia is an ever-present risk in diabetes treated with insulin injections (see Chapter 12).

Insulinomas are very rare, making the differential diagnosis important (see Boxes 10.1 and 10.2). Some individuals develop hypoglycaemic symptoms a few hours after a large meal when large carbohydrate loads, particularly those containing refined sugars, in the intestine are thought to over-stimulate insulin secretion, causing a 'reactive hypoglycaemia' (Case history 10.1). This can occur in patients with dumping syndrome which may also be a complication of bariatric surgery (Chapter 15) and in patients with co-existing cortisol deficiency (Addison disease; see Chapter 6 and Case history 10.2).

In patients who are usually clearly unwell (e.g. cachectic) with large solid mesenchymal tumours, an alternative IGF-II protein (called big IGF-II) can cause non-islet cell tumour hypoglycaemia (NICTH) by failing to bind IGF binding proteins with consequent excessive hormone action. In contrast to insulinoma, serum insulin is undetectable. Surgical removal of the tumour is the treatment of choice but if this is impossible, glucocorticoids or growth hormone (GH) can prevent the hypoglycaemia.

In children, GH deficiency can present with hypoglycaemia.

Investigation and diagnosis

The diagnosis of hypoglycaemia is made by demonstrating serum glucose <2.2 mmol/L (40 mg/dL) by laboratory assay (i.e. not by capillary glucose monitor as used in diabetes; see Chapter 12). This can be precipitated by admission to hospital for a 72-h fast when plasma glucose is measured regularly and, if hypoglycaemia occurs, a simultaneous sample can be assayed for insulin and C-peptide. Detecting the latter alongside insulin indicates endogenous β-cell overactivity rather than injection of synthetic insulin. Sulphonylureas, which stimulate the β-cell, are used to treat type 2 diabetes (see Chapter 13) and can also cause hypoglycaemia; they can be detected in toxicological screens of urine and blood. It is exceptional for reactive hypoglycaemia in otherwise well individuals to lower blood glucose below 2.2 mmol/L (40 mg/dL) (Box 10.1).

Once a biochemical diagnosis of hypoglycaemia secondary to endogenous insulin has been made, the search for an insulinoma is performed by magnetic resonance imaging (MRI) or computed tomography (CT). Imaging facilitates surgery yet can be challenging because tumours may be small and multiple. Arteriography and endoscopic ultrasound can be used. Insulinomas occur more frequently in the pancreatic tail where most β-cells reside.

Box 10.1 Differential diagnosis of hypoglycaemia

Inappropriate levels of insulin and C-peptide
- Insulinoma
- Sulphonylurea overdose
- Congenital hyperinsulinism
- Neonatal consequence of maternal diabetes in pregnancy
- Reactive hypoglycaemia [highly unlikely to lower serum glucose <2.2 mmol/L (40 mg/dL) if patient otherwise well]

Inappropriate level of insulin, low C-peptide
- Exogenous insulin overdose – accidental (common in diabetes, Chapter 12) or deliberate/malicious

Low insulin
- Non-islet cell tumour hypoglycaemia
- Hypoadrenalism (can exacerbate reactive hypoglycaemia)
- GH deficiency (in children)

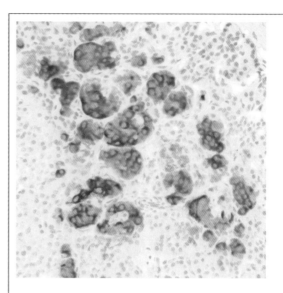

Figure 10.2 Congenital hyperinsulinism (diffuse form). Immunohistochemistry for insulin (brown staining) shows widespread clusters of β-cells in the pancreas resected from an infant who presented with hypoglycaemia. Image courtesy of Rachel Salisbury, University of Manchester.

Treatment

Treatment is by surgery, but where this is impossible, diazoxide may ameliorate hypoglycaemia. Somatostatin analogues, such as octreotide, may also be useful in preventing hypoglycaemia by inhibiting insulin secretion.

Congenital hyperinsulinism and neonatal hypoglycaemia

Excessive and inappropriate insulin secretion can also arise from genetic defects in components of the glucose-sensing/insulin secretion pathway, such as constitutive activity of the ATP-sensitive K^+ channel (see Figure 11.9). This congenital hyperinsulinism presents in infancy as either focal or diffuse pancreatic disease and is treated by diazoxide and surgical resection (Figure 10.2). The latter is inherited as an autosomal recessive disorder. Conversely neonatal diabetes, which affects 1 in 100,000–200,000 live births, may result from inactivating mutations of the ATP-sensitive K^+ channel (type 1 diabetes is rare before 1 year).

Transient hypoglycaemia can also occur in neonates of mothers with diabetes; fetal hypergly-caemia increases fetal insulin secretion in late gestation that persists transiently at inappropriately high levels after birth (see Chapter 14).

Case history 10.1

An overweight 37-year-old woman consulted her doctor because 2–3 h after a meal she became light-headed, sweaty and felt faint. Her symptoms improved with food. She has a family history of type 2 diabetes. She mentioned that once when she felt unwell, she borrowed her mother's blood glucose meter and found that the reading was 3.2 mmol/L (~60 mg/dL).

What is the most likely diagnosis?
How might you investigate the cause of her symptoms?

Answers, see p. 231

Case history 10.2

A 34-year-old man presented as an emergency to hospital having fainted upon standing up. A passerby who had diabetes used her glucose monitor and obtained a reading of 1.9 mmol/L (~34 mg/dL). She called an ambulance. The man recovered quickly and on questioning reported that he had a mother who took thyroxine. He was tanned. A blood result from hospital revealed serum K^+ of 5.6 mmol/L (5.6 mEq/L).

What is the diagnosis until proven otherwise?
What other examination and investigations would you perform?
What emergency treatment is needed?

Answers, see p. 231

Glucagon

α-cells are arranged around the β-cells in pancreatic islets and secrete glucagon (see Table 10.1 and Figure 11.7). Glucagon is antagonistic to insulin, acting to mobilize the liver's stored carbohydrate and raise serum glucose (see Chapter 11). It acts via its cell surface G-protein–coupled receptor and is used by injection in an emergency to treat hypoglycaemia in diabetes (see Chapter 12).

Glucagonomas are tumours of the pancreatic α-cells secreting excess glucagon, the hallmark of which is secondary diabetes (Box 10.2). In addition, there can be an unusual migratory skin rash associated with amino acid and zinc deficiency (necrolytic migratory erythema). Glucagonomas may also lead to hypertrophy of the intestinal villi and mucosal thickening, which may be noted during gastroscopy or CT scanning of the abdomen. Treatment is by surgery wherever possible.

Somatostatin

Somatostatin is secreted by δ-cells scattered in the pancreatic islets where it inhibits secretion of insulin

Box 10.2 Gastrointestinal hormone-secreting tumours

Gastrinoma
- Profound reduction in gastric pH causing severe ulceration of stomach and duodenum
- Treated by proton pump inhibitors or surgery

Insulinoma
- Causes hypoglycaemia (Box 10.1)
- Treated by surgery but may be improved with diazoxide or somatostatin analogues

Glucagonoma
- Causes secondary diabetes (+ typical skin rash)
- Villous hypertrophy on gastroscopy
- Treated by surgery

Somatostatinoma
- Causes secondary diabetes, reduced gastric acid secretion, gallstones, steatorrhoea and weight loss
- Treated by surgery

VIPoma/Verner–Morrison syndrome
- Presents with severe watery diarrhoea, hypokalaemia and skin flushing
- Treated by surgery or somatostatin analogues

Carcinoid tumour
- See Box 10.3

and glucagon (Table 10.1). It is also synthesized by hypothalamic neurones to regulate growth hormone (GH) (see Figure 5.5) and in other endocrine cell types throughout the gastrointestinal tract, where it has multiple inhibitory effects on gut motility and exocrine secretion.

Rare tumours of the pancreatic δ-cells are called somatostatinomas and present variably, but tend to cause diabetes, reduced gastric acid secretion, gallstones, steatorrhoea and weight loss (Box 10.2). Treatment is by surgery wherever possible.

Pancreatic polypeptide

The pancreatic polypeptide cells of the islet secrete pancreatic polypeptide (see Table 10.1). The function of this hormone remains somewhat unclear and tumours secreting it are exceptionally rare.

Ghrelin

Ghrelin is secreted by ε-cells of the pancreatic islet and by cells in the body of the stomach. It inhibits GH secretion and is involved in appetite control (see Chapters 5 and 15; Figure 5.5). No syndrome has been described from its excess or inappropriate action.

Gastrointestinal endocrinology

Intestinal hormone-secreting cells scattered throughout the stomach wall and at the bottom of intestinal crypts are termed 'enteroendocrine'. They secrete a multitude of hormones that regulate gastrointestinal function and metabolism (see Table 10.1). Some of the hormones, such as vasoactive intestinal polypeptide (VIP), are actually released from the enteric nervous system and function as neurotransmitters (review Figure 1.1). Not all of the cells and hormones are associated with tumour syndromes.

Gastrin

Gastrin is secreted as peptides of three sizes from G-cells in the duodenum, pancreas and antral part of the gastric mucosa following distension of the stomach by food or by the presence of small peptides or amino acids within the stomach (see Table 10.1). Anticipation of eating also increases gastrin secretion via the vagus nerve. Gastrin increases stomach acid secretion and blood flow to the gastric mucosa. Gastrin is thought to play a role in gastric motility and peristalsis. Once the pH of the stomach falls below 2.5, negative feedback inhibits further gastrin release. Its secretion is also inhibited by somatostatin, glucagon and VIP.

Zollinger–Ellison syndrome

Gastrinomas, first described by Zollinger and Ellison, over-secrete gastrin and tend to arise in the duodenum or the pancreas (Box 10.2). Profound gastric acidity causes severe ulceration of the stomach and duodenum (Case history 10.3). From its original description, Zollinger-Ellison syndrome refers to the triad of peptic ulceration, excess gastric acid and a pancreatic islet tumour secreting gastrin. Diagnosis is made by assaying fasting levels of serum gastrin. Visualizing the tumour can be difficult, but MRI, CT and endoscopic ultrasound may be useful. Proton pump inhibitors (drug names ending with '-prazole') are effective in controlling the acid secretion. The ideal surgical treatment is discrete removal of the tumour or, if this is not possible, partial gastrectomy.

🔍 Case history 10.3

A 64-year-old man presented to the emergency surgery team with sudden onset of severe upper abdominal pain. On examination, his abdomen was rigid. Serum amylase was normal. Erect abdominal X-ray revealed air under the diaphragm. He took no medications. At operation there was a perforated duodenal ulcer. Five years previously he had had emergency endoscopy to control a bleeding duodenal ulcer. A doctor measured a fasting level of a gastrointestinal hormone that could account for the repeated ulceration. The hormone was elevated.

What was the hormone?
What further investigations are warranted to investigate this elevated hormone level?

Answers, see p. 231

Vasoactive intestinal polypeptide

VIP is a 28-amino acid peptide neurotransmitter in the gut and central nervous system. At pharmacological doses, VIP increases hepatic glucose release, insulin secretion and pancreatic bicarbonate production, while inhibiting stomach acid production, partly through relaxation of gastric blood vessels and smooth muscle. These actions are similar to those of glucagon, secretin and glucose-dependent insulinotrophic peptide (GIP; also known as gastric inhibitory peptide). GIP and VIP may have evolved from a single gene.

VIPomas and Verner–Morrison syndrome

VIPomas, first described by Verner and Morrison, are enteric neural gangliomas over-secreting VIP and causing severe watery diarrhoea and flushing of the skin (Box 10.2). The diarrhoea may provoke dehydration and severe hypokalaemia (see Box 6.14). Diagnosis is by detecting raised fasting serum VIP levels and visualization by MRI or CT. The somatostatin analogue, octreotide, can help identify the tumour when labelled (review Chapter 4) or treat its symptoms if tumour resection is not possible.

Glucagon-like peptide-1 and glucose-dependent insulinotropic peptide

Alternative cleavage of proglucagon gives rise to hormones other than glucagon; PC1/3 (the enzyme that cleaves insulin from proinsulin and ACTH from POMC) generates glucagon-like peptide 1 (GLP-1) (see Table 10.1). GLP-1 is released in response to nutrients by L-cells, which are predominantly located in the terminal ileum and large bowel but are also found elsewhere. It also seems increasingly likely that some GLP-1 is produced by α-cells in the pancreatic islet.

GLP-1 acts as an incretin, magnifying insulin secretion from stimulated β-cells. Its secretion from the gut is the main reason why insulin secretion after oral glucose is greater than from an equivalent dose of intravenous glucose. L-cell tumours have not been described, but it has been questioned whether reactive hypoglycaemia in dumping syndrome (Box 10.1) is mediated by GLP-1 (and GIP) overactivity. GLP-1 analogues and inhibitors of the enzyme dipeptidyl peptidase 4 (DPP-4) that degrades GLP-1 are now in widespread use as treatments for diabetes (see Chapter 13).

GIP is also an incretin (see Table 10.1). It is secreted higher up in the gut than GLP-1 by K-cells in the duodenum and jejunum, but acts similarly to enhance glucose-stimulated insulin secretion by pancreatic β-cells.

Cholecystokinin, secretin and motilin

Cholecystokinin (CCK), secretin and motilin are all peptide hormones secreted by the small intestine in response to a variety of stimulants and act via cell surface G-protein–coupled receptors (Table 10.1). CCK increases gallbladder contraction and stimulates pancreatic exocrine secretion. Secretin is released in response to stomach acid entering the duodenum and stimulates the pancreas to secrete bicarbonate-rich fluid that neutralizes the acidity. Motilin, synthesized in duodenal and jejunal M-cells, enhances gut peristalsis and pepsin secretion.

Carcinoid syndrome

Pancreatic islet tumours or those secreting gastrin or VIP all appear 'neuroendocrine' on histology (i.e. they contain secretory granules). However, in addition to these tumour types defined by hormone product, there is another broad category of tumour called 'carcinoid'. Most are non-functioning without detectable hormone secretion. Functional tumours can cause 'carcinoid syndrome', the hallmark of which is symptoms and signs from the release of serotonin (5-hydroxytryptamine) and its metabolites (plus other factors) into the systemic circulation (Figure 10.3). Systemic detection is more prevalent with tumours that lie outside the portal circulation, such as lung carcinoids or intestinal tumours that have metastasized to the liver.

Carcinoid tumours can be classified according to embryological origin of tumour location (Table 10.2). Foregut carcinoids lie proximal to the second part of the duodenum and include those in lung, thymus, pancreas and thyroid. Midgut ones arise between the distal duodenum and transverse colon with hindgut tumours situated more distally. Colonic and ileal carcinoids are more prone to metastasize. Distant deposits in either the liver or lymph nodes are observed in ~70% of colonic carcinoids compared with only 2–5% of those in the

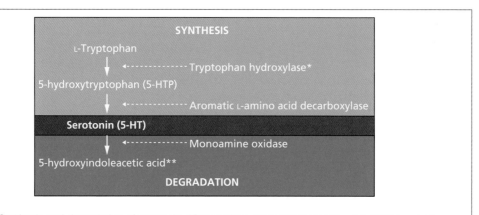

Figure 10.3 Synthesis and degradation of serotonin. *Rate-limiting step: two isoforms exist. **Measured in urine in carcinoid syndrome.

Table 10.2 Distribution of carcinoid tumours

Site	Frequency (%)
Foregut	
Thymus	<1
Lung	10
Stomach	2
Duodenum	2
Midgut	
Ileum	11
Jejunum	1
Appendix	44
Caecum	3
Hindgut	
Colon	5
Rectum	15

Carcinoids constitute around a third of all tumours in the small intestine but only 1% of those in the stomach, colon or rectum. In total, carcinoid tumours constitute around 2% of all malignant tumours. The incidence is approximately 1 in 100,000 and may occur at all ages, including in children.

Symptoms and signs

The majority of carcinoids are asymptomatic and only detected at post-mortem examination. Carcinoid syndrome has distinctive symptoms and signs (Box 10.3 and Case history 10.4). Pellagra-like skin lesions reflect tryptophan deficiency from consumption of the amino acid in serotonin synthesis (Figure 10.3).

Investigation and diagnosis

Carcinoid syndrome is diagnosed by detection of excessive 5-hydroxyindoleacetic acid (5-HIAA) in a 24-h urine sample (Figure 10.3). An acidified container is necessary (see Box 4.1) and avocadoes, bananas, tomatoes, plums, walnuts, pineapples, aubergines and chocolate need to be avoided for the preceding 24 h and during the collection period. The collection starts after the first micturition of the day is discarded and continues for the next 24 h up to and including the first urination of the following day. The assay has a sensitivity of ~70% and specificity of 100% in carcinoid syndrome. Serum chromogranin A can also be raised but is relatively non-specific as it is a component of all secretory granules. After making

appendix, the commonest tumour location in young patients when it is an incidental finding at appendicectomy. The risk of metastasis increases with the size of the tumour. In older patients, carcinoids are more frequently found in the ileum and jejunum.

Box 10.3 Clinical features of carcinoid syndrome

- Flushing
- Diarrhoea
- Abdominal pain
- Bronchoconstriction and asthma-like episodes
- Tricuspid or pulmonary valve abnormalities:
  - Occur in 60–70%
  - May be complicated by right heart failure
  - Fibrotic change in mural and valvular endocardium
  - Seem unrelated to tumour mass or duration; possibly related to secretion of serotonin and tachykinins
- Pellagra-like skin lesions
- Treated by somatostatin analogues, surgery, chemotherapy, or, potentially, interferon-α

Case history 10.4

A 65-year-old man presents with breathlessness, rash, flushing, abdominal pain and diarrhoea. Examination revealed a wheeze and his peak flow rate was reduced. A chest X-ray was unremarkable but abdominal ultrasound showed a single mass in his liver. A barium meal and follow through demonstrated an ileal mass. Urinary 5-HIAA was markedly raised upon 24-h collection.

What is the likely diagnosis?
What are the treatment options?
What factors are likely to affect his prognosis?

Answers, see p. 232

Box 10.4 Warning signs for neoplasia syndromes

- Family history of tumours
- Unusually early age of onset
- History of multiple tumours

a biochemical diagnosis, the tumour is potentially localized by a range of techniques, including endoscopy, barium enema, chest radiograph, ultrasound, CT, MRI, angiography, selective venous sampling and labelled somatostatin scanning.

Treatment

Surgical resection of carcinoid tumours may be curative for local disease. Even with more extensive metastatic disease, aggressive surgery to debulk tumour mass can improve symptoms markedly. Carcinoid tumours express somatostatin receptors and medical treatment with somatostatin analogues can be highly effective. Other treatment includes chemotherapy and, potentially, interferon-α.

Outcome from carcinoid tumours can be good with some patients living for 10–15 years with metastatic disease. However, overall 5-year survival rates, when liver metastases are present, are 18–38% with a median survival time of ~23 months. Approximately one-third of patients die from carcinoid heart disease and heart valve replacement can be important to prevent this. 24–hour urinary 5-HIAA and serum chromogranin assay allow monitoring of disease activity.

Familial endocrine neoplasia

Inheritance of endocrine tumour predisposition syndromes is usually dominant (i.e. mutation in only one of the two alleles is sufficient to predispose to tumour formation). Four different categories are discernible (Table 10.3). By inheriting a tumour-promoting mutation in every cell in the body, tumours tend to be familial, multiple and occur at an earlier age than usual; all warning signs for familial tumour predisposition syndromes (Box 10.4).

In general, neoplasms arise through sequential acquisition of mutations in four types of gene, giving a cell a proliferative or survival advantage over its neighbours to produce clonal growth (Box 10.5). Two of these, proto-oncogenes and tumour suppressor genes, are associated with familial endocrine neoplasia syndromes. Inheritance of a mutated proto-oncogene usually leads to hyperplasia of all cells in which the gene is expressed (e.g. mutations

Table 10.3 Categories of endocrine tumour pre-disposition syndromes

Category	Primarily endocrine	Description	Example
Multiple endocrine neoplasia (MEN)	Yes	Multiple tumours in multiple endocrine glands	MEN-1
Single organ	Yes	Multiple tumours in one endocrine gland	Familial parathyroid tumours
Non-endocrine tumour with minor endocrine component	No	Only a minority develop endocrine tumours	Neurofibromatosis
Other syndrome	No	Diverse dysfunction with some endocrine abnormality	McCune–Albright (review Figure 3.14)

Box 10.5 Four types of tumour-promoting mutation

- Proto-oncogenes – mutation confers a positive growth advantage and hyperplasia of the affected cell type
- Tumour suppressor genes – mutation de-restricts clonal cell growth
- DNA repair genes – mutation increases likelihood of further mutations
- Cell adhesion and invasion genes – mutation increases chance of metastasis

---

in the *RET* oncogene, which causes MEN-2; Figure 10.4). On this background, tumour development then depends on the chance acquisition of tumour-promoting mutations in other genes. In contrast, inheriting a mutation in one copy of a tumour suppressor gene (e.g. *NF1* in neurofibromatosis) tends not to cause hyperplasia. However, losing function of the other normal allele (i.e. by mutation or silencing) can lead to a tumour; the 'second hit' in Knudsen's two-hit hypothesis.

Multiple endocrine neoplasia

There are two types of MEN (Table 10.4). Although both are rare outside of tertiary referral centres, management is time-intensive and morbidity and mortality are significantly increased. Both may be familial or sporadic [i.e. the occurrence of a new ('*de novo*') mutation; note most endocrine tumours are sporadic]. Multidisciplinary teams of clinical genet-

ics alongside endocrinology professionals are important for tracing relatives, counselling, screening, diagnosis, treatment and management.

MEN-1

Tumours characterizing MEN-1 are listed in Table 10.4; carcinoids, lipomas, VIPomas and adrenocortical tumours are more unusual. It is caused by inactivating mutations in *MEN1*, the gene encoding the MENIN tumour suppressor protein.

Clinical features and treatment of MEN-1 are related to tumour site (Table 10.4). Having ascertained a diagnosis genetically or, failing that, by a history of tumours in at least two organs, regular screening is vital for the index case and asymptomatic family members, as early diagnosis and treatment of new tumours reduces mortality and morbidity. A genetic diagnosis can be established in ~80% of cases and allows easy identification of affected or discharge of unaffected family members.

Frequency of screening is debated and influenced by detection of ever-smaller lesions of unclear significance by high-resolution imaging. Arguably it should commence in early childhood and continue for life as some individuals have developed first manifestations as early as 5 years or as late as the eighth decade. However, virtually all affected individuals have primary hyperparathyroidism by age 50 years. Somewhat unusually as MENIN is a tumour suppressor, this can be from hyperplasia of all glands as well as individual tumours.

In addition to history and examination, serum calcium (Ca^{2+}), fasting gastrointestinal hormones

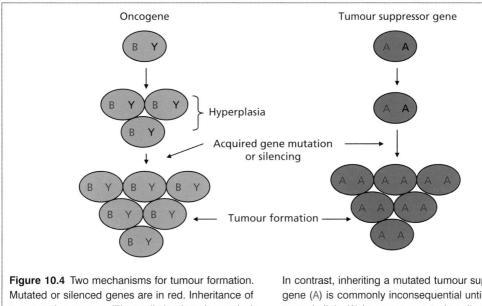

Figure 10.4 Two mechanisms for tumour formation. Mutated or silenced genes are in red. Inheritance of a mutated oncogene (B) usually leads to hyperplasia of all cells where gene B is normally expressed. On this background, a second predisposing 'hit' (e.g. mutation of gene Y to Y) causes tumour formation.

In contrast, inheriting a mutated tumour suppressor gene (A) is commonly inconsequential until the normal allele (A) becomes mutated or silenced (A). At this point, complete loss of gene A function causes tumour development.

Table 10.4 Features of multiple endocrine neoplasia			
Type	**Organ affected**	**Endocrine consequence**	**See chapter**
MEN-1 (*MEN1* gene) (~1:35,000)	Parathyroid	Primary hyperparathyroidism (virtually all patients by age 50 years)	9
	Pancreas	Islet cell tumour, gastrinoma or non-functioning	10
	Anterior pituitary	Prolactinoma, acromegaly, Cushing disease or non-functioning	5
MEN-2 (*RET* gene) (~1:40,000)	Thyroid	Medullary thyroid cancer (MTC*)	8
	Adrenal medulla	Phaeochromocytoma or non-functioning	6
	Parathyroid	Primary hyperparathyroidism (MEN-2A)	9
	Mucosa	Neurofibromata (MEN-2B)	
	Skeleton	Marfanoid appearance (MEN-2B)	

*Can occur in families in isolation as familial MTC.
Inheritance of MEN is autosomal dominant or sporadic.

and pituitary assessment [e.g. prolactin, insulin-like growth factor I (IGF-I), exclusion of Cushing disease and thyroid function tests] should be performed annually. MRI of the anterior pituitary (e.g. every few years) and pancreas (arguably annually) complements biochemical screening and allows detection of non-functioning tumours. Most tumours are benign but can be malignant, especially in the pancreas. Some published guidelines suggest more frequent imaging surveillance; however, as with all screening, outcome benefits (e.g. mortality) need to justify intrusiveness and cost. This remains contentious, especially for asymptomatic pancreatic tumours that can require very intensive surgery, leaving the patient with life-long insulin-requiring diabetes. CT scanning should not be used for surveillance as the cumulative lifetime dose of radiation itself becomes a tumour risk factor.

Familial isolated hyperparathyroidism

Primary hyperparathyroidism can run in families. In 20% of kindreds, mutations can be identified in *MEN1*.

🔍 Case history 10.5

A 35-year-old active fit man was referred with hypercalcaemia and hypertension. He had also been suffering with palpitations and headaches. He had been well previously. There was no family history of endocrine disease. Investigations confirmed raised serum Ca^{2+} and the doctor went on to detect elevated serum parathyroid hormone (PTH) and normal vitamin D levels. In addition, the doctor prescribed a β-blocker for the hypertension and palpitations. Five days later, the man was admitted collapsed with a blood pressure of 230/110.

What diagnosis did the doctor detect?
What diagnosis was missed?
Why was he admitted?
What other condition needs urgent consideration for him and his family?

Answers, see p. 232

MEN-2

The tumours characterizing MEN-2 are listed in Table 10.4, with reference to relevant chapters elsewhere. Phaeochromocytomas (adrenal medulla) and medullary thyroid cancer (MTC; thyroid C cells) are both derived embryologically from the same source, neural crest cells. Clinically, MEN-2 can be further sub-divided into 2A (including parathyroid disease; Case history 10.5) or 2B (including neurofibromata and Marfanoid habitus where arm span is greater than height). Both are autosomal dominant, highly penetrant and caused by inactivating mutations in the *RET* proto-oncogene, which encodes a cell-surface receptor with tyrosine kinase activity (review Chapter 3). Mutations lead to potent growth stimulation and hyperplasia, predisposing to 'second hit' tumour formation.

Genetic screening for MEN-2 is more effective than for MEN-1 because, in most cases, the causative mutation can be identified within the *RET* coding region (review Figure 2.2 on gene structure and Figure 4.5 on polymerase chain reaction). Those without the mutation can be reassured, while a definitive diagnosis can be made in affected individuals during early childhood and biochemical monitoring commenced.

For MTC or its preceding C-cell hyperplasia (see Chapter 8), surveillance is done by annual measurement of calcitonin either without stimulation or less commonly during a pentagastrin stimulation test. Once over the age of 5–6 years, prophylactic thyroidectomy should be considered as the tumour almost inevitably develops in affected individuals (>90% by 30 years). Absolute risk and timing of surgery depend on which codon is mutated. If surveillance and prophylaxis fails (which should not happen in familial cases), presentation is with goitre (see Chapter 8).

Screening for phaeochromocytoma is increasingly done by annual measurement of serum metanephrine and, especially, normetanephrine as a normal result practically excludes the tumour (see Chapter 6). Periodic measurement of serum Ca^{2+} screens for primary hyperparathyroidism due to parathyroid adenomas (note that calcitonin secreted from MTC does not alter serum Ca^{2+}). Interestingly, some *RET* mutations have never been associated with phaeochromocytoma, emphasizing the value of careful genotype–phenotype correlations and research.

Familial medullary thyroid cancer

Familial MTC, still caused by mutations in the *RET* proto-oncogene, can occur without the other manifestations of MEN-2. However, its management is the same as if it were part of MEN-2.

Other familial endocrine tumour predisposition syndromes

Familial phaeochromocytoma syndromes

Approximately one-quarter of phaeochromocytomas occur because of germline (i.e. potentially heritable) mutations in one of several tumour suppressor genes, all inherited as autosomal dominant disorders (Table 10.5). Management and screening are detailed in Chapter 6 with additional imaging surveillance required for relevant extra-adrenal manifestations (e.g. annual MRI for head and neck paragangliomas).

Phaeochromocytomas are unusual in Von Hippel Lindau (VHL) and neurofibromatosis type 1 (NF1) syndromes. *SDHB* and *SDHD* genes encode subunits of the succinate dehydrogenase enzyme complex. Phaeochromocytomas or paragangliomas associated with *SDHB* mutations are commonly malignant whereas those due to *SDHD* mutations tend to be benign. Some mutations have also been identified in the SDHC subunit. *VHL* and *SDH* mutations (especially *SDHB*) are associated with extra-adrenal phaeochromocytomas when

norepinephrine secretion can predominate over epinephrine (see Chapter 6).

McCune-Albright syndrome

McCune-Albright syndrome is caused by gain-of-function mutations in Gsα (review Box 3.8 and Figure 3.14) in somatic cells partway through development. This gives rise to a sporadic syndrome of endocrine overactivity and other features, including café-au-lait spots and fibrous dysplasia of the bones. It is a cause of isosexual gonadotrophin-independent precocious puberty (see Table 7.5). Although distinct from true neoplasia, it can give rise to hyperfunctioning nodules in the adrenal cortex, thyroid and pituitary, respectively giving rise to Cushing syndrome (see Chapter 6), thyrotoxicosis (see Chapter 8) and acromegaly (see Chapter 5).

Carney complex

Carney complex is an autosomal dominant condition caused by mutations in the *PRKAR1α* gene, giving rise to adrenocortical overactivity (Cushing syndrome; see Chapter 6), hyperpigmentation and rare atrial myxoma tumours.

Ectopic hormone syndromes

Some solid tumours unexpectedly secrete peptide hormones (ectopic hormone secretion) (Table 10.6 and Case history 10.6). Various mechanisms have been proposed: the tumour might derive from neural crest cells with some endocrine capacity;

Table 10.5 Familial phaeochromocytoma syndromes		
Mutated gene	**Wider syndrome**	**Other features**
*SDHB**	Hereditary paragangliomas	Paragangliomas
*SDHD**	Hereditary paragangliomas	Paragangliomas
VHL	Von Hippel Lindau syndrome	Haemangiomas, renal cell carcinoma, café-au-lait spots
NF1	Neurofibromatosis (type 1)	Neurofibromas, café-au-lait spots, axillary freckling, optic glioma

SDHB/D encode the B and D subunits of succinate dehydrogenase.

Table 10.6 Examples of ectopic hormone secretion

Tumour	Hormone	Endocrine abnormality
Small cell carcinoma of the lung, medullary thyroid cancer, thymic carcinoma, islet cell tumours	ACTH or ACTH-like peptides (see Chapter 5)	Cushing syndrome; sometimes isolated hypokalaemia (see Chapter 6)
Small cell carcinoma of the lung, gastrointestinal tumour	Vasopressin (see Chapter 5)	SIADH/ hyponatraemia (see Box 5.12)
Carcinoma of the bronchus, liver or kidney	Human placental lactogen, oestrogen, testosterone	Gynaecomastia (ultimately due to oestrogen activity; see Chapter 7)
Hepatomas, large mesenchymal tumours	Insulin-like activity, big IGF-II	Hypoglycaemia (see Box 10.1)
Carcinoma of the bronchus or kidney	Prolactin	Galactorrhoea (see Chapter 5)
Squamous cell carcinoma of the bronchus, breast carcinoma	Parathyroid hormone-related peptide (PTHrP)	Hypercalcaemia (see Chapter 9)
Carcinoma of the kidney and uterus	Erythropoietin	Polycythaemia

ACTH, adrenocorticotrophic hormone; IGF, insulin-like growth factor; SIADH, syndrome of inappropriate antidiuretic hormone.

🔍 Case history 10.6

A 76-year-old lifelong smoker was referred during winter to the respiratory clinic because of failure to resolve bronchitis, haemoptysis, and opacities on chest X-ray in the upper zone of the left lung and left hilum. His serum sodium was 152 mmol/L (152 mEq/L) and serum potassium was 2.4 mmol/L (2.4 mEq/L). An overnight dexamethasone suppression test produced serum cortisol of 134 nmol/L (~4.8 µg/dL). The man looked tanned and had lost 10 kg (22 lb) during the last 6 months without dieting.

What diagnosis is of concern from the history and chest investigations?
What endocrine complication seems likely?
What is the prognosis?

Answers, see p. 232

---

malignant cells have lost their differentiated phenotype allowing expression of normally repressed genes, some of which encode hormones; or specific oncogenes might activate hormone expression.

Hormone-sensitive solid tumours

Hormone and growth factor stimulation of both normal and tumour cells is a major mechanism regulating cell growth. Antagonizing these stimuli can provide valuable therapeutic options.

Prostate cancer

Prostate cancer accounts for ~8% of all cancers in men and is the fourth commonest malignant cause of male death in England and Wales. Carcinoma of the prostate becomes increasingly common with age such that by 80 years, 80% of men have malignant foci within the gland, although most seem clinically insignificant. Androgenic hormones play an important role in the aetiology and progression of the tumour and consequently endocrine manipulation is an important treatment (Box 10.6).

> ## Box 10.6 Endocrine treatments of prostate cancer
>
> - Continuous GnRH analogues (see Chapter 7) – leuprorelin or goserelin
> - Androgen receptor antagonists – cyproterone acetate
> - Bilateral orchidectomy

Surgical prostatectomy is the first line of therapy; other options include radiotherapy, chemotherapy and cryotherapy. However, endocrine manipulation can be used to reduce or inhibit androgen action. Continuous gonadotrophin-releasing hormone (GnRH) analogues, such as leuprorelin or goserelin, cause a secondary hypogonadism (review Chapter 7). Around 30% of prostate tumours respond to this therapy, which can be combined with the androgen receptor antagonist, cyproterone acetate. 5α-reductase inhibitors can also be used to block formation of dihydrotestosterone (see Figure 7.7); finasteride is already used clinically to control prostatic hypertrophy and related urinary symptoms. Surgical removal of the testes (bilateral orchidectomy) is also possible to remove androgen supply to the tumour.

Breast cancer

Breast cancer is the commonest tumour in women. Its incidence has increased in recent years to 54 per 100,000 women per year. Hormone and growth factor-related treatment of breast cancer is important (Box 10.7). A major factor is whether the oestrogen receptor (ER) is present in the tumour cells: if it is, 60% of these tumours respond to antioestrogen therapy; if ER-negative, this falls to only 10%. Around 60% of breast cancers are ER-positive. Endocrine treatment aims to decrease oestrogen supply or antagonize ER action.

Tamoxifen is the most commonly prescribed hormone-related therapy. It acts as an ER antagonist in breast cancer cells while acting as a weak agonist in other tissues. It has a low incidence of side-effects, is effective in both pre- and post-menopausal women and can be used for metastatic disease as well as adjuvant therapy.

Progestins, such as medroxyprogesterone acetate or megestrol acetate, help to diminish oestrogen

> ## Box 10.7 Endocrine treatments of breast cancer
>
> *Oestrogen antagonist*
> - Tamoxifen
> - Effective in both pre- and post-menopausal women
>
> *Blockade of oestrogen production*
> - Continuous GnRH analogues or bilateral oophorectomy – both induce premature menopause
> - Aromatase (CYP19) inhibitors – anastrozole or letrozole; used in post-menopausal women
>
> *Progestins*
> - E.g. medroxyprogesterone acetate or megestrol acetate
> - Effective in both pre- and post-menopausal women
> - Second-line therapy
>
> *HER2 antagonists (human epidermal growth factor 2)*

action in breast cancers and are effective in both pre- and post-menopausal women. They are considered second-line agents and are helpful in ~50% of women who have previously responded to endocrine therapy.

In pre-menopausal women, drugs that block ovarian oestrogen production, such as continuous GnRH analogues, lead to a significant fall in oestrogen concentrations (see Chapter 7). The unavoidable 'side-effect' (= desired effect) of these drugs is that they induce a premature menopause. An alternative is bilateral oophorectomy (surgical removal of the ovaries).

In post-menopausal women, oestrogens are mainly formed through the peripheral conversion of androgens by the action of aromatase (CYP19; see Figure 7.12). Inhibition of this enzyme with drugs such as anastrozole or letrozole leads to a significant fall in oestrogen levels.

More recently, there has been much interest in monoclonal antibodies that block the epidermal growth factor receptor (HER2 antagonists, e.g.

trastuzumab) and limit signalling through tyrosine kinase pathways.

Other tumours of relevance to endocrinology

Ovarian cancer

Excluding the breast, ovarian cancer is the commonest malignancy of an endocrine organ, accounting for 4–6% of all cancers in women. There are three types of ovarian neoplasm: epithelial, germ cell and sex cord stromal tumours. The vast majority of malignant tumours are epithelial. Ovarian cancer is generally more common in developed countries with incidence rates in northern Europe and North America of 8–12/100,000 per year.

The cause of ovarian cancer remains unclear, but hormonal factors appear to be important as risk relates to the lifetime number of ovulations. Nulliparity, low parity and older age at menopause all increase risk, while use of the oral contraceptive pill is protective. Thus, it appears that total oestrogen exposure is important to some degree. Despite this, no hormonal therapy has been approved for ovarian cancer.

Endometrial cancer

Endometrial cancer affects ~142,000 women worldwide each year, with an estimated 42,000 women dying from this cancer. Most cases are diagnosed after the menopause, with the highest incidence around the seventh decade of life. Readily detected symptoms, such as post-menopausal bleeding, explain why most women with endometrial cancer are diagnosed with early-stage disease. Overall, the 5-year survival is ~80%.

The most common lesions are hormone sensitive and low grade, and have an excellent prognosis. First-line treatment is hysterectomy, which is important for staging and enables appropriate tailoring of adjuvant treatment in high-risk patients. Currently, there is no proof that adjuvant hormone therapy improves outcome in early cancers but progestagens may have a place in the treatment of metastatic endometrial cancer. The response rate is 15–20%, related to expression of steroid-hormone receptors. Tamoxifen has a small benefit in this setting. Progesterone is certainly important in preventing endometrial carcinoma; chronic unopposed oestrogen increases risk ~six-fold, explaining the need for a withdrawal bleed every 4 months or so in polycystic ovarian syndrome (see Chapter 7).

Testicular cancer

Testicular cancer is uncommon but increasing with incidence rates of 3–9/100,000 per year in white men and much lower rates in Africans and Asians. The majority of testicular cancer is of germ cell origin and can be divided into seminoma and non-seminomatous tumours. Most testicular cancer presents before the age of 40 years. Incidence increases modestly after the age of 65 years (see Box 7.13).

A major, established risk factor is maldescent of the testis. The mechanism is unknown but it appears that risk is only raised for the maldescended testis and not the opposite side. Increased exposure to environmental oestrogens has also been proposed as a cause, but as yet there is no definite evidence to support this hypothesis. At present, hormonal treatments are not available for testicular cancer, but measurement of the hormonal marker, human chorionic gonadotrophin, is important in monitoring the treatment of non-seminomatous germ cell tumours.

🔑 Key points

- The pancreas and gastrointestinal tract contain cell types that release many important hormones and are vulnerable to tumour formation
- Endocrine neoplasms can occur sporadically or as inherited syndromes
- For most inherited endocrine tumours, the genetic cause is known, allowing precise diagnoses that influence subsequent management of the patient and relatives
- Familial syndromes should be considered in those with multiple endocrine tumours, those diagnosed at an early age, or in those with a positive family history
- Prostate and breast cancer are hormone-responsive tumours

Answers to case histories

Case history 10.1

The symptoms are those of hypoglycaemia and are relieved by food. Even without venesection, biochemical hypoglycaemia is unlikely with this monitor reading. The differential diagnosis of hypoglycaemia is given in Box 10.1. Given her family history, the most likely diagnosis is reactive hypoglycaemia (or potential sulphonylurea misuse of her mother's tablets).

A 72-h fast could be performed, which in all likelihood would exclude true hypoglycaemia and rule out insulinoma. A prolonged 75-g oral glucose tolerance test could assess the possibility of reactive hypoglycaemia. Low glucose after 3h [but almost certainly >2.2 mmol/L (>40 mg/dL)] with detectable insulin and C-peptide concentrations would support the diagnosis. Management would be dietary advice on low glycaemic index, high fibre foods and weight loss.

Case history 10.2

The diagnosis until proven otherwise is hypoadrenalism, most likely Addison disease (see Chapter 6). The reasoning is as follows. The man has hypoglycaemia (see Box 10.1); had fainted on standing (postural hypotension); was tanned (excess ACTH due to loss of negative feedback from cortisol; see Chapter 5); and has a family history consistent with autoimmune endocrinopathy (see Box 8.8). The final major clue is raised serum K[+]. This is hypoadrenalism until proven otherwise because it is the most important, potentially life-threatening consideration in the differential diagnosis.

Lying and standing blood pressure, and signs of Addison disease and other autoimmune endocrinopathies should be assessed. Laboratory serum glucose should be measured and if low, contemporaneous insulin and C-peptide should be assayed. Ideally, prior to starting hydrocortisone

therapy, an ACTH stimulation test should be done with ACTH measured on the time 0 sample. If hydrocortisone has been started, the test can be done later if preceding dose(s) of hydrocortisone are withheld (see Chapter 6). Random cortisol could be requested on the original blood sample; if <100 nmol/L (~3.6 µg/dL) during the morning, it is supportive evidence for hypoadrenalism. Serum renin could also be measured and would likely be raised in Addison disease. If primary hypoadrenalism is confirmed, other potential autoimmune endocrinopathy should be investigated (see Box 8.8).

As hypoadrenalism is potentially life-threatening, treatment with hydrocortisone is warranted, and should be started if investigation to confirm the diagnosis is not immediate. As the man had recovered quickly, this could be given orally at the hospital with a prescription for 10 mg twice daily oral hydrocortisone thereafter. He may also require oral fludrocortisone (e.g. 100 µg daily). The man should also eat and should not be discharged until the diagnosis is clear and his blood glucose is consistently normal.

Case history 10.3

The hormone was gastrin.

Repeat ulceration and a raised serum gastrin raise concern over gastrinoma. He is not on H_2 antagonists or proton pump inhibitors, both of which can raise gastrin levels (stomach acid suppresses gastrin production; this effect is lost with medication that lowers acid production). MRI is warranted to look for a gastrinoma in the pancreas (where there is a higher risk of malignancy) or duodenum. Scintigraphy with labelled somatostatin may also be useful. A duodenal abnormality may also have been observed at operation or by subsequent endoscopy. Some consideration should be given to the possibility of MEN-1.

Case history 10.4

The diagnosis is likely to be a carcinoid tumour with hepatic metastasis.

The primary treatment is surgical. The presence of hepatic spread is not a contraindication to surgery. Indeed surgical removal of the hepatic tumour may even be curative. If he is unfit for surgery, treatment with somatostatin analogues, interferon-α and chemotherapy should be considered.

His prognosis is reduced by the metastasis, but nevertheless he may still live for a considerable time. Although bronchoconstriction would appear to be causing his breathlessness, it is important to consider carcinoid heart disease, which has a poorer prognosis. High levels of tumour markers, particularly post surgery, would worsen his prognosis.

Case history 10.5

The doctor had diagnosed primary hyperparathyroidism.

A phaeochromocytoma was missed. Although this is a rare diagnosis, hypertension in a fit young man is unusual.

He was admitted in hypertensive crisis because of excessive unopposed catecholamine action on α-receptors after β-receptor blockade (see Chapter 6).

The combination of a primary hyperparathyroidism and

phaeochromocytoma should suggest MEN-2. He requires urgent investigation for medullary thyroid cancer, which, if the patient has a mutation in the *RET* proto-oncogene, is highly likely to be present by the age of 35 years. Calcitonin should be measured. The patient should be referred to a clinical geneticist and the *RET* proto-oncogene sequenced. The case may be sporadic; however, if a *RET* mutation is found, genetic screening should be offered to family members. Unaffected family members can be reassured and discharged. Those with the mutation or, if the mutation remains cryptic, all first-degree relatives, should be encouraged to undertake screening as described in the chapter text.

Case history 10.6

The features are all consistent with lung cancer.

The man failed a 1-mg dexamethasone suppression test [serum cortisol the following morning >50 nmol/L (~1.8 μg/dL)] and so may well have Cushing syndrome. The most likely underlying cause is ectopic secretion of ACTH causing inappropriate skin pigmentation from a small cell carcinoma of the lung.

The prognosis is poor because of the hilar mass, weight loss and ectopic hormone secretion.

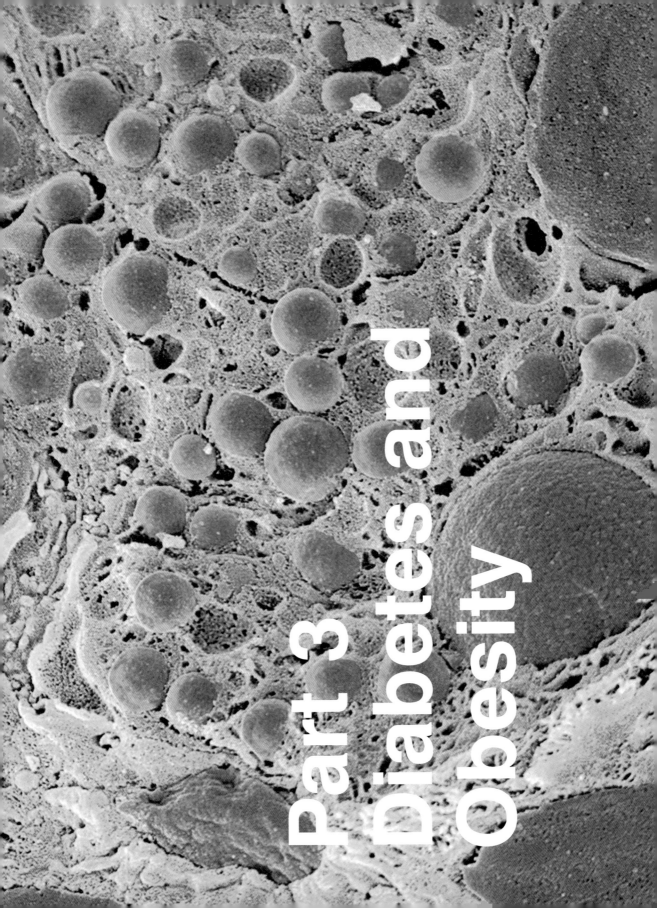

Part 3
Diabetes and Obesity

CHAPTER 11
Overview of diabetes

Key topics

- A brief history of diabetes and its classification   238
- Classification of diabetes   240
- Diagnosis of diabetes   241
- Insulin   243
- Glucagon   254
- Key points   255
- Answers to case histories   255

Learning objectives

- To understand what diabetes is and how it is diagnosed and classified
- To understand the physiology of insulin and the counter-regulatory hormone glucagon

This chapter provides an overview of the commonest of all endocrine disorders – diabetes mellitus

To recap

- The biosynthesis of protein hormones that is relevant to the production of insulin and glucagon is covered in Chapter 2
- Both insulin and glucagon act through cell-surface receptors. The physiology of cell-surface hormone receptors is covered in Chapter 3

Essential Endocrinology and Diabetes, Sixth Edition. Richard IG Holt, Neil A Hanley.
© 2012 Richard IG Holt and Neil A Hanley. Publlished 2012 by Blackwell Publishing Ltd.

Cross-reference

■ Several hormones influence the action of insulin and exert an effect on glucose control. These include growth hormone (GH) (see Chapter 5), cortisol and catecholamines (see Chapter 6)

■ There are other hormones produced in the pancreas that can lead to endocrine disease; these are covered in Chapter 10

■ The clinical aspects of diabetes are covered in Chapters 12–14

Diabetes mellitus is a complex metabolic disorder characterized by persistent hyperglycaemia (higher than normal blood glucose levels) resulting from defects in insulin secretion, insulin action or both.

The two main types of diabetes are type 1 (formerly known as insulin-dependent diabetes) and type 2 (formerly known as non–insulin-dependent diabetes). Type 1 diabetes is caused predominantly by the autoimmune destruction of the insulin-producing β-cells of the pancreatic islets, while type 2 diabetes results from both impaired insulin secretion and resistance to the action of insulin.

Diabetes is a major global health problem and in 2010 was estimated to affect 285 million individuals worldwide; this figure is projected to rise to more than 400 million over the next two decades as a result of changing population demographics, such as ageing and urbanization, and changes in lifestyle, such as diet and exercise, and the associated increase in obesity (Figure 11.1). The increase

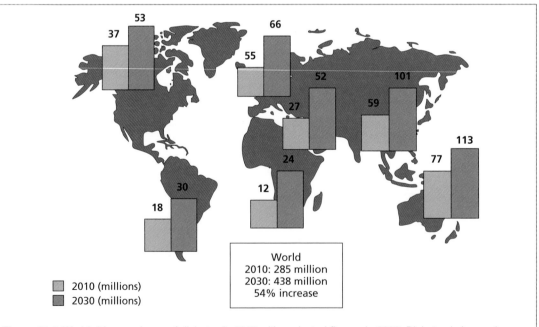

World
2010: 285 million
2030: 438 million
54% increase

■ 2010 (millions)
■ 2030 (millions)

Figure 11.1 Worldwide prevalence of diabetes in 2010 with projected figures in 2030. Diabetes is increasing in every continent. Figures are number of people with diabetes in millions. Source *IDF Atlas 2009* (http://www.idf.org/diabetesatlas/downloads).

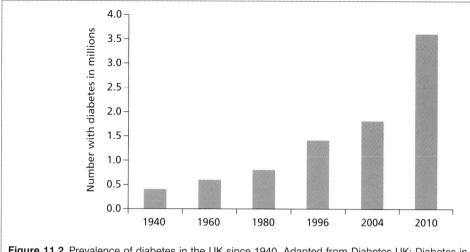

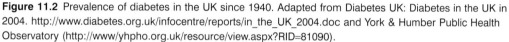

Figure 11.2 Prevalence of diabetes in the UK since 1940. Adapted from Diabetes UK: Diabetes in the UK in 2004. http://www.diabetes.org.uk/infocentre/reports/in_the_UK_2004.doc and York & Humber Public Health Observatory (http://www.yhpho.org.uk/resource/view.aspx?RID=81090).

largely represents an increase in the prevalence of type 2 diabetes, which accounts for ~90% of all cases of diabetes, but the prevalence of type 1 diabetes is also increasing.

The prevalence of diabetes in the USA in 2010 was almost 27 million (12.3%), while 3.6 million people are affected by diabetes in the UK (7.4%). The prevalence of diabetes has doubled in the UK every 20 years since the end of the Second World War (Figure 11.2). It is now recognized that low- and middle-income countries face the greatest burden of diabetes, with around two-thirds of those affected by diabetes living in these areas of the world. Eight of the top 10 countries with the highest absolute numbers of people with diabetes have developing or transitioning economies (Table 11.1). Similarly many of the countries with the highest percentage of the population with diabetes are also from resource-poor nations (Table 11.2).

Type 2 diabetes has a slow and gradual onset and the diagnosis is frequently delayed for many years; so many people with diabetes are undiagnosed but still develop diabetic complications. This may lead to underestimates of the true global burden of disease (Case history 11.1).

Case history 11.1

The local public health consultant would like to know the prevalence of diabetes in your region and if it differs from the national average.

What are the difficulties they may encounter?
How might these be overcome?

Answers, see p. 255

Diabetes is the fifth leading cause of death worldwide, accounting for 4 million deaths annually and outnumbering the global deaths from human immunodeficiency virus (HIV)/acquired immune deficiency syndrome (AIDS). The premature mortality is predominantly driven by an increase in atherosclerotic vascular disease, but diabetes also causes considerable morbidity through its microvascular complications, which affect the eye, nerve and kidney (Case history 11.2).

(icon) Case history 11.2

An overweight 58-year-old man attended for a routine occupational health medical. Generally he had been well but had noticed some tiredness in the previous year, which he attributed to his long hours at work. His blood pressure was elevated (155/87 mmHg) and a routine blood test showed that his fasting glucose was 9.7 mmol/L (174 mg/dL). Repeat testing confirmed the diagnosis of diabetes. Retinal photography showed that he had bilateral background retinopathy (described in Chapter 14).

Is it unusual for diabetes to be detected on routine testing?
Is it unusual that this man was found to have retinopathy at diagnosis?

Answers, see p. 255

Table 11.1 Prevalence of diabetes in people aged 20–79 years in 2010 and projected prevalence in 2030.*

2010		2030	
Country/ territory	**Millions**	**Country/ territory**	**Millions**
India	50.8	India	87.0
China	43.2	China	62.6
USA	26.8	USA	36.0
Russian Federation	9.6	Pakistan	13.8
Brazil	7.6	Brazil	12.7
Germany	7.5	Indonesia	12.0
Pakistan	7.1	Mexico	11.9
Japan	7.1	Bangladesh	10.4
Indonesia	7.0	Russian Federation	10.3
Mexico	6.8	Egypt	8.6

*The 10 countries with the highest numbers of people with diabetes are listed.
Data from *IDF Atlas 2009* (http://www.idf.org/diabetesatlas/downloads)

The economic and social costs of diabetes are enormous, both for healthcare services and through loss of productivity. In developed countries, 10% or more of the total health budget is spent on the management of diabetes and its complications.

A brief history of diabetes and its classification

Diabetes was first described in ancient Egyptian times (Box 11.1). Throughout history there has been a focus on sugars or glucose, first from a recognition of excess sugar in the urine and then in the blood. This 'glucocentric' view of diabetes has shaped our current means of diagnosis and treatment.

Although there has been an awareness of different degrees of severity of diabetes for many centuries, the possibility of distinct types of diabetes only emerged at the beginning of the 20th century.

The original World Health Organization (WHO) classification of diabetes in 1980 and its revision in 1985 were based on clinical characteristics. The two commonest types of diabetes were termed insulin-dependent diabetes mellitus (IDDM) and non–insulin-dependent diabetes mellitus (NIDDM), reflecting the body's need for insulin to survive. The WHO classification also recognized malnutrition-related diabetes mellitus, other types of diabetes mellitus associated with specific conditions (Case history 11.3) and gestational diabetes, which is diabetes diagnosed for the first time during pregnancy.

In 1997, the American Diabetes Association (ADA) proposed a classification that distinguished the types of diabetes according to aetiology and clinical stages of the disease as it was hoped that this would be more clinically useful. The classification was subsequently adopted by the WHO in 1999

Table 11.2 Prevalence of diabetes in people aged 20–79 years in 2010 as a percentage and projected percentage in 2030.*

2010		2030	
Country/territory	**Percentage**	**Country/territory**	**Percentage**
Nauru	20.4	Nauru	21.5
Singapore	18.8	Bahrain	20.1
Bahrain	18.8	UAE	20.1
United Arab Emirates	18.8	Singapore	19.8
Kiribati	17.3	Kiribati	18.3
Poland	15.3	Poland	16.5
Ghana	14.1	Syria	15.3
Mauritius	13.5	Mauritius	14.3
Tonga	13.1	Tonga	14.0
Syria	13.0	Denmark	13.8

*The 10 countries with the highest percentage of people with diabetes are listed.
Data from *IDF Atlas 2009* (http://www.idf.org/diabetesatlas/downloads)

Box 11.1 A brief history of diabetes

1550 BC	The oldest description of diabetes as a polyuric state in ancient Egypt
5th/6th century BC	Indian physicians, such as Susrata and Charak, recognized the sweet, honey-like taste of urine from polyuric patients, which attracted ants and insects The descriptions of diabetes also recognized the distinction between two forms of diabetes, one in older, fatter people, and the other in thin people who rapidly succumbed to their illness
2nd century AD	Because of the urinary symptoms, Aretaeus of Cappadocia first used the term 'diabetes', coming from Greek meaning 'siphon' or 'pass through'
10th century AD	Avicenna, living in Arabia, recognized the sugary urine and complications of gangrene and erectile dysfunction
17th century AD	Thomas Willis, physician to King Charles II, re-discovered sweetness in urine. He also noted the importance of lifestyle when he remarked that the prevalence of diabetes was increasing because of '*good fellowship and gusling down chiefly of unalloyed wine*'. Willis was the first to recognize the link with mental illness '*Diabetes is a consequence of prolonged sorrow*'
1776	Matthew Dobson showed that urinary sweetness was caused by sugar and was associated with a rise in blood sugar

End 18th century	John Rollo first used the term 'diabetes mellitus' (honey) to distinguish the condition from 'diabetes insipidus' (insipid = tasteless), a deficiency of vasopressin, see Chapter 5
19th century	Claude Bernard, a French physiologist, discovered that: • Sugar is stored as glycogen in the liver • Transfixation of the medulla in conscious rabbits caused hyperglycaemia
1869	Paul Langerhans discovered the pancreatic islets
1889	Oskar Minkowski removed the pancreas from a dog and discovered that the animal developed diabetes
1893	Edouard Laguesse showed islets were the endocrine tissue of the pancreas
1921	Frederick Banting, Charles Best, James Collip and JJR Macleod discovered insulin in Toronto
1920s	First patients treated with insulin by physicians such as Elliot P Joslin, who introduced systematic diabetes education in the USA, and Robin D Lawrence, who had diabetes himself and founded the British Diabetic Association (now Diabetes UK)
1955	Primary structure of insulin elucidated by Frederick Sanger
1966	First transplant of human pancreas to treat type 1 diabetes by Kelly, Lillehei, Goetz and Merkel at the University of Minnesota
1969	Dorothy Hodgkin described the three-dimensional structure of insulin using X-ray crystallography
1980	Introduction of recombinant human insulin
1994	First implantation of pancreatic islets to treat type 1 diabetes by Pipeleers and colleagues in Belgium
1996	Introduction of insulin analogues
2000	James Shapiro and colleagues establish the 'Edmonton protocol' revitalizing efforts to cure type 1 diabetes by transplantation

(see Box 11.2). The terms IDDM and NIDDM were replaced with type 1 diabetes and type 2 diabetes respectively. Malnutrition-related diabetes was omitted from the new classification because its aetiology was uncertain and it was unclear whether it is a separate type of diabetes. The classification was reassessed by the WHO in 2006 when no changes were made. It is currently under discussion again.

Classification of diabetes

The current classification of diabetes is shown in Box 11.2. Type 1 and type 2 diabetes are covered in Chapters 12 and 13 respectively and gestational diabetes in Chapter 14. A number of secondary causes of diabetes are listed in Box 11.2 and include genetic mutations as well as other pathologies such as chronic pancreatitis.

Approximately 2–5% of cases of diabetes are caused by mutations in a single gene (monogenic mutation). For instance, maturity-onset diabetes of the young (MODY) is inherited as an autosomal dominant condition and is caused in most cases by a mutation in one of six genes, most commonly the one encoding hepatocyte nuclear family 1α (HNF1α) (Table 11.3 and review Chapter 2).

Box 11.2 1999 World Health Organization classification of diabetes

Type 1 diabetes (β-cell destruction)
- Immune mediated
- Idiopathic
- Formerly insulin-dependent diabetes

Type 2 diabetes
- Insulin resistance with inadequate insulin secretion
- Formerly non–insulin-dependent diabetes

Secondary diabetes
- Diabetes secondary to pancreatic disease:
  - Chronic pancreatitis
  - Haemochromatosis
  - Pancreatic surgery or trauma
  - Cystic fibrosis
- Diabetes secondary to endocrine disease:
  - Acromegaly
  - Cushing syndrome
  - Phaeochromocytoma
- Diabetes secondary to drugs and chemicals:
  - Glucocorticoids
  - Diuretics
  - Antipsychotics
  - β-blockers

- Diabetes secondary to genetic abnormalities:
  - Genetic defects of β-cell function:
    - MODY (maturity-onset diabetes of the young):
      Glucokinase mutations
      Hepatic nuclear factor mutations
      Insulin promoter factor 1 mutations
    - GATA6 mutations (neonatal diabetes)
    - Mitochondrial DNA 3243 mutation
  - Genetic defects of insulin action:
    - Leprechaunism
    - Type A insulin resistance
    - Rabson–Mendenhall syndrome
    - Lipoatrophic diabetes
  - Other genetic syndromes:
    - Down syndrome
    - Prader–Willi syndrome
    - DIDMOAD (Wolfram) syndrome
- Infections:
  - Congenital rubella
  - Cytomegalovirus
  - Mumps

Gestational diabetes

Table 11.3 Genetic mutations in maturity-onset diabetes of the young (MODY)

	Gene	MODY type
Glucokinase	GCK	2
Hepatic nuclear factor 1α Also known as transcription factor 1	HNF1α	3
Hepatic nuclear factor 4α	HNF4α	1
Hepatic nuclear factor 1β Also known as transcription factor 2	HNF1β	5
Insulin promoter factor 1 Also known as pancreatic duodenum homeobox gene 1	IPF1	4
Neurogenic differentiation-1/β2	NEUROD1	6

Diagnosis of diabetes

A diagnosis of diabetes is made if the fasting plasma glucose is 7.0 mmol/L (126 mg/dL) or greater or if the random or 2-h glucose tolerance test plasma glucose is 11.1 mmol/L (200 mg/dL) or greater (Table 11.4). The WHO diagnostic criteria also recognize two further categories of abnormal glucose concentrations: impaired fasting glycaemia (IFG) and impaired glucose tolerance (IGT), the latter of which can only be diagnosed following a 75-g oral glucose tolerance test (OGTT). The ADA definition of impaired fasting glycaemia differs slightly from the WHO criteria in that the threshold for IFG is 100 mg/dL (5.6 mmol/L).

Only one abnormal glucose value is required in a patient with classical diabetic symptoms, such as polydipsia (increased thirst) or polyuria (increased volume of micturition), but a supplementary test is required in asymptomatic individuals (Case history 11.4). The gold standard test for diabetes, endorsed

(Q) Case history 11.3

An 18-year-old woman with a strong family history of diabetes was diagnosed with insulin-dependent diabetes in 1990 after she presented with classical hyperglycaemic symptoms. Insulin therapy was commenced and her glycaemic control during the early stages of diabetes was excellent with no significant hypoglycaemia or diabetic complications. Fifteen years later she decided to start a family and requested genetic testing. She was found to have MODY caused by an inactivating mutation in the gene encoding HNF1α.

Does this diagnosis matter?
Are there any therapeutic implications to the revised diagnosis?

Answers, see p. 256

Table 11.4 The 1999 WHO diagnostic criteria for diabetes

		Fasting plasma glucose (mmol/L or *mg/dL*)		
		<6.1 *<110*	≥6.1–6.9 *≥110–125*	≥7.0 *≥126*
2-h plasma glucose following a 75-g oral glucose tolerance test (mmol/L or *mg/dL*)	<7.8 *<140*	Normal	Impaired fasting glycaemia*	Diabetes
	≥7.8–11.0 *≥140–200*	Impaired glucose tolerance	Impaired fasting glycaemia and impaired glucose tolerance	Diabetes
	≥11.1 *≥200*	Diabetes	Diabetes	Diabetes

*The American Diabetes Association defines impaired fasting glucose as between 110 and 125 mg/dL (5.6–6.9 mmol/L). Diabetes may also be diagnosed if a random plasma glucose is ≥11.1 mmol/L (200 mg/dL).

by the WHO, is currently the OGTT, which requires an overnight fast followed by a 75-g glucose drink, with blood samples taken for plasma glucose concentrations before the drink and 2 h afterwards (Box 11.3).

(Q) Case history 11.4

An asymptomatic 80-year-old frail woman is found to have a random plasma glucose of 11.3 mmol/L (203 mg/dL).

Does she have diabetes?

Answer, see p. 256

The criteria for the diagnosis of diabetes are constantly being reviewed and it is instructive to consider why there has been so much debate about the diagnosis. Plasma glucose concentrations show a skewed normal distribution in the general population and, as such, the delineation of abnormal from normal becomes arbitrary (Figure 11.3). An analogy to this would be height within the population. Height is normally distributed and so any distinction between short, normal and tall is subjective. For example, many would suggest a tall man is someone over 6′ tall (~180 cm), but in reality there is little difference in height between this man and another man who is 5′ 11″ (178 cm). The fact that this analogy does not work for those using metric measurements illustrates the point. The same is true for glucose and so it is important to consider why the WHO and ADA have chosen the cut-off values that they have. The reason is that the diagnostic criteria reflect the concentration of plasma glucose at which there is an association with the development of microvascular complications, particularly retinopathy. A clear threshold exists below which microvascular diabetic complications have not been identified. By contrast, the relationship between hyperglycaemia and macrovascular complications extends across the normal range with no threshold for the development of cardiovascular disease (Figure 11.4). This implies that cardiovascular risk also rises with increases in plasma glucose across the normal population.

Impaired fasting glycaemia (IFG) and impaired glucose tolerance (IGT) are not distinct clinical entities, but rather risk factors for future diabetes and cardiovascular disease. Indeed, the new term

'pre-diabetes' has been advocated to describe IGT and IFG. As many people with IFG or IGT do not develop diabetes, however, 'intermediate hyperglycaemia' is probably a better term. Other terminology has also been used to describe this situation.

A diagnosis of diabetes has important social, legal and medical implications for the patient and it is therefore essential that any diagnosis is secure and handled sensitively. The diagnosis of diabetes should never be made on the basis of glycosuria, and the glucose concentration should be measured on a venous plasma sample in an accredited laboratory.

Glycated haemoglobin

Although glucose has been used for many years to diagnose diabetes, there are on-going discussions about the use of glycated haemoglobin (HbA_{1c}) as an alternative method (Box 11.4). The major advantage is that the person does not need to fast, but HbA_{1c} is also more reproducible than a non-fasting glucose value. The reliability of HbA_{1c} may, however, be affected by a number of conditions such as anaemia and haemoglobinopathy. Both the WHO and ADA have endorsed the use of HbA_{1c} [≥6.5% (48 mmol/mol)] as a diagnostic test for diabetes, while the ADA also recognizes that HbA_{1c} levels of 5.7–6.4% (39–47 mmol/mol) indicate increased risk for future diabetes.

Insulin

Insulin is a 51-amino acid peptide hormone comprising two polypeptide chains, the A and B chains,

---

Box 11.3 How a glucose tolerance test is performed

- The patient should ensure that they have consumed >150 g of carbohydrate in the day prior to the test:
  - One slice of bread has 12 g of carbohydrate
  - 100 g of uncooked pasta contains 75 g of carbohydrate
- The patient should fast overnight, although water may be drunk
- The patient should refrain from smoking for 12 h prior to the test
- After collection of the fasting blood sample, the patient should drink 75 g of anhydrous glucose in 250–300 mL of water over 5 min
- A second blood sample should be collected exactly 2 h after the glucose challenge

As glucose should stimulate insulin secretion, it also acts as a metabolic negative feedback stimulus to suppress growth hormone (GH) secretion. Thus, this test is also used with more frequent blood sampling to diagnose acromegaly when GH fails to be suppressed (see Chapter 5).

Box 11.4 What is glycated haemoglobin?

Glycated haemoglobin (HbA_{1c}) is a measure of integrated glycaemic control over the preceding 2–3 months, reflecting the average lifespan of erythrocytes (red blood cells). Glucose becomes attached to adult haemoglobin in a non-enzymatic fashion that is dependent on the average concentration of blood glucose (Figure 11.5). This process is known as the Amadori reaction.

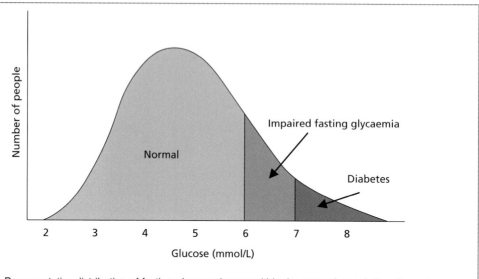

Figure 11.3 Representative distribution of fasting plasma glucose within the general population. It can be seen that people with impaired fasting glycaemia and diabetes are not discretely different from the rest of the population. As such, the diagnostic cut-off limits are somewhat arbitrary, but are largely based on the risk of developing microvascular complications.

which are linked by disulphide bridges (Figure 11.6). Insulin is synthesized in the β-cells of the islets of Langerhans in the pancreas (Figure 11.7). The other endocrine cell types of the islet are the α-cells producing glucagon, the δ-cells producing somatostatin, the ε-cells producing ghrelin and the pancreatic polypeptide (PP) cells producing pancreatic polypeptide. The β-cells are the most numerous, tend to be located more centrally in islet structures and are surrounded by the other cell types.

Insulin is synthesized on the ribosomes of the rough endoplasmic reticulum (RER) as a single amino acid chain precursor molecule called pre-proinsulin (review Chapter 2 and Figures 2.3 and 2.4). After removal of the signal peptide, proinsulin is transferred from the RER to the Golgi apparatus, where soluble zinc-containing proinsulin hexamers are formed. The prohormone convertase enzyme, PC1/3, finally acts outside the Golgi apparatus to produce the mature insulin and connecting peptide (C-peptide). The same enzyme cleaves adrenocorticotrophic hormone (ACTH) from pro-opiomelanocortin (POMC) in the anterior pituitary (see Chapter 5); hence, inactivating mutations

in PC1/3 cause both secondary hypoadrenalism and diabetes. In the pancreatic islet, both insulin and C-peptide are released simultaneously in equimolar quantities by exocytosis in response to a number of stimuli, including glucose and amino acids (Table 11.5).

Secretion

In response to nutrients following a meal, insulin is secreted in a coordinated pulsatile fashion from the β-cells into the portal vein in a characteristic biphasic pattern (Figure 11.8); first there is an acute rapid 'first phase' release of insulin, lasting for a few minutes, followed by a less intense more sustained 'second phase'. Pancreatic β-cells also secrete 0.25–1.5 units of insulin/h during the fasting state. Although at a low-level, this background secretion accounts for over 50% of total daily insulin production.

Glucose is the principal stimulus for insulin secretion, though other macronutrients, and hormonal and neuronal factors may alter this response (Table 11.5). When glucose enters the β-cell via a family of high-capacity glucose transporters (GLUT

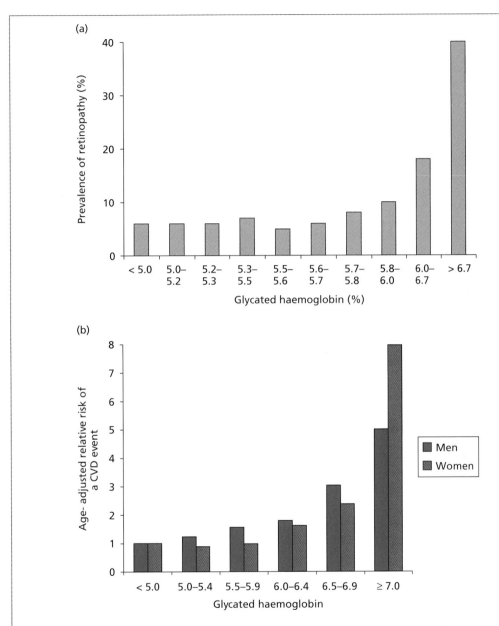

Figure 11.4 Relationship between plasma glucose and microvascular and macrovascular complications. (a) The prevalence of retinopathy according to glycated haemoglobin (measured as a %) in the US National Health and Nutrition Examination Survey. Data from Cheng YJ et al. *Diabetes Care* 2009;32:2027–32. (b) The age-adjusted relative risk of a cardiovascular (CVD) event according to glycated haemoglobin (measured as a %) in men and women in the European Prospective Investigation into Cancer in Norfolk. Data from Khaw KT et al. *Ann Intern Med* 2004;141:413–20. Note how the risk of macrovascular disease increases with increasing glycated haemoglobin across the normal range, particularly in men. In contrast, there is a threshold for the diagnosis of retinopathy.

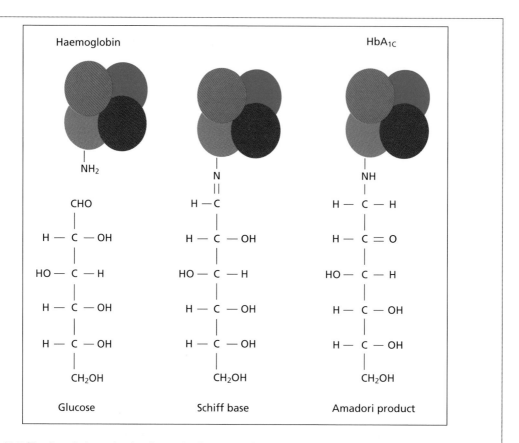

Figure 11.5 The Amadori reaction leading to the formation of glycated haemoglobin (HbA$_{1C}$). Haemoglobin reacts in a non-enzymatic manner with glucose to form glycated derivatives. The extent of glycation depends on the concentration of glucose and duration of exposure. Reproduced from Holt RIG *et al.*, eds. *Textbook of Diabetes: A Clinical Approach*, 4th edn. Oxford: Wiley-Blackwell, 2010, Chapter 25.

1–3, mainly GLUT-2), it undergoes phosphorylation by the enzyme glucokinase and metabolism by glycolysis to produce ATP (Figure 11.9). The rise in ATP closes a type of potassium channel, the potassium inward rectifying channel type 6.2 (KIR6.2), on the cell surface, leading to depolarization of the membrane. This is followed by an influx of calcium ions which triggers insulin granule translocation to the cell surface and the hormone's release by exocytosis. The mechanism of action of sulphonylureas, a class of oral hypoglycaemic agents (see Chapter 13), is by binding to a receptor, the sulphonylurea receptor 1 (SUR1), in close apposition to the KIR6.2 channels and resulting in their closure. This process can be divided in two: glucose sensing

and insulin secretion. Normal β-cell function is dependent on the exquisite coupling of glucose sensing and insulin secretion. For instance, inactivating mutations in glucokinase causes a form of MODY and activating mutations in KIR6.2 or SUR1 can cause permanent neonatal diabetes. In contrast, inactivation of KIR6.2 or SUR1 can uncouple secretion from glucose sensing and cause a rare syndrome of excessive insulin production and hypoglycaemia, called congenital hyperinsulinism.

Action

Insulin exerts its biological actions by binding to the insulin receptor on the target cell surface. The

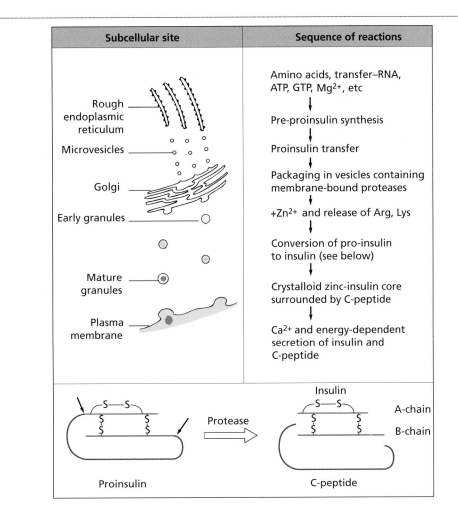

Subcellular site	Sequence of reactions

Figure 11.6 Insulin synthesis and secretion from the β-cells of pancreatic islets of Langerhans. Protein synthesis on the rough endoplasmic reticulum yields pre-proinsulin, which is transferred into the lumen of the endoplasmic reticulum (see also Figures 2.3 and 2.4). Hydrolysis yields proinsulin, which is then transferred to the Golgi apparatus approximately 20 min after the initiation of protein synthesis. Proinsulin is enclosed in vesicles that carry specific proteases bound to the membrane. Over a period of 30 min to 2 h, the specific proteases act on proinsulin to release C-peptide and insulin within the granule. Progressive maturation and crystallization of the zinc 1–insulin complex yields a dense crystalloid region surrounded by a clear space containing C-peptide. When the cells are stimulated, e.g. by a rise in blood glucose, an energy-dependent and Ca^{2+}-dependent fusion of the granules with the cell membrane releases the contents into the bloodstream. Insulin and C-peptide are released in approximately equimolar amounts. The lower portion of the illustration shows a schematic diagram of the structures of proinsulin and insulin. Proinsulin, on the left, is cleaved at two points (arrows) by specific proteases packaged into early β-cell granules. The C-peptide is cleaved from a single-chain peptide to leave insulin, which then has two chains, A and B, linked by two disulphide bridges, with the A chain also carrying an intrachain disulphide bridge. Proinsulin contains 86 amino acids, while insulin has 21 amino acids in the A chain and 30 in the B chain.

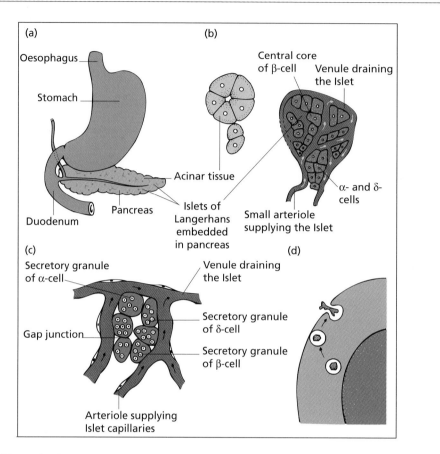

Figure 11.7 The endocrine pancreas. (a) Small clusters of cells, the islets of Langerhans, are embedded in the exocrine acinar tissue. (b) Each islet consists of a core mainly of β-cells surrounded by α- and δ-cells. The islet is supplied with one or more small arterioles that penetrate the centre of the islet and then break up into capillaries. These first supply the central β-cells and then flow to the more peripherally located α- and δ-cells. The capillaries leave the islet and form the draining venules. In this way, the circulation ensures that the β-cell rich core of the islet is the first to be exposed to high glucose concentrations, and the peripheral α- and δ-cells are exposed to high insulin concentrations from the inner β-cells. (c) The different cell types of the islet have distinctive secretory granules, which enable them to be easily identified under the electron microscope. The islet cells are also coupled to each other via gap junctions. (d) Part of a β-cell, showing a secretory granule discharging its contents in the process of exocytosis, leading to the release of insulin.

insulin receptor is a heterotetramer consisting of two α- and two β-glycoprotein subunits linked by disulphide bonds. Insulin binds to the extracellular α-sub-units, resulting in conformational change enabling ATP to bind to the intracellular component of the β-subunit; this triggers phosphorylation of the β-subunit, conferring tyrosine kinase activity (Figure 3.6). Tyrosine phosphorylation of intracellular substrate proteins, known as insulin responsive substrates (IRSs), ensues, and these can then bind other signalling molecules that in turn mediate further cellular actions of insulin (Figure 11.10).

Effects on intermediate metabolism

Insulin may be considered as a hormone that signals the 'post-meal' fed state. During this period, insulin is pivotal in regulating cellular energy supply and macronutrient balance, and directing anabolic processes (Figure 11.11).

Table 11.5 Factors regulating insulin release from the β-cells of the pancreatic islets

Insulin secertion increased by	Insulin secretion decreased by
Nutrients	Nutrients
Raised glucose	Low glucose
Amino acids	Hormones
Hormones	Somatostatin
Glucagon	NPY
Gastrin, secretin	Ghrelin
Cholecystokinin	Pancreatic innervation
GIP	Signalling via
GLP-1	sympathetic β
Pancreatic innervation	receptors
Signalling via	Adipokines
sympathetic	Leptin
α-receptors	Resistin
Parasympathetic	Stress
stimulation	Exercise
Adipokines	Hypoxia
Adiponectin	Hypothermia
	Surgery
	Severe burns

GIP, glucose-dependent insulinotrophic peptide (previously known as 'gastric inhibitory peptide'); GLP-1, glucagon-like peptide 1; NPY, neuropeptide Y.

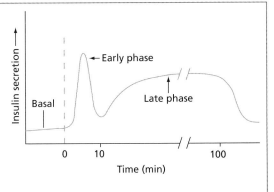

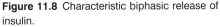

Figure 11.8 Characteristic biphasic release of insulin.

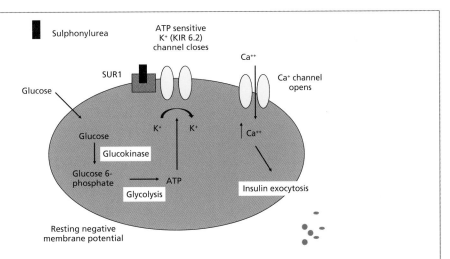

Figure 11.9 Mechanism of insulin secretion. After uptake, glucose is metabolized within the β-cell to generate ATP. The increase in ATP closes ATP-sensitive potassium (KIR 6.2) channels in the cell membrane and prevents potassium ions from leaving the cell. This depolarizes the cell membrane, which in turn opens voltage-gated calcium channels in the membrane allowing calcium ions to enter the cell and be released from intracellular stores. The increase in intracellular calcium initiates insulin granule exocytosis. Sulphonylureas act by binding to the SUR1 which is a component of the K$^+$-ATP channel.

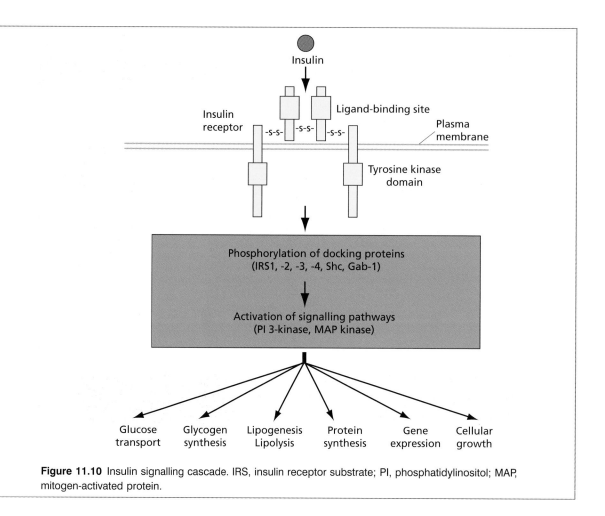

Figure 11.10 Insulin signalling cascade. IRS, insulin receptor substrate; PI, phosphatidylinositol; MAP, mitogen-activated protein.

Insulin has major anabolic actions on intermediate metabolism, affecting glucose, lipid and protein metabolism. The most important insulin-sensitive tissues are the liver, skeletal muscle and adipose tissue. Following secretion of insulin, 60% is subsequently removed by the liver; so portal vein insulin concentrations reaching the liver are almost three-fold higher than in the peripheral circulation. Insulin plays a major role in regulating hepatic glucose output by inhibiting gluconeogenesis and promoting glycogen storage. Similarly in muscle cells, insulin-mediated glucose uptake enables glycogen to be synthesized and stored, and for carbohydrates, rather than fatty acids or amino acids, to be utilized as the immediately available energy source for muscle contraction. Adipose tissue fat breakdown is suppressed and fat synthesis is promoted.

Glucose metabolism

Normally plasma glucose concentration is maintained within a narrow range despite wide fluctuations in nutrient supply and demand. Under normal physiological conditions, insulin, together with its principal counter-regulatory hormone glucagon, is the prime controller of glucose metabolism.

Insulin is involved in the regulation of carbohydrate metabolism at many steps (Table 11.6). As already mentioned, insulin increases glucose uptake into key insulin-sensitive tissues. As in the β-cell (see earlier), glucose is carried into cells across the cell membrane by glucose transporters (GLUTs). GLUT-1 is involved in basal and non–insulin-mediated glucose uptake by cells, while GLUT-2 is important in the β-cell for glucose sensing. GLUT-3 is involved in non–insulin-mediated glucose

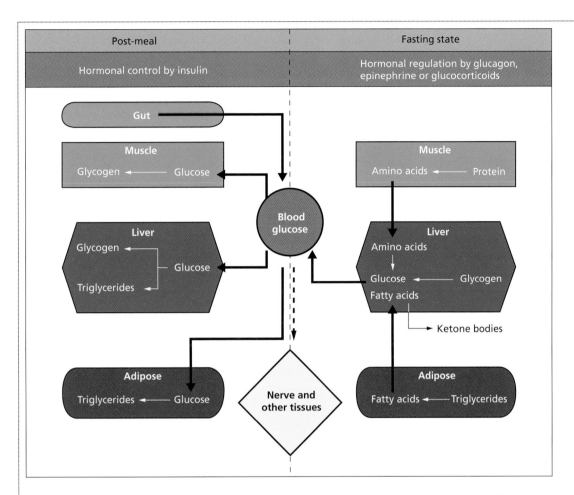

Figure 11.11 Regulation of blood glucose concentration. Tissue utilization of metabolites after a meal and in a fasting state are contrasted. Food is absorbed from the gut and increases the blood glucose concentration. Insulin facilitates absorption and stimulates the synthesis of glycogen and triglyceride storage in liver and adipose tissues. Approximately 90% of stored glucose is in the form of lipids. In the fasting state, amino acids are mobilized from muscle proteins to yield pyruvate in the liver, where gluconeogenesis and glycogenolysis are capable of maintaining the plasma glucose levels for utilization by brain, nerves and other tissues. Various hormones, including epinephrine, glucagon and glucocorticoids, exert a regulatory action at different sites in these tissues. Fatty acids, mobilized from adipose tissues under the control of a number of hormones (epinephrine, adrenocorticotrophic hormone, glucagon, growth hormone), provide a substrate for liver and muscle metabolism. Ketone bodies produced in the liver provide an energy source for muscle and brain during long periods of fasting.

uptake into the brain and GLUT-4 is responsible for insulin-stimulated glucose uptake into muscle and adipose tissue. GLUT-4 is normally located within vesicles in the cytoplasm, but following binding of insulin to its receptor, it is translocated to the cell surface where it creates a pore for glucose entry.

Insulin acts to increase glycogen synthesis and inhibit glycogen breakdown. The control of glycogen metabolism is dependent on the

Table 11.6 Insulin actions on carbohydrate metabolism

Action	Mechanism
Increases glucose uptake into cells	Translocation of glucose transporter (GLUT)-4 to the cell surface
Increases glycogen synthesis	Activates glycogen synthase by dephosphorylation
Inhibits glycogen breakdown	Inactivates glycogen phosphorylase and its activating kinase by dephosphorylation
Inhibits gluconeogenesis	Dephosphorylation of pyruvate kinase and 2,6-biphosphate kinase
Increases glycolysis	Dephosphorylation of pyruvate kinase and 2,6-biphosphate kinase
Converts pyruvate to acetyl CoA	Activates the intramitochondrial enzyme complex pyruvate dehydrogenase

phosphorylation and dephosphorylation of the enzymes controlling glycogenolysis and glycogen synthesis (Figure 11.12). The rate-limiting enzymes are the catabolic enzyme glycogen phosphorylase and the anabolic enzyme glycogen synthase. Insulin increases glycogen synthesis by activating glycogen synthase, while inhibiting glycogenolysis by dephosphorylating glycogen phosphorylase kinase. Glycolysis is stimulated and gluconeogenesis inhibited by dephosphorylation of pyruvate kinase (PK) and 2,6-biphosphate kinase. Insulin also enhances the irreversible conversion of pyruvate to acetyl CoA by activation of the intramitochondrial enzyme complex pyruvate dehydrogenase. Acetyl CoA may then be directly oxidized via the tricarboxylic acid (Krebs') cycle, or used for fatty acid synthesis (Figure 11.13).

Lipid metabolism

Insulin increases the rate of lipogenesis in several ways in adipose tissue and liver, and controls the formation and storage of triglyceride. The critical step in lipogenesis is the activation of the insulin-sensitive lipoprotein lipase in the capillaries. Fatty acids are then released from circulating chylomicrons or very low-density lipoproteins and taken up into the adipose tissue. Fatty acid synthesis is increased by activation and increased phosphorylation of acetyl CoA carboxylase, while fat oxidation is suppressed by inhibition of carnitine acyltransferase (Table 11.7). Lipogenesis is also facilitated by glucose uptake, because its metabo-

lism by the pentose phosphate pathway provides nicotinamide adenine dinucleotide phosphate (NADPH), which is needed for fatty acid synthesis.

Triglyceride synthesis is stimulated by ester-ification of glycerol phosphate, while triglyceride breakdown is suppressed by dephosphorylation of hormone-sensitive lipase.

Cholesterol synthesis is increased by activation and dephosphorylation of hydroxymethylglutaryl co-enzyme A (HMGCoA) reductase, while choles-terol ester breakdown appears to be inhibited by dephosphorylation of cholesterol esterase. Phospholipid metabolism is also influenced by insulin.

Protein metabolism

Insulin stimulates the uptake of amino acid into cells and promotes protein synthesis in a range of tissues. There are effects on the transcription of specific mRNA, as well as their translation into proteins on the ribosomes (review Chapter 2 and Figure 2.2). Examples of enhanced mRNA tran-scription include glucokinase and fatty acid syn-thase. By contrast, insulin decreases mRNA encoding liver enzymes such as carbamoyl phos-phate synthetase, which is a key enzyme in the urea cycle. However, the major action of insulin on protein metabolism is to inhibit the breakdown of proteins (Figure 11.14). In this way it acts synergis-tically with GH and insulin-like growth factor I (IGF-I) to increase protein anabolism.

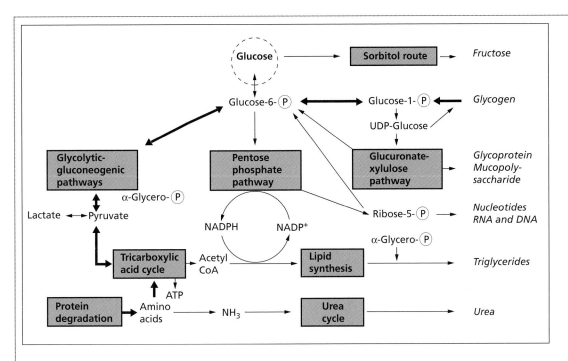

Figure 11.12 Inter-relationships among alternative routes of glucose metabolism. The central role of glucose in carbohydrate, fat and protein metabolism is summarized. The principal metabolic pathways are shown enclosed in boxes in order to simplify the diagram; some key intermediates and products of metabolic interconversions are shown. The reversibility of certain reaction sequences implied by double-headed arrows is not necessarily intended to suggest that the same enzymes are involved in both the forward and reverse reactions. The principal reversible pathways that are activated during fasting are marked with heavy arrows.

Table 11.7 Insulin actions on fatty acid metabolism	
Action	**Mechanism**
Releases fatty acids from circulating chylomicrons or very low-density lipoproteins	Activates lipoprotein lipase
Increases fatty acid synthesis	Activates acetyl CoA carboxylase
Suppresses fatty acid oxidation	Inhibits carnitine acyltransferase
Increases triglyceride synthesis	Stimulates esterification of glycerol phosphate
Inhibits triglyceride breakdown	Dephosphorylates hormone-sensitive lipase
Increases cholesterol synthesis	Activates and dephosphorylates HMGCoA reductase
Inhibits cholesterol ester breakdown	Dephosphorylates cholesterol esterase

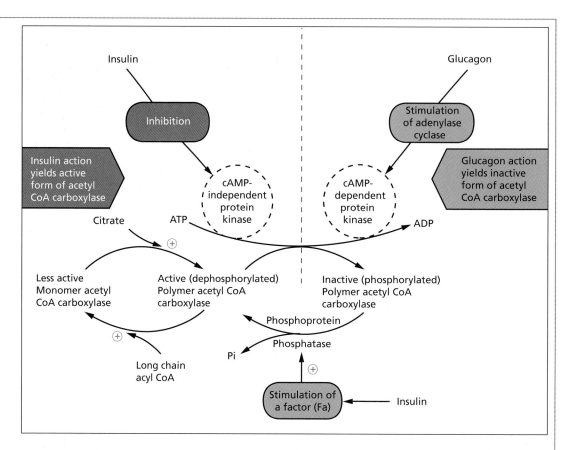

Figure 11.13 Regulation of acetyl co-enzyme A (CoA) carboxylase by allosteric regulators and by phosphorylation–dephosphorylation mechanisms. Acetyl CoA carboxylase, which is involved in fatty acid synthesis, exists as a monomer and in two polymeric forms, which are interconvertible by dephosphorylation. Citrate and long-chain acyl CoA control the relative proportions of the less active monomer and the active polymeric form of acetyl CoA carboxylase by allosteric mechanisms. As in the case of glycogen synthetase, two protein kinase enzymes are capable of regulating the conversion of active polymer acetyl CoA carboxylase to the inactive phosphorylated form of the enzyme. The cyclic adenosine 5′-monophosphate (cAMP)-dependent protein kinase may be activated by glucagon (top right), while the cAMP-independent protein kinase is inhibited by insulin action on the target cell (top left). As fatty acid synthesis is increased by activation and increased phosphorylation of acetyl CoA carboxylase, glucagon action on the cell decreases lipogenesis, while insulin stimulates fatty acid synthesis.

Glucagon

Glucagon is a polypeptide with a molecular weight of ~3.5 kD. It is synthesized as a large precursor, pre-proglucagon, and is cleaved within the α-cells to the active hormone.

Its secretion is stimulated by a fall in blood glucose and by amino acids. Release of glucagon is also under neural control; sympathetic adrenergic activation increases glucagon release.

Glucagon plays an important part in preventing significant hypoglycaemia during fasting by antagonizing the actions of insulin. Its primary site of action is the liver where it binds to specific G-protein–coupled glucagon receptors that are linked to adenylate cyclase (review Chapter 3). This leads to the mobilization of glycogen and to the production of glucose from non-carbohydrate precursors by gluconeogenesis.

Key points

- Diabetes is the commonest endocrine condition and its prevalence is increasing rapidly worldwide
- Diabetes is a major clinical specialty in its own right alongside endocrinology
- The commonest types of diabetes are type 1 and type 2 diabetes
- Diabetes is defined by elevations in blood glucose
- Insulin is the pivotal hormone regulating cellular energy supply and macronutrient balance during the fed 'post-meal' state

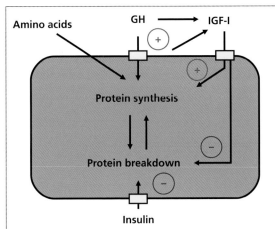

Figure 11.14 The synergistic actions of insulin, IGF-I, and GH on protein synthesis. GH and IGF-I stimulate protein synthesis directly, while insulin is mainly anabolic through the inhibition of protein breakdown. The anabolic action of both GH and IGF-I appears to be mediated through induction of amino acid transporters in the cell membrane. IGF-I may act in a local autocrine or paracrine fashion as well as in an endocrine manner.

Answers to case histories

Case history 11.1

There is a large burden of diabetes in every community, with 20–50% of all cases of diabetes remaining undiagnosed. Diabetes prevalence varies from region to region according to the demographics of the region, and therefore estimates from other regions may be inappropriate. Any questionnaire survey of diabetes prevalence may significantly underestimate the true prevalence as many people do not know they have the disorder. Similarly, extrapolation from historical publications may underestimate the prevalence as this is increasing more rapidly than previously.

Establishing registers of patients with diabetes is one way of obtaining a reasonable estimate of known cases of diabetes. Epidemiologists have developed models based on published studies that can be used to estimate the burden of diabetes locally. One such example is the York & Humber Public Health Observatory (http://www.yhpho.org.uk/resource/view.aspx?RID=81090).

Case history 11.2

No. Type 2 diabetes is frequently found in asymptomatic individuals. There is an increasing drive towards screening for type 2 diabetes, especially in high-risk individuals, which is relatively straightforward in the era of automated biochemical testing. This man is overweight, which increases the risk of diabetes. Hypertension is also associated with an increased risk of diabetes. Symptoms of diabetes usually only begin when the blood glucose exceeds the renal capacity to re-absorb glucose from the proximal tubules. Although this varies between individuals, this is usually greater than 11 mmol/L (200 mg/dL). The gradual insidious onset of diabetes means that people frequently are asymptomatic and may have had diabetes for many years before the development of symptoms.

Again no. Even though the person with diabetes is asymptomatic, the hyperglycaemia is still damaging and so complications can occur in people with previously undiagnosed diabetes. In the UK Prospective Diabetes Study, around 50% of people with newly diagnosed diabetes had one or more diabetic complications. It is hoped that with increased awareness and targeted screening of high-risk individuals, this proportion will decrease, and this is one of the major rationales for screening for diabetes.

Case history 11.3

Yes. At an individual level, a precise diagnosis is important to predict clinical course, explain other associated clinical features, enable genetic counselling and diagnosis of family members, and guide appropriate treatment. For instance, some forms of MODY, such as inactivating glucokinase mutations, tend to have a more benign course and do not appear to be associated with the development of diabetic complications. Some other forms have extra-pancreatic features, such as renal cysts, lipodystrophy or deafness. She is only 33 years old and wishes to have a family. As well as predicting the risk to her future children, the management of MODY during pregnancy differs from that of type 1 or type 2 diabetes. MODY should be considered when there is an autosomal dominant family history of early-onset diabetes; when the presentation or course is atypical for type 1 or type 2 diabetes; when diabetes is diagnosed in the first 6 months of life; or when there are associated extra-pancreatic clinical features. More broadly, diagnostic precision is always critical for understanding epidemiological and other clinical features.

Yes. This woman was treated with insulin for 15 years. Diabetes caused by HNF1α mutations often responds better to sulphonylureas than insulin and this would have saved her ~20,000 injections!

Case history 11.4

We do not know. In order to make a diagnosis of diabetes in an asymptomatic person, two values above the internationally agreed criteria are required. A random blood glucose of 11.2 mmol/L (201 mg/dL) is in the diagnostic range for diabetes, but a second confirmatory test is required. The WHO recommends that the gold standard confirmatory test is a 75-g OGTT, although if the fasting glucose was ≥7.0 mmol/L (126 mg/dL), this would be sufficient. An alternative would be to consider the use of glycated haemoglobin.

CHAPTER 12

Type 1 diabetes

Key topics

- What is type 1 diabetes?   258
- Management   264
- Acute metabolic emergencies   274
- Key points   283
- Answers to case histories   283

Learning objectives

- To discuss the epidemiology, aetiology and pathology of type 1 diabetes
- To understand the clinical features of type 1 diabetes and, in particular, recognize the importance of diabetic ketoacidosis
- To understand the principles of insulin therapy and its pitfalls
- To manage the acute metabolic complications:
  - □ Hypoglycaemia
  - □ Diabetic ketoacidosis

This chapter describes type 1 diabetes

To recap

- Genetic abnormalities may affect pancreatic β-cell function and lead to a presentation of diabetes that is similar to autoimmune type 1 diabetes. A description of the structure of genes and their transcription and translation is given in Chapter 2
- An overview of diabetes is given in Chapter 11

Essential Endocrinology and Diabetes, Sixth Edition. Richard IG Holt, Neil A Hanley.
© 2012 Richard IG Holt and Neil A Hanley. Publlished 2012 by Blackwell Publishing Ltd.

Cross-reference

- Several hormones influence the action of insulin and exert an effect on glucose control. These include growth hormone (see Chapter 5), cortisol and catecholamines (see Chapter 6)

- The pathogenesis of type 1 diabetes involves a selective autoimmune destruction of the pancreatic β-cells. Individuals with type 1 diabetes are at increased risk of other autoimmune diseases, such as thyroid disease, which is covered in Chapter 8

- Exercise plays an important part in the management of both type 1 and type 2 diabetes. Exercise is discussed in greater detail in Chapter 13

- Diabetes can lead to the development of a number of complications, which are discussed in Chapter 14

Although type 1 diabetes only accounts for around 10% of all cases of diabetes, its presentation, particularly in children and young adults, and acute complications are the most dramatic. Prior to the discovery of insulin, type 1 diabetes rapidly led to the death of the patient; consequently, the use of insulin to treat people with type 1 diabetes can rightly be considered as one of the greatest advances in medicine in the 20th century. Insulin has saved and transformed the lives of millions of people worldwide and continues to do so.

What is type 1 diabetes?

Type 1 diabetes is caused by an absolute deficiency of insulin. In populations of white Northern European ancestry, it usually occurs as the result of a T-cell–mediated autoimmune destruction of the β-cells of the pancreas (Box 12.1).

By contrast, autoimmune type 1 diabetes is uncommon in non-Caucasian populations. With a better understanding of the pathogenesis of diabetes, it is recognized that other genetic or acquired factors affecting pancreatic β-cell function can result in diabetes that presents in the same way as autoimmune type 1 diabetes (Box 12.2). Furthermore, there may be a broad range of clinical manifestations that overlap between type 1 and type 2 diabetes (Chapter 13).

Epidemiology

Approximately 20 million people have type 1 diabetes worldwide. Although type 1 diabetes may

---

Box 12.1 What is autoimmunity?

Under normal circumstances, the immune system does not react against the body's cells, tissues and organs. This is known as immune tolerance. Autoimmunity is caused by a breakdown of this normal immune tolerance of self. See Box 8.8 for other examples of organ-specific autoimmune diseases with shared genetic predisposition.

Box 12.2 Genetic and acquired factors that can affect pancreatic β-cell function leading to a presentation of diabetes that is similar to autoimmune type 1 diabetes

- Mitochondrial gene mutations
- Amylin gene mutations
- Maturity-onset diabetes of the young (MODY)
- Latent autoimmune diabetes of adults (LADA)
- Viral infection

---

affect all age groups, most are diagnosed as children, adolescents or young adults. According to a large European study, the incidence is increasing and age of onset is becoming younger. Type 1 diabetes is rare in children younger than 1 year old and if diabetes occurs at this age, maturity onset diabetes of the young (MODY) or other monogenic cause of diabetes should be considered (Box 12.3 and Table 11.3). There is a steady rise in incidence throughout childhood with the peak occurring slightly earlier in girls (~11 years) than boys (~14 years), suggesting an influence of puberty. There is also a smaller peak at the age of 4–5 years.

The incidence of type 1 diabetes varies dramatically throughout the world. The highest incidence rates are in northern Europe, where the rates are up to 500-fold greater than in China, Pakistan or Venezuela (Figure 12.1). Some of this difference may reflect ethnic heterogeneity between populations, but this does not explain all the difference, e.g. the rates of diabetes in Sardinia are three- to six-fold higher than in mainland Italy.

Box 12.3 The difference between monogenic and polygenic disorders

Monogenic
- Caused by a mutation in one gene
  - E.g. MODY and permanent neonatal diabetes

Polygenic
- Caused by many genes
  - E.g. type 2 diabetes

Worldwide the incidence and prevalence of type 1 diabetes increased markedly during the second half of the 20th century. Overall, the incidence rate increased between 3.2% and 5.3% per year during the 1990s, with the most pronounced increase seen in pre-school children. The only global regions with a decreasing trend were Central America and the West Indies.

During the 1970s, diabetes was slightly commoner in European boys and in populations of European origin while in contrast, in African or Asian populations, girls were more commonly affected. However, during the 1990s the sex-specific pattern changed and the male excess has disappeared from many but not all populations.

Pathogenesis

The pathogenesis of type 1 diabetes remains poorly understood, but the most likely scenario is that an environmental factor triggers a selective autoimmune destruction of the β-cells in the pancreas of a genetically predisposed individual.

The autoimmune process develops as a result of a loss of immunological tolerance and involves both cellular and humoral immune pathways. Histological examination of the pancreas from an individual with type 1 diabetes reveals a chronic inflammatory mononuclear cell infiltrate of CD4+ and CD8+ T lymphocytes and macrophages in the islets (insulitis).

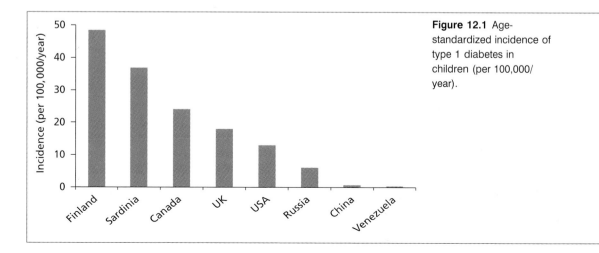

Figure 12.1 Age-standardized incidence of type 1 diabetes in children (per 100,000/year).

Table 12.1 Islet cell auto-antibodies involved in the pathogenesis of type 1 diabetes

Antigen	Antibody abbreviation	Function	Proportion with antibody at diagnosis (%)	Age	Gender
Glutamic acid decarboxylase	GAD65Ab	GABA production	70–80	Frequency increases with increasing age	Female preponderance if onset is <10 years
Islet antigen-2	IA-2Ab	Unknown	60–70	Frequency decreases with increasing age	Male preponderance
Insulin	IAA	Regulates glucose	50	Better predictive value in children	No difference
ZnT8 transporter	ZnT8Ab	Zinc transport and accumulation in β-cells	60–80	Better predictive value with age	No difference

The CD8+ T lymphocytes are thought to be responsible for the selective and specific killing of the β-cells.

The presence of circulating islet-related auto-antibodies in the period preceding the clinical onset of diabetes adds further evidence for an autoimmune process (Table 12.1). These antibodies may be present for many months prior to the onset of diabetes and have been used to predict which individuals will develop diabetes with considerable accuracy (up to 98%). It was previously thought that the development of type 1 diabetes occurred rapidly over a period of several weeks. Having followed individuals with islet cell antibodies, it is now known that β-cell loss can be slow and some individuals do not develop diabetes until many years after the appearance of the auto-antibodies (Figure 12.2). Furthermore, not all individuals with auto-antibodies develop diabetes, suggesting that autoimmunity against the islet cells does not necessarily progress to sufficient β-cell loss to cause diabetes.

The autoimmune basis for type 1 diabetes is also suggested by its association with a number of other organ-specific autoimmune diseases, such as autoimmune thyroid disease, coeliac disease, pernicious anaemia and Addison disease (Case history 12.1; see Box 8.8).

Case history 12.1

A 24-year-old woman with previously well-controlled type 1 diabetes presents with tiredness and lethargy. She also remarks that she has had many more hypoglycaemic episodes than previously and has had to cut her insulin dose by 50%. She mentions that she often feels dizzy when she stands up and has noticed that she is more 'tanned' than usual.

What is the possible explanation for her symptoms?
How would you confirm your diagnosis?

Answers, see p. 283

Aetiology

It is apparent that both genetic and environmental factors are important in the development of type 1 diabetes.

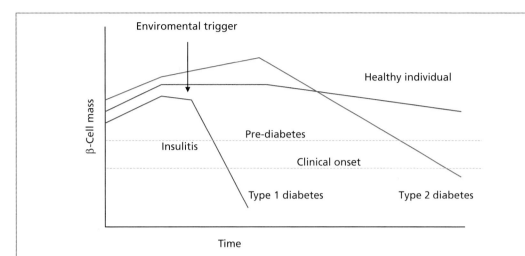

Figure 12.2 The natural history of diabetes. β-Cell mass increases during childhood and reaches a peak in early adulthood. Thereafter there is a progressive loss of β-cell mass of approximately 1%/year. In type 2 diabetes, the rate of β-cell loss is accelerated to approximately 4%. One model for the natural history of type 1 diabetes is that certain individuals are genetically pre-disposed to develop diabetes. Environmental factors act as triggers or regulators of the autoimmune destructive process that results in insulitis, β-cell injury and finally loss of β-cell mass. As β-cell function falls, first-phase insulin secretion is lost, followed by the development of intermediate hyperglycaemia and eventually overt diabetes. At the onset of diabetes, some β-cells will remain and their presence can be identified by the presence of circulating C-peptide. With time, however, these remaining cells will also be destroyed, leading to absolute insulin deficiency. The difference between type 1 and type 2 diabetes appears to be one of tempo and there has been debate recently about whether the division into two types is wholly justified. An alternative view is that they are opposite ends of a spectrum of β-cell loss.

Genetic factors

Evidence for the importance of genetic factors comes from twin and family studies. The risk of developing diabetes increases with the number of family members with the condition. The background risk in the population is 0.4%, but this increases to around 65–70% for a monozygotic twin whose other twin developed type 1 diabetes under the age of 5 years (Table 12.2).

The risk of diabetes is modified markedly by genes in the class II region of the human leucocyte antigen (HLA) system (Box 12.4). Over 95% of white European people with type 1 diabetes have HLA-DR-3 and/or DR-4 class II HLA antigens, as compared with only 50% of individuals without diabetes. By contrast, certain HLA haplotypes, such as HLA DQ-5 and DQ-6, may protect against diabetes. In Europe, around 5–6% of siblings of children with type 1 diabetes will develop diabetes themselves by the age of 15 years. However, if the HLA genotype is identical to the sibling with diabetes, the risk of developing diabetes increases to 16–20%, while siblings who share one HLA gene have a risk of 9% (Table 12.2).

Recently, genome-wide association studies have identified a number of additional 'non-HLA' loci that are associated with the development of type 1 diabetes. The strongest associations seem to link to the following nearby genes:

• INSULIN (*INS*), the association is particularly localized to the variable number of tandem repeat (VNTR) polymorphisms in the *INS* promoter (*INS VNTR*; review gene structure in Figure 2.2)
• Protein tyrosine phosphatase non-receptor type 2 (*PTPN2*)
• Interleukin-2 receptor, α chain (*IL2RA*).

Table 12.2 Risk of developing type 1 diabetes for relatives of people with type 1 diabetes

Family member	Risk
Monozygotic twin	30–50% in other twin 65–70% if twin diagnosed before age of 5 years
Dizygotic twin	15%
Sibling with HLA genotype that is identical to the affected sibling	16-20%
Sibling who shares one HLA gene	9%
HLA non-identical sibling	3%
Mother	2%
Father	8%
Both parents	30%
General population	0.4%

Environmental factors

Although the genetic susceptibility to type 1 diabetes is inherited, only 12–15% of type 1 diabetes occurs in families with a history of diabetes and only 10% of HLA-susceptible individuals develop type 1 diabetes. This indicates that genetic factors do not account entirely for the development of type 1 diabetes, and several environmental triggers have been suggested (Box 12.5).

How these factors affect the autoimmune response is unclear and it should be noted that none of the environmental factors is either necessary or sufficient to cause type 1 diabetes.

There are several overlapping hypotheses to explain the environmental effect on the risk of diabetes:

• An environmental trigger leads to an abnormal production of co-stimulatory molecules and up-regulation of the HLA antigens in susceptible people. This may lead to self-antigens being presented to T-helper cells and triggering an autoimmune response.

Box 12.4 What are HLA molecules?

• HLA antigens are glycoproteins found on the cell surface that are involved in the immune process
• There are two classes (I and II), which differ in their structure
• Class I molecules are found on all nucleated cells, while class II molecules are only found on antigen-presenting cells, such as macrophages
• Class II molecules bind foreign antigen peptides and present them to T-helper lymphocytes
• There are three types of class II molecule – DP, DQ and DR. Each of these is sub-classified by numbers

Box 12.5 Putative, but unproven, environmental triggers of type 1 diabetes

• Chemicals:
  ○ N-nitro compounds:
    □ Streptozotocin
    □ Nitrosamines
    □ Nitrosamides
• Viruses:
  ○ Mumps
  ○ Rubella
  ○ Cytomegalovirus
  ○ Enteroviruses
  ○ Retroviruses
• Bacteria:
  ○ Streptomyces
• Vaccination
• Puberty
• Stress
• Perinatal factors:
  ○ Maternal rubella
  ○ Blood group incompatibility
  ○ Maternal age
  ○ Pre-eclampsia
  ○ Caesarean section
  ○ Birth weight
  ○ Gestational age
  ○ Birth order
• Food components
  ○ Milk protein
  ○ Wheat protein
  ○ Vitamin D deficiency
• High energy intake and weight gain

• Self-antigens may be modified and become antigenic.
• An immune response against a dietary or infective agent may cross-react with self-antigens, so-called 'molecular mimicry'.

• Reduced exposure to pathogens and their products. The 'hygiene hypothesis' proposes that better sanitation has led to a relatively immature immune system prone to autoimmunity.

Clinical features

People with type 1 diabetes usually present with a short duration of illness of 1–4 weeks. Although there is diversity in the clinical presentation, the classical triad of thirst, polydipsia and polyuria together with weight loss are the commonest symptoms (Box 12.6).

Symptoms related to the osmotic effect of the hyperglycaemia

Many of the presenting symptoms are linked to the osmotic effect of the hyperglycaemia. These symptoms are common to all types of diabetes, but they are usually more severe and the time course is usually shorter in type 1 diabetes.

Under normal physiological conditions, the renal tubule re-absorbs filtered glucose in the proximal tubule; however, once the plasma glucose exceeds the renal resorption capacity, glucose is excreted in the urine. There is considerable variability in the renal threshold above which glucose enters the urine between individuals. It averages 11 mmol/L (200 mg/dL) but ranges from ~6 to 14 mmol/L (110–250 mg/dL). Once present in the urine, glucose exerts an osmotic effect that can lead to profound dehydration and hypovolaemia as water leaves the cells along the osmotic gradient, only to be lost in the urine. Changes in osmotic pressure in the eye as a result of changing intraocular and plasma glucose concentration may distort the shape of the eye and lens and cause blurred vision.

Symptoms related to the failure of anabolism

The profound weight loss that often accompanies the development of type 1 diabetes occurs because of the loss of the anabolic actions of insulin. There is a failure to transport fuel substrates into the cells and protein breakdown occurs because of the loss of insulin action.

> ## Box 12.6 Presenting features of type 1 diabetes
>
> • Symptoms related to the osmotic effect of the hyperglycaemia:
>   ○ Increased thirst and polydipsia
>   ○ Polyuria and nocturia
>   ○ Blurred vision
>   ○ Drowsiness and dehydration
> • Cutaneous candidal infection:
>   ○ Vulva (pruritus vulvae)
>   ○ Foreskin (balanitis)
> • Symptoms related to the inability or inappropriate transport of fuel substrates:
>   ○ Extreme fatigue
>   ○ Muscle wasting through protein breakdown
>   ○ Weight loss
> • Diabetic ketoacidosis

Diabetic ketoacidosis

Diabetic ketoacidosis (DKA) occurs as a result of marked insulin deficiency and elevated counter-regulatory hormones. It is a potentially fatal condition that is a medical emergency requiring prompt diagnosis and treatment. In a European study, 8.6% of people with type 1 diabetes had been admitted with DKA in the previous year; 25% of the cases occurred in people without a prior history of diabetes.

Prognosis

Prior to the discovery of insulin in 1921, the development of type 1 diabetes meant an almost certain death shortly after diagnosis. Since then, the prognosis for people with type 1 diabetes has improved dramatically, but despite this, type 1 diabetes remains associated with a two- to 10-fold increased risk of premature mortality compared with the general population.

A significant proportion of early deaths are attributable to DKA, while later deaths are more commonly associated with cardiovascular disease and nephropathy (described in more detail in

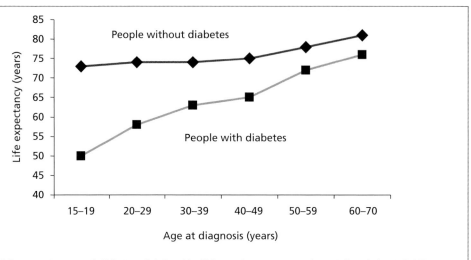

Figure 12.3 Life-expectancy and diabetes. Adults with diabetes have an annual mortality of about 5.4%, double the rate for adults without diabetes. Life-expectancy is decreased by 5–10 years.

Chapter 14). Mortality rates for cardiovascular disease are eight- to 40-fold higher in people with type 1 diabetes than in the general population.

It used to be said that on the day that a person is diagnosed with diabetes, their life-expectancy is reduced by around one-third (Figure 12.3). Consequently the greatest burden of diabetes falls on those who are diagnosed during childhood. However, these data reflect older cohorts and there is evidence that better control of hyperglycaemia and other cardiovascular risk factors, such as hypertension and lipids, is being translated into improved survival.

It is salutary to remember that in some low-income countries, where there is a lack of access to diagnostic equipment and basic supplies of insulin, the life-expectancy of a child with new-onset type 1 diabetes is only 3–4 months, similar to pre-1922 mortality rates in the developed world.

Diagnosis

The diagnosis of type 1 diabetes is relatively straightforward once it is considered in a person with weight loss and the classical triad of thirst, polydipsia and polyuria. As the patients have symptoms, only one plasma glucose concentration above the diagnostic cut-off is needed to confirm the diagnosis (review Chapter 11).

When the clinical features are less clear-cut, it may be difficult to distinguish between type 1 and type 2 diabetes (Table 12.3). The detection of islet auto-antibodies is indicative of type 1 diabetes but not pathognomonic (Box 12.7). With time the precise diagnosis usually becomes clearer, but at the initial presentation is less important than the practical question about whether insulin is necessary. Unlike type 2 diabetes, type 1 diabetes must be treated with insulin.

A catch for the unwary is the person with MODY (see Chapter 11, Table 11.3 and Case history 11.3). These are inherited monogenic forms of diabetes. As they often present in childhood, they may be mistaken for type 1 diabetes. An autosomal dominant family history of early-onset diabetes should alert the clinician to this possibility.

Management

Type 1 diabetes is a life-long condition that is currently incurable. For most of the time, the person with diabetes will manage their diabetes themselves with only a minority of the time spent in contact with their healthcare professionals. As such, the person with diabetes needs to be supported to assume much of the responsibility for their diabetes.

Table 12.3 Comparison of presenting features of type 1 diabetes, type 2 diabetes, monogenic diabetes and secondary diabetes

	Type 1	Type 2	Monogenic	Secondary
Weight loss	Usually present	No	No	Depends on underlying cause
Ketonuria	Usually present	No or minimal if recent fasting	No or minimal if recent fasting	May be present
Duration of symptoms	Few weeks	Months	Months	Weeks or months
Severity of symptoms	Can be marked	Variable but usually mild	Not usually severe	Depends on underlying cause
Family history	Possible (see Table 12.2)	Present in 30% with onset in adulthood	Present in almost all with onset in early adulthood or (more commonly) earlier	Unusual unless diabetes secondary to conditions such as haemochromatosis
Age	Peak incidence is during pre-school and adolescent years, but can affect any age	Usually after age of 20 years, but becoming commoner in children	Neonates to early adulthood	Usually middle or older age

---

Box 12.7 Definition of pathognomic

A particular symptom or sign whose presence means that a particular disease is present beyond any doubt.

The aims of diabetes care and management are four-fold:

• Life-threatening diabetes emergencies, such as DKA and hypoglycaemia, should be managed effectively, ideally by preventative measures
• Symptoms relating to the osmotic effects of hyperglycaemia should be addressed
• Long-term complications should be minimized through screening and effective control of hyperglycaemia and other cardiovascular risk factors
• Iatrogenic side-effects, such as hypoglycaemia, should be avoided.

Insulin

The discovery of insulin in 1921 transformed the management of type 1 diabetes (Figure 12.4). Prior to its introduction, people with diabetes were left with a choice of death by DKA or death by 'inanition', the exhausting condition resulting from want or insufficiency of nourishment. People with type 1 diabetes could survive for several years on diets of ~500–700 calories/day, but had a miserable existence and inevitable weight loss until either the patient broke their diet or died from starvation.

In people without diabetes, insulin is secreted at a slow basal rate throughout the day, which gives rise to a low plasma insulin concentration between meals and during the night. Following a meal there is a rapid rise and peak in plasma insulin concentration, which falls back to baseline within 2 h (Figure 12.5). The philosophy of managing the insulin replacement in people with diabetes is to mimic this pattern as closely as possible (Box 12.8).

Although the introduction of insulin transformed the lives of many with diabetes and is one of the most significant advances in medicine, it became apparent that subcutaneous insulin delivery is not ideal and many developments have happened since the 1920s to allow the replacement of insulin in a more physiological pattern (Box 12.9). The use of insulin should be tailored to meet individual

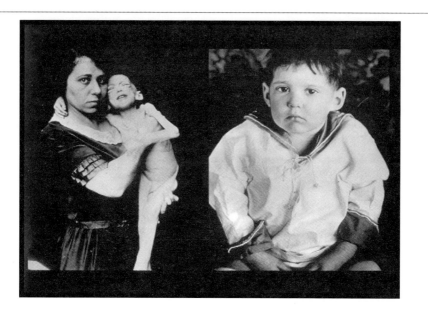

Figure 12.4 Pictures of one of the first people with diabetes to receive insulin in the 1920s. The photographs illustrate the dramatic effect of diabetes before treatment and the remarkable recovery with insulin. Images reproduced with kind permission of Eli Lilly & Co.

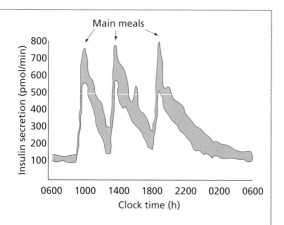

Figure 12.5 Normal insulin secretion throughout a 24-h period. There is background (basal) insulin secretion throughout the day superimposed on which are mealtime-related peaks of insulin (mimicked by the bolus insulin injections of the basal-bolus regimen). Re-drawn from O'Meara *et al. Am J Med* 1990;89:11S–16S.

Box 12.8 Principle of insulin replacement

Insulin replacement in people with diabetes should mimic the normal physiological pattern of secretion of healthy individuals as closely as possible.

requirements in order to achieve the best possible control without the risk of disabling and dangerous hypoglycaemia.

Types of insulin

There are three main types of insulin.

Soluble insulin

This was first introduced in 1922 and still plays an important part in the management of type 1 diabetes (Figure 12.6). Usually it is administered subcutaneously but may also be given intravenously or occasionally intramuscularly whilst managing diabetic emergencies. Initially insulin was isolated

Box 12.9 Disadvantages of subcutaneous insulin administration compared with endogenous insulin production from the pancreas

- Insulin must be given by injection
- Insulin is delivered into the systemic rather than portal circulation:
  - The physiological delivery of insulin to the liver is compromised resulting in lower insulin transport to the liver while peripheral tissues such as adipose tissue receive a higher concentration
  - Insulin has a number of actions in the liver that are not normalized by subcutaneous administration, e.g. production of insulin-like growth factor I (IGF-I)
- Loss of normal feedback mechanism between glucose concentration and insulin secretion
- Pharmacodynamics are altered, making it difficult to match insulin supply to requirement

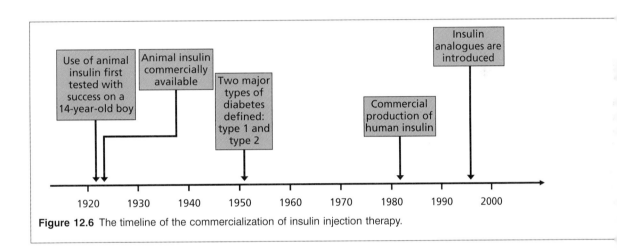

Figure 12.6 The timeline of the commercialization of insulin injection therapy.

from pigs or cattle but since the 1980s, insulin has been produced biosynthetically using recombinant DNA technology whereby the *INSULIN* coding sequence is inserted into bacteria such as *Escherichia coli*. This technology has allowed large amounts of insulin to be produced in a highly purified manner under 'Good Manufacturing Practice'. Some people are still treated with animal insulin but the numbers are becoming progressively fewer.

Protamine insulin and insulin zinc suspensions

Protamine insulin and insulin zinc suspensions were introduced to form isophane insulin in the 1930s and 1950s respectively. These preparations prolong the action of insulin to provide a sustained basal level of insulin.

Insulin analogues

Most recently, in the mid-1990s, short- and long-acting insulin analogues have been introduced, allowing injections to mimic more closely the daily changes in physiological insulin secretion. When soluble insulin is injected subcutaneously it forms a hexamer that delays its absorption from the injection site. For this reason it acts more slowly than endogenously secreted insulin. To combat this, newer rapid-acting insulin analogues (insulin lispro, insulin aspart, insulin glulisine) that are less likely to form hexamers were developed and consequently are more rapidly absorbed. Long-acting insulin analogues (insulin glargine or insulin detemir) have been introduced to provide a more stable basal plasma insulin concentration. Newer analogues in ongoing development are likely to be introduced in the near future.

Insulin regimens

In theory any combination of insulin can be used as long as the person with diabetes achieves good glycaemic control; however, there are several regimens that are more commonly used.

One of the simplest regimens is twice-daily mixed insulin. The mixed insulin contains both short- and intermediate-acting insulin and is given shortly before breakfast and the evening meal (Figure 12.7a). While the advantage of this regimen is that only two injections a day are needed, there are several disadvantages, such as inflexibility and relatively poorer control. Basal bolus regimens are the treatment of choice for most individuals with type 1 diabetes (Figure 12.7b and c; Table 12.4; Case history 12.2).

> ### 🔍 Case history 12.2
>
> A 35-year-old man who has had type 1 diabetes for 10 years attends the clinic complaining of late morning 'hypos'. He is currently treated with twice-daily pre-mixed insulin containing 30% soluble insulin and 70% isophane insulin. He mentions that work is hectic and he does not always know when he is going to eat lunch.
>
> **What possible changes to his insulin regimen could you make?**
>
> *Answer, see p. 283*

Injection sites and technology

Insulin is given subcutaneously by intermittent injection or by continuous infusion. Although it can be injected almost anywhere if there is enough flesh, the best sites are the front and side of the thigh, lower abdominal wall, buttocks and upper arms (Figure 12.8).

Intermittent insulin injections may be given by needle and syringes but more commonly insulin pen devices are used (Figure 12.9). Pens may be disposable with pre-filled insulin or may be re-used by changing the insulin cartridge when empty. They

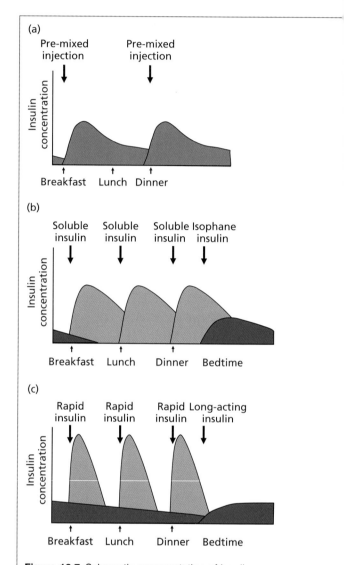

Figure 12.7 Schematic representation of insulin profiles with different regimens. (a) Pre-mixed insulin; (b) basal bolus regimen with soluble and isophane insulin; (c) basal bolus regimen with analogue insulin. Soluble insulin is in light blue; pre-mixed, mid blue; longer-acting insulin, dark blue.

are portable, use a fine needle and have a simplified procedure for measuring the insulin; the pens allow the user to dial up and dispense their required doses. The many advantages of insulin pens include convenience, easier injection and less pain. Insulin pen needles were initially 12 mm in length but as manufacturing has improved, progressively shorter

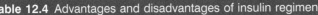

Table 12.4 Advantages and disadvantages of insulin regimens

	Twice daily insulin mixture	Basal bolus regimen using soluble insulin	Basal bolus regimen using analogue insulin
Number of injections	2	Usually 4	Usually 4
Timing	5–30 min before breakfast and evening meal	20–30 min before each meal (bolus) and pre-bedtime (basal)	5–10 min before each meal (bolus) and pre-bedtime (basal)
Flexibility of mealtimes	No – patient must eat regularly at pre-determined times	Yes – injection given before meal	Yes – injection given before meal. If basal insulin is provided by long-acting analogues, meals may be missed and bolus insulin omitted
Variable meal sizes	Lunch insulin is delivered at breakfast time, therefore little flexibility	Yes – meal doses can be adjusted according to need	Yes – meal doses can be adjusted according to need
Need for mid-meal snack	Yes	Yes	No
Risk of hypoglycaemia	High	Lower	Lowest
Glycaemic control	Achievable	Better control than twice-daily insulin	Best control
Insulin allergy	Possible	Possible	Reduced risk

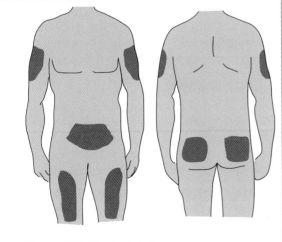

Figure 12.8 Sites for injection.

needles have become available. The shortest available needles are now 4 mm in length and their use is associated with fewer inadvertent intramuscular injections than longer needles.

Continuous subcutaneous insulin infusion (CSII) or insulin pumps are an alternative form of insulin delivery that was first introduced over 30 years ago. CSII comprises an insulin reservoir and delivery catheter that continuously infuses insulin into the subcutaneous tissue (Figure 12.10). The technology has steadily improved and allows the user to give a basal infusion throughout the day with boluses at mealtimes. The latest models also include software to help the user calculate the most appropriate insulin dose. When used by well-motivated people, CSII leads to improved control with fewer episodes of hypoglycaemia and improved quality of life compared with multiple daily insulin injections. Given these results, it is unsurprising

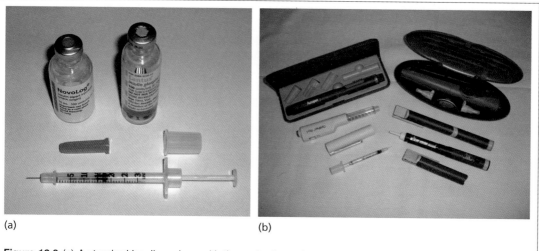

(a)   (b)

Figure 12.9 (a) A standard insulin syringe with the protective safety cap removed. At the top are two vials of insulin, both are 10 mL and contain 100 units/mL each. From http://en.wikipedia.org/wiki/File:Standard_insulin_syringe.JPG, accessed 20 August 2010. (b) A variety of insulin pen devices and carrying cases.

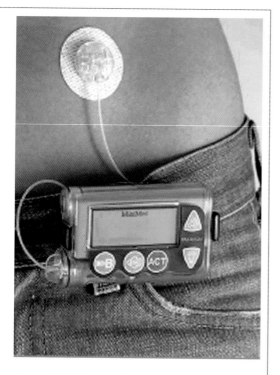

Figure 12.10 Person with type 1 diabetes wearing a Medtronic Paradigm insulin pump.

that there are an increasing number of people with type 1 diabetes who are using CSII.

Lipohypertrophy and lipoatrophy

When insulin is repeatedly injected into the same subcutaneous sites, it can lead to an accumulation of fat, lipohypertrophy, because of the local trophic effects of insulin. This can be unsightly and also increases the variability of insulin absorption. The affected sites are often painless and therefore may be favoured by the patient. The best way to avoid lipohypertrophy is to rotate the site of injection within any given anatomical area.

Now that highly purified insulin is available, insulin allergy is rare. However, immunoglobulin G immune complexes against the insulin can be formed that can produce local atrophy of fat tissue (lipoatrophy) as well as compromising insulin action.

Education

Diabetes education is an important cornerstone of diabetes care and improves the long-term outcomes for people with diabetes. Many different educational models have been used to meet the learning styles of different people. The education process,

Box 12.10 Areas covered by diabetes education

- Description of the diabetes disease process and treatment options
- Diet
- Physical activity
- Medication(s) including insulin – effectiveness and safety
- Self-monitoring of blood glucose
- Preventing, detecting and treating acute complications
- Preventing, detecting and treating chronic complications
- Personal strategies to address psychosocial issues and concerns
- Personal strategies to promote health and behaviour change

Box 12.11 Dietary advice for people with diabetes

Fats
- Restrict the intake of saturated fatty acids and *trans*-fats
- Vegetable oils, nuts and seeds are preferred
- Consume oily fish two to three times per week

Fibre and micronutrients
- Consume foods rich in dietary fibre and micronutrients
- Consume five servings of fresh fruit and vegetables per day
- Legumes and whole-grain products are recommended

Carbohydrates
- Eating complex carbohydrates such as bread, potatoes, pasta and rice in moderate amounts with each meal should be encouraged
- Low glycaemic index (GI) carbohydrates are preferred because they cause a slower rise in blood glucose concentration
- Sugar is not forbidden but excessive intake is not desirable
- Non-caloric sweeteners are safe

Alcohol
- Alcoholic beverages should only be taken in moderation

Other
- Special diabetic foods are unnecessary
- Meals, snacks and food choices should match individual therapeutic needs, preferences and culture

which is equally applicable to people with type 2 diabetes, embraces a 'patient-centred approach' and encompasses all aspects of diabetes care (Box 12.10).

Only when a person with diabetes is informed about their condition and the treatment options can they take control of their diabetes and make an informed judgement about their care.

Although diabetes education is an on-going process, structured educational programmes, such as the 'Dose Adjustment For Normal Eating (DAFNE)', at the time of or shortly after diagnosis are important to equip the person with knowledge and skills for their life with diabetes. Structured education has been shown to lead to improvements in glycaemic control and improved quality of life.

Diabetes and diet

It is important to encourage patterns of healthy eating (Box 12.11). Ideally 60% of total caloric intake should be provided by carbohydrate, with no more than 30% coming from fat. It should be recognized, however, that the real dietary limitations are dictated by the inadequacy of the available insulin regimens rather than the diabetes itself. Historically people with diabetes were taught to count their carbohydrate intake so that the carbohydrate content in each meal or snack could be prescribed to match the insulin dose. The rigidity of this approach became unpopular and was replaced by more general advice advocating healthy eating. The pendulum is now swinging back towards the use of carbohydrate counting; however, it is now being used to adjust the meal bolus of insulin to match the carbohydrate intake rather than *vice versa*. This approach promotes good glycaemic control while allowing flexible eating; in effect, the aim is to mimic the response of healthy β-cells when confronted by meals of varying size and composition.

Diabetes and exercise

Exercise is an important component of a healthy lifestyle and is discussed again in Chapter 13. It brings a number of special considerations for people with type 1 diabetes because of the need to maintain normal glucose concentration during exercise (Box 12.12). A reduction in insulin dose together with a snack before and during exercise may be needed.

Monitoring diabetic control

People with diabetes have to achieve a balance between maintaining as near normal glucose concentration as possible to prevent the long-term complications of diabetes (see Chapter 14), while preventing the acute complication of hypoglycaemia (see below). As people with diabetes have lost the normal homeostatic mechanisms to control glucose, it is necessary to monitor plasma glucose concentration to allow people with diabetes to understand the nature of their disease and guide the day-to-day adjustment of diabetes treatments.

Measurements of plasma glucose can be divided into short-term measures that provide an almost instantaneous record of the current glucose concentration and long-term measures that provide an assessment of average glucose concentration over the preceding weeks or months (Box 12.13).

Capillary blood glucose monitoring

The availability of hand-held meters has allowed people with diabetes to measure their capillary blood glucose concentration themselves regularly throughout the day wherever they are (Figure 12.11). Single blood glucose concentrations are of little use because of their wide variability, but serial glucose measurements allow patterns to be recognized and appropriate adjustment of insulin to be made according to the readings.

At present most blood samples are obtained by finger-prick but alternative site testing and non-invasive methods are being developed. People with

---

Box 12.12 Effect of exercise on blood glucose in people with type 1 diabetes

Glucose concentration will tend to decrease if:
- Too much insulin or too little carbohydrate is taken before exercise
- Exercise is prolonged (>30–60 min)

Glucose concentration will tend to remain unchanged if:
- Exercise is short in duration or mild in intensity
- Appropriate snacks are eaten or insulin adjustments are made before exercise

Glucose concentration will tend to increase if:
- Too little insulin or too much carbohydrate is taken prior to exercise
- The exercise is very intense: this occurs because high-intensity exercise increases catecholamine (and cortisol) secretion, which act as insulin antagonists

---

Box 12.13 Methods of monitoring glycaemic control

Blood glucose (instant)
- Intermittent capillary
- Continuous monitoring

Integrated measures of long-term glycaemic control (weeks, months)
- Glycated haemoglobin (HbA$_{1c}$)
- Fructosamine

---

diabetes are usually advised to monitor their blood glucose immediately pre-meal or approximately 2 h after a meal between two and four times a day to assess the effectiveness of both basal and mealtime bolus insulin. Although self-monitoring of blood glucose is an important tool for achieving good glycaemic control, the principle that any investigation should lead to a change in management should be followed; therefore, if patients are unable or

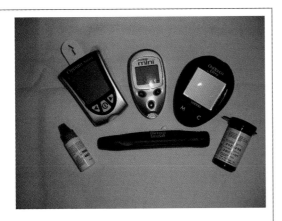

Figure 12.11 Variety of meters used for self-monitoring capillary blood glucose.

unwilling to adjust their insulin or diet then 'testing for testing's sake' should be discouraged (Case history 12.3).

Urinary glucose can be used as a crude index of blood glucose but because of its lack of sensitivity, it should be a last resort.

🔍 Case history 12.3

A 47-year-old man who is being treated with soluble insulin three times a day and isophane insulin before bed presents with the following set of blood results:

	Before breakfast	Before lunch	Before evening meal	Before bed
Insulin dose (units)	10	12	18	30
Home glucose readings (mmol/L or *mg/dL*)	4.0–7.8 *72–140*	2.3–5.2 *41–94*	9.4–13.0 *169–234*	5.0–7.8 *90–140*

What advice would you give?

Answer, see p. 283

Integrated measures of glycaemic control

Glycated haemoglobin (HbA_{1c}) is a measure of integrated glycaemic control over the preceding 2–3 months and reflects the mean lifespan of 117 days of a normal red blood cell. Glucose becomes attached to adult haemoglobin in a non-enzymatic fashion that is dependent on the average concentration of blood glucose (see Figure 11.5).

The measurement and interpretation of HbA_{1c} as the major longer term monitor of glycaemic control has become the currency of most diabetologists' daily work. The HbA_{1c} concentration correlates with the risk of development of microvascular diabetic complications and clinical studies have confirmed the direct benefits of lowering HbA_{1c}. Target HbA_{1c} values are typically between 6.5% and 7.5% (48–58 mmol/mol), but this must be judged on an individual basis according to the patient's clinical situation and risk of hypoglycaemia. Nevertheless HbA_{1c} has a number of limitations and so should be seen as just one of a number of tools that can be used to improve the lives of people with diabetes (Box 12.14). HbA_{1c} reduction is a means to an end and not an end in itself.

Traditionally HbA_{1c} has been measured as a percentage of total haemoglobin. Until recently there was no international reference standard and consequently there are small numerical differences between assays. In order to allow comparison between centres, the results from different assays are aligned to the results obtained during the Diabetes Control and Complications Trial. So, many laboratories report results as DCCT-aligned HbA_{1c}. Following the development of an international standard by the International Federation of Clinical Chemistry and Laboratory Medicine (IFCC), it is possible to measure the quantity of HbA_{1c} and so new results are being reported as mmol/mol. The conversion is shown in Table 12.5. In some countries, HbA_{1c} values are converted to provide a measure of estimated average glucose.

An alternative to HbA_{1c} is fructosamine which is a measure of glycated serum proteins. It is an index of glycaemic control over the previous 2–3 weeks, reflecting the shorter half-life of albumin compared with haemoglobin. As HbA_{1c} assays have

Box 12.14 Limitations of HbA$_{1c}$

Analytical variability
- Different methods for HbA$_{1c}$ may give different results, but this has been largely addressed by reference method standardization
- Molecular variants of haemoglobin:
  - Fetal haemoglobin

Biological variability
- Interindividual variability:
  - An individual with a mean glucose of 10 mmol/L (180 mg/dL) may have an HbA$_{1c}$ value which ranges from 6.0% to 9.0% (42–75 mmol/mol)
  - Probably reflects differences in the rates of protein glycation
- Variation in erythrocyte lifespan:
  - Shortened lifespan can give spuriously low results
  - Haemolytic anaemia
  - Acute or chronic blood loss
  - Pregnancy
  - Diabetes may shorten lifespan of red blood cells

Clinical variability
- Predictive link between HbA$_{1c}$ and clinical outcomes is not clear-cut

Table 12.5 IFCC and DCCT aligned values for HbA$_{1c}$

Current DCCT aligned HbA$_{1c}$ (%)	IFCC HbA$_{1c}$ (mmol/mol)
4.0	20
5.0	31
6.0	42
6.5	48
7.0	53
7.5	59
8.0	64
9.0	75
10.0	86

IFCC-HbA$_{1c}$ (mmol/mol) =
[DCCT-HbA$_{1c}$(%) − 2.15] × 10.929.
IFCC, International Federation of Clinical Chemistry and Laboratory Medicine; DCCT, Diabetes Control and Complications Trial.

improved, the use of fructosamine has declined and is only used rarely now; however, it may have a theoretical place in pregnancy, where changes in average plasma glucose can occur rapidly, and in those with haemoglobinopathies.

Acute metabolic emergencies

Hypoglycaemia

Hypoglycaemia occurs when the blood glucose falls below 3.5 mmol/L (63 mg/dL). It is worth noting that this is a higher threshold for the day-to-day lives of people with diabetes than the 2.2 mmol/L (40 mg/dL) used in the insulin tolerance test of anterior pituitary function (see Table 5.4). It is the commonest side-effect of insulin therapy and the major barrier to obtaining optimal glycaemic control. Most people with type 1 diabetes will experience several episodes of mild hypoglycaemia per week and one to two severe episodes per year where external help is needed. Hypoglycaemia is commoner in people with type 1 diabetes, where there is absolute insulin deficiency, compared with type 2 diabetes. It occurs more frequently in young children and those receiving intensive insulin treatment to achieve tight glycaemic control.

Hypoglycaemia significantly affects the quality of life of people with type 1 diabetes. It may put them at risk of harm, e.g. if they are driving at the time, and may have physical health consequences, e.g. cardiac arrhythmias and sudden death. It is caused by inappropriate insulin action and may result from hyperinsulinaemia or an enhanced insulin effect. This may occur when there is poor matching of the insulin requirement to the person's lifestyle (Case history 12.4; Box 12.15).

Case history 12.4

A 35-year-old builder with well-controlled type 1 diabetes was admitted to hospital with diarrhoea and vomiting. He was initially treated with intravenous fluids and insulin but was subsequently changed back to his normal insulin regimen. The doctors noticed that his normal doses were not controlling his glucose concentration adequately and so they increased his doses substantially.

Two days after discharge, the man had a severe hypoglycaemic episode and was admitted back to hospital.

What is the most likely reason this man became profoundly hypoglycaemic on discharge?
Could this have been prevented?

Answers, see p. 283

Box 12.15 Causes of hypoglycaemia

- Excessive insulin administration:
  - Error by doctor, pharmacist or person with diabetes:
    - Dose
    - Type of insulin
  - Deliberate overdose as self-harm or from carer
- Unpredictable insulin absorption:
  - Insulin is absorbed more rapidly from the abdomen
  - Lipohypertrophy
- Altered clearance of insulin:
  - Decreased insulin clearance in renal failure
- Decreased insulin requirement:
  - Missed, small or delayed meals
  - Alcohol:
    - Inhibits hepatic glucose output
  - Vomiting:
    - May occur with gastroparesis (a loss of normal stomach motility; see Chapter 14), a long-term complication of diabetes
  - Weight loss
  - Physical activity*:
    - Also increases rate of insulin absorption
- Recurrent hypoglycaemia and unawareness

*Not just exercise, such as sport; a common cause of hypoglycaemia is an increase in everyday activity, e.g. from a new job.

Physiological response to hypoglycaemia

In people without diabetes, the initial response to falling blood glucose is a decrease in pancreatic insulin secretion. This occurs within the physiological range of plasma glucose. As glucose concentration falls below the normal range, secretion of the insulin antagonist, glucagon, increases from the α-cells of the pancreatic islets. At the same time, a number of other insulin antagonists or 'counter-regulatory' hormones are released. The major ones are norepinephrine (noradrenaline), cortisol and growth hormone (review Chapters 5 and 6).

In diabetes these combined protective mechanisms are unavailable because of abnormal islet cell function or defective counter-regulatory hormone secretion. The only circulating insulin comes from subcutaneous delivery that cannot be reduced in response to hypoglycaemia. Once insulin has been given subcutaneously, the only way to prevent this from entering the circulation is by surgical removal, which is impractical in most situations. In addition,

with recurrent hypoglycaemia and longer duration of diabetes, the magnitude of the counter-regulatory hormone response and other sympathetic nervous system responses to hypoglycaemia become diminished.

Symptoms and signs

The physiological responses to hypoglycaemia produce a range of symptoms and signs that are

Table 12.6 Symptoms and signs of hypoglycaemia		
Autonomic	**Neuroglycopaenic**	**Non-specific**
Sweating	Difficulty speaking	Nausea
Paraesthesia (pins and needles)	Loss of concentration	Hunger
Feeling hot	Drowsiness	Weakness
Shakiness	Dizziness	
Anxiety	Hemiplegia	
Palpitations	Fits	
Pallor	Coma	
	Death (rare)	

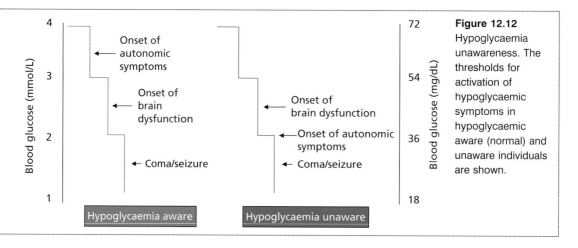

Figure 12.12 Hypoglycaemia unawareness. The thresholds for activation of hypoglycaemic symptoms in hypoglycaemic aware (normal) and unaware individuals are shown.

relieved by the restoration of plasma glucose concentration. The symptoms are important as they alert the individual to hypoglycaemia and prompt them to take corrective action. They can be divided into two main categories, autonomic and neuroglycopaenic, although non-specific symptoms may be also be experienced (Table 12.6). Autonomic symptoms occur because of activation of both the adrenergic and cholinergic parts of the autonomic nervous system, while neuroglycopaenic symptoms result from inadequate glucose supply to the brain, leading to neurological dysfunction. Glucose is an obligate fuel for the brain under physiological conditions and the brain accounts for 50% of whole-body glucose utilization. As the brain cannot synthesize or store glucose, it requires a constant supply of glucose from the circulation.

Under usual circumstances the development of autonomic symptoms precedes cognitive impairment. This is clinically important as it prompts corrective action before cognitive impairment begins; however, if these autonomic signals are diminished and if the counter-regulatory hormone response is reduced, awareness of hypoglycaemia becomes impaired and the person is at risk of severe hypoglycaemia (Figure 12.12).

Treatment

Suspected hypoglycaemia should be treated immediately with oral glucose if possible. If the patient is unconscious or unable to swallow safely, intramuscular or subcutaneous glucagon or intravenous glucose can be administered. As glucagon causes mobilization of hepatic glycogen stores when it is used to treat hypoglycaemia, these stores become diminished. So, once the patient is able to eat longer-acting carbohydrate, it is also important that they do so to replenish the glycogen stores.

The patient usually recovers within minutes, after which it is important to ascertain the cause of the hypoglycaemic episode to try to prevent this from happening in future.

If an individual with diabetes suffers from recurrent hypoglycaemia or is experiencing 'hypo' unawareness, it is necessary to avoid hypoglycaemia. This allows recovery of the counter-regulatory hormone response and the patient to regain their awareness of falling blood glucose (Case history 12.5).

🔍 Case history 12.5

A 28-year-old woman has recently tried hard to improve her glycaemic control, but unfortunately had a car accident when she was hypoglycaemic. She mentions that her usual warning has disappeared and when you look at her glucose monitoring records, you find she is having frequent 'hypos'.

How can you help her?

Answer, see p. 284

Diabetic ketoacidosis

Diabetic ketoacidosis is the most severe diabetic emergency and is still associated with a significant mortality (~1–2% in western countries, but particularly in developing countries where mortality is substantially higher). It is a state of severe uncontrolled diabetes caused by insulin deficiency and requires urgent treatment with insulin and fluids to prevent death. DKA occurs more commonly in younger people, but the mortality is higher in the elderly. It is estimated that 2–8% of hospital admissions in children occur because of DKA and there are ~5–8 episodes per year per 1000 people with type 1 diabetes.

Many factors can precipitate DKA. Infections account for 30–40% of cases and new cases of diabetes for 10–20%. Other acute stressful illnesses, such as myocardial infarction, may also trigger DKA by increasing the production of counter-regulatory hormones. Insulin errors, omissions and non-adherence are also common (15–30%) (Case history 12.6). A common mistake is for patients to stop insulin when they become unwell. Their appetite falls and they reduce the insulin in order to prevent hypoglycaemia; however, infection often increases insulin requirement, partly through the insulin antagonistic actions of cytokines and cortisol (see Chapter 6). The challenge of matching insulin injection to calorie intake during illness may be complicated further by nausea and vomiting, and admission may be needed for intravenous glucose and insulin. The golden rule is *never stop insulin*.

🔍 Case history 12.6

A 15-year-old girl with a 6-year history of type 1 diabetes was admitted to hospital following a short illness during which she had developed vomiting and general malaise. Her admission pH was 7.0, plasma glucose 27.6 mmol/L (496 mg/dL) and plasma ketones 5.2 mmol/L (5.6 mg/dL).

She was treated appropriately and discharged, but during the next few months she was re-admitted with a similar presentation on three separate occasions.

She had been previously well controlled with an HbA_{1c} of 7.2% (55 mmol/mol) but had lost weight recently. When questioned she admitted that she had been feeling unhappy about her diabetes, not least because several of her schoolmates had teased her about her weight.

What was the diagnosis during her first admission?
Why may this and the subsequent admissions have occurred?

Answers, see p. 284

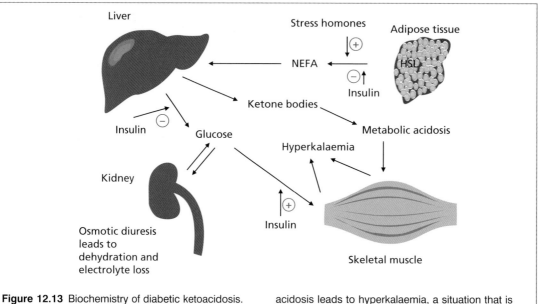

Figure 12.13 Biochemistry of diabetic ketoacidosis. Hormone-sensitive lipase (HSL) is sensitive to inhibition by insulin. Insulin deficiency leads to activation of HSL and break down of adipose tissue triglyceride to non-esterified fatty acid (NEFA), a process that is augmented by stress hormones. The NEFAs are transported to the liver where they are converted to acidosis-promoting ketone bodies. The acidosis leads to hyperkalaemia, a situation that is worsened because insulin usually leads to transport of potassium into cells with glucose. Hyperglycaemia occurs because of a failure to inhibit hepatic glucose output and a reduction in insulin-mediated glucose uptake. Renal gluconeogenesis is also increased. This leads to an osmotic diuresis and profound electrolyte loss.

Biochemistry

Diabetic ketoacidosis is characterized by hyperglycaemia, metabolic acidosis and hyperketonaemia (Figure 12.13).

Hyperglycaemia – the 'diabetic' part of diabetic ketoacidosis

The absolute insulin deficiency usually leads to hyperglycaemia secondary to increased hepatic glucose output and diminished peripheral insulin-mediated glucose uptake. It should be noted that DKA is predominantly caused by deranged lipid metabolism and therefore DKA may occur in people with normal or only moderately elevated glucose concentration.

Hyperglycaemia is accelerated by the presence of catabolic counter-regulatory stress hormones, in particular glucagon and catecholamines, but also growth hormone and cortisol. Renal gluconeogenesis is also enhanced in the presence of acidosis. The hyperglycaemia causes an osmotic diuresis and profound dehydration and loss of electrolytes. The latter is worsened by the insulin deficiency which impairs renal sodium re-absorption.

Hyperketonaemia – the 'keto' part of diabetic ketoacidosis

The most important biochemical abnormality in DKA is uncontrolled lipolysis in adipose tissue and uncontrolled ketogenesis in the liver. Insulin is a potent inhibitor of the enzyme hormone-sensitive lipase, which breaks down adipose triglycerides to non-esterified fatty acids (NEFAs). By contrast, this process is accelerated by the presence of catabolic counter-regulatory hormones. Consequently, the absence of insulin and increased counter-regulatory hormones leads to a marked increase in lipolysis.

NEFAs are transported to the liver where they are partially oxidized to acidic ketones bodies, such as acetoacetic acid and 3-hydroxybutyric acid, and acetone. This occurs because hepatic re-esterification of NEFA to triglyceride is impaired in the absence of insulin and presence of increased glucagon. The ketone bodies are exported from the liver as an alternative fuel supply, but build up in the circulation because of impaired uptake into peripheral tissues such as muscle and brain secondary to lack of insulin. Plasma ketone body concentration is commonly elevated 200–300 times above normal fasting values.

Acidosis – the 'acidosis' part of diabetic ketoacidosis

Ketones bodies are strong organic acids that associate at physiological pH and generate a high concentration of H^+ ions. This rapidly exceeds the body's buffering capacity and leads to severe metabolic acidosis.

In order to compensate for the acidosis, respiratory rate and depth increase (Kussmaul breathing) and ketone bodies may be smelt on the breath (similar to nail varnish remover). Ketone bodies are nauseating and many patients will vomit, worsening the dehydration and potassium loss. The metabolic acidosis has a negative inotropic effect on the heart and exacerbates peripheral vasodilatation. It may also cause respiratory depression and contribute to insulin resistance.

Metabolic acidosis leads to extracellular export of potassium in exchange for hydrogen ions moving into the cell. This causes hyperkalaemia. Insulin promotes the co-transport of potassium along with glucose into cells. Thus, lack of insulin further exacerbates the hyperkalaemia. Significant quantities of potassium are lost in vomit and urine. Therefore, although serum potassium may be elevated, there is a severe whole-body potassium deficiency. Potassium alterations may lead to cardiac arrhythmias.

Diagnosis

Some patients' first presentation of diabetes is DKA. The clinical features of DKA are similar to those of type 1 diabetes but tend to be more severe (Box 12.16).

> **Box 12.16 Clinical features of diabetic ketoacidosis**
>
> - Polyuria and nocturia
> - Thirst and polydipsia
> - Nausea and vomiting
> - General malaise and weakness
> - Abdominal pain and leg cramps
> - 'Air hunger' with Kussmaul breathing (deep, sighing breathing)
> - Odour of ketones on the breath (pear drops or nail varnish remover)
> - Altered conscious level
> - Postural hypotension and dehydration

> **Box 12.17 Diagnosis of diabetic ketoacidosis**
>
> - Ketonaemia ≥ 3 mmol/L (31.2 mg/dL) *or* significant ketonuria (≥2 on standard urine sticks)
> - Blood glucose >11 mmol/L (200 mg/dL) *or* known diabetes mellitus
> - Bicarbonate (HCO_3^-) below 15 mmol/L (15 mEq/L) *and/or* venous pH < 7.3

Making the diagnosis requires diabetes, ketosis and acidosis (Box 12.17). Hyperglycaemia should be determined by a blood sample. Ketosis can be detected by measuring urinary or blood ketones. Previously, metabolic acidosis was always determined by arterial blood gases, but the pH difference between venous and arterial blood is only 0.02–0.15 pH units and this is not of sufficient magnitude to change either the diagnosis or subsequent management. A low venous plasma bicarbonate concentration provides further evidence of the acidosis.

A common mistake is to describe a hyperglycaemic patient without ketosis as having DKA. These two situations have different management strategies and therefore it is important to distinguish patients with DKA correctly.

At presentation, it is also important to measure serum electrolytes to look for hyperkalaemia and to investigate the underlying cause of the DKA.

Management

The treatment of DKA is a medical emergency and patients frequently require admission to an intensive care unit or high-dependency ward with high clinical staff to patient ratios. It is important to involve the diabetes specialist team at the earliest opportunity. Treatment of DKA involves intravenous rehydration (the most important first step), insulin administration and correction of electrolytes. Treatment should be initiated without delay with the overall goal of controlled, gradual correction of metabolic abnormalities and fluid and electrolyte deficiencies over the next 24 h. It is important to treat the precipitating cause.

The management of children differs from adults because of their increased risk of cerebral oedema; it is particularly important to avoid too rapid fluid replacement and overload.

Previously, guidelines for the management of DKA have focused on lowering the elevated blood glucose with fluids and insulin, together with the use of arterial pH and serum bicarbonate to assess the rate of metabolic improvement (Table 12.7). It should be recognized, however, that the use of

Table 12.7 A management regimen for diabetic ketoacidosis

Fluid

Up to 10 L of fluid may be needed in the first 24 h:
    1 L over first h
    3 L over the next 6 h
    1 L every 6–8 h depending on fluid deficit
Use isotonic (normal – 0.9%) saline
10% glucose (125 mL/h) should be administered once the blood glucose falls below 14 mmol/L (~250 mg/dL) alongside the saline
More fluid may be needed if the patient is hypotensive on admission

Potassium replacement

On average, 40 mmol/L (40 mEq/L) KCl should be added to each litre of fluid depending on serum potassium concentration. Saline with pre-added KCl reduces the chance of user-error

Plasma potassium	Potassium added
<3.5 mmol/L (<3.5 mEq/L)	↑ Fluid rate or ↑ KCl concentration (senior advice required)
3.5–5.5 mmol/L (3.5–5.5 mEq/L)	40 mmol/L (40 mEq/L)
>5.5 mmol/L (>5.5 mEq/L)	None

Insulin

Insulin should be given by continuous infusion at a dose of 0.1 unit/kg/h
Continue long-acting basal insulin analogue

Acidosis

50 mL 8.4% bicarbonate should only be given if there is severe acidosis (pH < 7.0) despite adequate fluid and insulin replacement (senior advice required)

Other measures

Search for the precipitating cause
Insert nasogatric tube in those with impaired conscious level
Consider central venous pressure line, especially in the elderly or those with cardiac disease, to help monitor circulatory status
Insert urinary catheter if no urine passed within 4 h to assess renal function accurately

blood glucose is only a surrogate marker for the underlying metabolic abnormality.

The advent of bedside testing for blood ketones (3β-hydroxybutyrate) allows timely and direct monitoring of the metabolic abnormality and has led to modern guidelines moving away from the use of glucose concentration to drive treatment decisions in the management of DKA. The resolution of DKA depends upon the suppression of ketonaemia; therefore, direct measurement of blood ketones is 'best practice' for monitoring the treatment response. If bedside ketone measurement is unavailable, bicarbonate concentration can be used to assess response during the first 6 h, although it may be less reliable thereafter. Blood glucose monitoring still remains an option.

Fluid and electrolyte administration

Patients may lose up to 10% of their circulating volume together with significant electrolytes (Box 12.18).

The main aims of fluid and electrolyte replacement are:

- Restoration of circulatory volume
- Promotion of ketone clearance
- Correction of the electrolyte imbalance.

Fluid should be replaced as crystalloid in the first 24 h, but care should be taken not to overload the patient (Box 12.19); this is particularly important in children, adolescents and the elderly, or those with overt or incipient renal failure or heart failure.

Isotonic (normal, 0.9%) sodium chloride saline has been used successfully for many decades, is readily available in most clinical settings and comes pre-mixed with potassium (see below). Glucose and compound sodium lactate (Hartmann's solution) is an acceptable alternative, although potassium must be added to treat the potassium loss adequately.

DKA is associated with potassium depletion despite the initial hyperkalaemia. As insulin is administered, potassium concentration can fall precipitously and may cause a fatal cardiac arrhythmia if unaddressed. Therefore, serum potassium concentration is monitored and replaced once the serum concentration has fallen below 5.5 mmol/L (5.5 mEq/L).

> **Box 12.18 Typical fluid and electrolytes losses in diabetic ketoacidosis**
>
> | | |
> |---|---|
> | Water | 100 mL/kg |
> | Sodium | 7–10 mmol/kg (7–10 mEq/kg) |
> | Chloride | 3–5 mmol/kg (3–5 mEq/kg) |
> | Potassium | 3–5 mmol/kg (3–5 mEq/kg) |

> **Box 12.19 Crystalloids and colloids**
>
> - *Crystalloids* are aqueous solutions of mineral salts or other water-soluble molecules
> - *Colloids* contain larger insoluble molecules, such as gelatine; blood is also a colloid

Dehydration in DKA may cause 'pre-renal' renal failure, making it important to monitor urine output; otherwise potassium may accumulate, leading to dangerous hyperkalaemia. There is debate about the need for a urinary catheter. As patients are significantly dehydrated on admission, it is unlikely that they will pass urine for several hours after the initiation of fluid replacement. It therefore seems reasonable to delay the insertion of a urinary catheter for up to 4 h. A central venous cannula may be required to monitor fluid balance in elderly patients and those with cardiac disease.

Once insulin treatment is initiated, blood glucose concentration will fall and care is necessary to prevent hypoglycaemia, which might precipitate cardiac arrhythmias, acute brain injury and death. Furthermore, it would increase secretion of counter-regulatory hormones that may prolong the ketosis. In order to prevent this, intravenous 10% glucose should be initiated alongside the saline once the glucose concentration has fallen below 14 mmol/L (~250 mg/dL).

Insulin replacement

Insulin should be administered intravenously to:

- Suppress ketogenesis
- Reduce blood glucose
- Correct electrolyte imbalance.

A continuous intravenous insulin infusion should be initiated at a rate of 0.1 units/kg/h as soon as possible *after* the fluid replacement has been started. Where the patient's weight is not known, this can be estimated. An initial loading dose is not needed unless there is considerable delay in setting up the infusion. Previously, the insulin dose was titrated according to the blood glucose (the so-called 'sliding scale'). From a pragmatic perspective, the fixed rate is simpler than the hourly dose adjustment and has been shown to be effective in the promotion of ketone clearance.

In recent years, the use of long-acting basal insulin analogues has become widespread. It is recommended that these are continued during treatment of DKA as this will prevent rebound hyperglycaemia when the intravenous insulin is discontinued and should reduce length of stay in hospital.

Sodium bicarbonate

Fluid and insulin replacement will frequently correct the acidosis and sodium bicarbonate should only be considered, with supervision by a senior doctor, if there is persistent acidosis (pH $\leq$ 7.0), as bicarbonate administration may worsen intracellular acidosis. Sodium bicarbonate may also predispose to cerebral oedema, an important cause of death in DKA. Repeat venous blood gas measurement can be used to monitor resolution of the acidosis.

Transfer to subcutaneous insulin

Unless there is good reason, the previous insulin regimen should be re-started once the acute metabolic abnormality has been corrected and the patient is ready for a meal. It is important to know how to do this and when to stop the intravenous insulin infusion. Bolus insulin is given with the meal (either by subcutaneous injection or as part of a CSII regimen) and the intravenous insulin infusion should be continued until some form of basal insulin has been re-instituted. For those who remained on their long-acting basal analogue insulin during the episode of DKA, the insulin infusion and fluids can be discontinued 30 min after the meal. If the long-acting insulin had been stopped, the intravenous insulin infusion and fluids should

---

> **Box 12.20 Complications of diabetic ketoacidosis**
>
> - Cerebral oedema
> - Adult respiratory distress syndrome
> - Aspiration of vomit
> - Thromboembolism

be continued until some form of background insulin has been given and for at least 30–60 min after the meal. For those on CSII, the basal pump rate should be re-introduced prior to discontinuing the intravenous insulin infusion. For those on twice-daily mixed insulin, this should only be re-introduced before breakfast or the evening meal.

Complications

Cerebral oedema is relatively uncommon in adults with DKA, but is more common in children (Box 12.20). It is potentially fatal and accounts for 70–80% of all deaths in children with DKA. The mechanisms responsible for the development of cerebral oedema are unclear, but one possibility is cerebral hypoperfusion with subsequent reperfusion. It is important to ensure that fluid replacement matches the patient's losses as excessive fluid replacement may be a further cause of cerebral oedema. If cerebral oedema occurs, intravenous mannitol and mechanical ventilation may be used.

A common cause of death in patients with DKA is aspiration of vomit. A nasogastric tube should be inserted to empty stomach secretions if the conscious level is impaired. Adult respiratory distress syndrome occasionally occurs in DKA. Features include shortness of breath, central cyanosis and hypoxaemia. The chest X-ray characteristically shows bilateral infiltrates that resemble pulmonary oedema. The management involves intermittent positive pressure ventilation and the avoidance of fluid overload.

Thromboembolism is a further potentially fatal complication of DKA, which arises from dehydration, increased blood viscosity and coagulability. The place of prophylactic anticoagulation remains controversial and routine anticoagulation is not recommended.

🔑 Key points

- Type 1 diabetes usually results from the autoimmune destruction of the β-cells in the islets of the pancreas
- It accounts for approximately 10% of all cases of diabetes in the western world
- Treatment is based on insulin replacement as physiologically as possible
- Blood glucose concentration is determined by the previous insulin injection and so, adjustment of insulin should be based more on the pattern of preceding blood glucose reading rather than the current level
- Insulin treatment is not perfect and may result in hypoglycaemia if more is given than is needed
- Diabetic ketoacidosis is the most serious acute complication of type 1 diabetes and is a medical emergency

👤 Answers to case histories

Case history 12.1

The most likely diagnosis is Addison disease, which is associated with type 1 diabetes (see Chapter 6 and Box 8.8). Tiredness, lethargy and postural hypotension are symptoms of hypoadrenalism. Corticosteroids are insulin antagonists; the onset of Addison disease is commonly associated with increased frequency and severity of hypoglycaemia, and necessitates a reduction in insulin dose. The increased skin pigmentation results from loss of negative feedback from cortisol, causing overexpression of the *POMC* gene and increased ACTH secretion, which stimulates the type 1 melanocortin receptor. A short synacthen test is needed to confirm the diagnosis.

Case history 12.2

The twice-daily regimen is not flexible enough for his lifestyle and so it would be appropriate to discuss whether he would like to go onto a basal-bolus insulin regimen, using four injections a day. This would give more flexibility for the timing and quantity of food he can eat. A rapid-acting analogue may be better for him as this should be given only 5–10 min before meals.

Case history 12.3

Blood glucose readings are determined by the previous insulin injection. Therefore, satisfactory breakfast readings suggest that his night-time insulin dose is fine. On a four times daily (basal bolus) regimen, getting the breakfast glucose right is the key as this implies good control overnight and sets up a solid platform for the meal-time bolus injections. His readings are too low before lunch, implying he is taking too much soluble insulin before breakfast. Unless there are major problems, it is usual to adjust the insulin doses by ~10% and so, it would be sensible for him to reduce his breakfast insulin dose to 9 units. Readings before his evening meal are too high, suggesting he is taking too little soluble insulin before lunch. A 10% increase to 13–14 units would be appropriate. His pre-bedtime readings are fine and so no adjustment is needed to the evening meal insulin injection.

Case history 12.4

It is almost certain that this man became hypoglycaemic because the dose of insulin was left inappropriately increased after his discharge from hospital. When the patient was ill and sedentary in bed, his insulin requirements increased. Thus, the dose required for perfect glycaemic control in hospital would almost certainly cause hypoglycaemia once the man became more active again after discharge.

This could have been prevented by reducing the insulin back to his pre-admission dose on discharge. We know he had good control prior to admission and so this dose was probably right for him.

Case history 12.5

The Diabetes Control and Complications Trial has shown that improved glycaemic control is often achieved at the expense of an increased frequency of severe 'hypos'. It is important that this woman avoids hypoglycaemia to allow the return of the usual autonomic symptoms of 'hypo' awareness. From a glycaemic control perspective, this is also important because 'hypos' are frequently followed by episodes of hyperglycaemia if the patient overtreats the 'hypo'. Frequent 'hypos' are often accompanied by large swings in blood glucose. It is also important to advise the woman not to drive until her awareness returns.

Case History 12.6

She has presented with general malaise and vomiting. Her biochemistry on admission confirms the presence of acidosis, hyperglycaemia and ketonaemia. She therefore has DKA.

It is unusual for a young girl with previously well-controlled diabetes to start to develop problems. The key is in the statement regarding her feelings about diabetes and weight. She has lost weight and the likelihood is that she has been omitting insulin as a means of weight control. This is not uncommon in young girls with type 1 diabetes, but is potentially dangerous, as illustrated by this case. She will need psychological support to help with this problem.

CHAPTER 13
Type 2 diabetes

Key topics

- What is type 2 diabetes?   286
- Prevention of diabetes   293
- Screening for diabetes   294
- Management   296
- Key points   309
- Answers to case histories   309

Learning objectives

- To discuss the epidemiology, aetiology and pathogenesis of type 2 diabetes
- To understand the clinical features of type 2 diabetes
- To discuss measures that might prevent or delay the onset of type 2 diabetes
- To understand the importance of screening for diabetes
- To understand the principles and pitfalls of oral hypoglycaemic therapy

This chapter describes type 2 diabetes

To recap

- The heritability of type 2 diabetes is estimated to account for 40–80% of its susceptibility and many patients have a family history of diabetes. The importance of genetic mutations to endocrine disease is covered in Chapter 2
- In order to understand the mechanisms underlying insulin resistance, it is important to review tyrosine kinase-mediated signalling (see Chapter 3)

- Thiazolidinediones are a class of oral antidiabetes drugs that act through binding to a nuclear hormone receptor; these receptors are described in detail in Chapter 3
- One of the two main abnormalities in type 2 diabetes is pancreatic β-cell failure. An understanding of normal insulin secretion is needed to appreciate the pathophysiology (see Chapter 11)

Cross-reference

- An overview of diabetes is given in Chapter 11
- Dietary management plays an important part in the management of both type 1 and type 2 diabetes. Dietary management is discussed in greater detail in Chapter 12
- Diabetes can lead to the development of a number of complications, which are discussed in Chapter 14
- The intrauterine environment may alter the risk of developing type 2 diabetes. The role of steroids in fetal growth and development is described in Chapter 6
- Sulphonylureas are a class of oral antidiabetes drugs. Some older sulphonylureas, such as chlorpropamide, are associated with hyponatraemia because they increase the sensitivity of the distal tubule to vasopressin (see Chapter 5)
- Other antidiabetes drugs act by manipulating prolactin, which is discussed in Chapter 5
- Incretins are hormones released by the gut in response to food ingestion. They augment insulin release and include glucagon-like peptide-1 (GLP-1) and glucose-dependent insulinotropic polypeptide (GIP). The physiology of these hormones is covered in Chapter 10.

Type 2 diabetes is the commonest type of diabetes, affecting around 285 million people worldwide. It is a heterogeneous disorder and this chapter examines what causes type 2 diabetes and why it is increasing at such an alarming rate. Although insulin can be used to treat type 2 diabetes, many patients are treated with lifestyle modification alone or in combination with oral antidiabetes drugs. Some of these treatments have been used for over 50 years, but in the last 20 years there have been major advances in the discovery of new drugs to treat type 2 diabetes with some recently introduced and others in late phase III trials.

What is type 2 diabetes?

Type 2 diabetes is a heterogeneous disorder that results from the interaction of genetic predisposition and environmental factors, creating a combination of insulin deficiency and insulin resistance (Figure 13.1).

Epidemiology

Type 2 diabetes accounts for around 90% of all cases of diabetes in western Europe and the USA. There are approximately 3 million people with diagnosed type 2 diabetes in the UK, with a further 800,000 estimated as having undiagnosed type 2 diabetes. The prevalence of diabetes is increasing rapidly; the World Health Organization (WHO) has predicted that by 2030, the number of adults with diabetes will have almost doubled worldwide, from 285 million in 2000 to 435 million. The incidence of type 2 diabetes increases with age, with most cases being diagnosed after the age of 40 years. This equates to a lifetime risk of developing diabetes of 1 in 10. The demographics of type 2 diabetes are changing, and it is now becoming increasingly common in children and young adults. In certain parts of the USA, the number of new cases of type 2 diabetes among teenagers is the same as for type 1 diabetes.

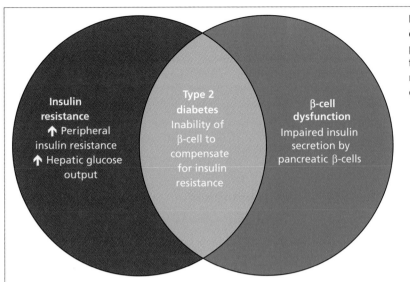

Figure 13.1 What is type 2 diabetes? The two main pathological components of type 2 diabetes are insulin resistance, and β-cell dysfunction and failure.

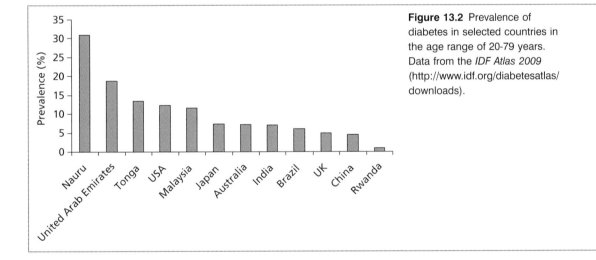

Figure 13.2 Prevalence of diabetes in selected countries in the age range of 20-79 years. Data from the *IDF Atlas 2009* (http://www.idf.org/diabetesatlas/downloads).

A marked geographical variation in the prevalence of type 2 diabetes exists (Figure 13.2). The highest rates of diabetes are found in the Pima Indians of Arizona and on the South Pacific Island of Nauru, where approximately 30–50% of the adult population has diabetes. By contrast, in the rural communities of China and Chile, the prevalence is <1%. In general, rates of type 2 diabetes are higher in urban populations than rural communities.

Regional and ethnic differences in the prevalence of type 2 diabetes reflect differences in both environ-ment and genetic susceptibility. For example, people from the Indian sub-continent living in Southall, UK have a rate of diabetes that is four times higher than that for the local white European population.

Aetiology

The risk factors for type 2 diabetes can be divided into those that are unmodifiable, and those that are environmental and therefore potentially changeable (Table 13.1).

Table 13.1 Risk factors for type 2 diabetes

Unmodifiable	Environmental
Family history – genetics	Obesity
Birth weight	Physical inactivity
Ethnicity	Diet
Age	Urbanization
Past history of diabetes in pregnancy (gestational diabetes)	Sleep apnoea

Table 13.2 Risk of developing type 2 diabetes for UK relatives of people with type 2 diabetes

Family member	Risk (%)
Monozygotic twin	90
Dizygotic twin	10
Sibling	10
Mother	15–20
Father	15
Both parents	75
General population	3

Genetic predisposition

The heritability of type 2 diabetes is greater than for type 1 diabetes, and is estimated to account for 40–80% of total disease susceptibility (Table 13.2). Many patients have a family history of diabetes, and monozygotic twin studies show a high concordance rate (60–90%). A maternal history of diabetes confers a higher risk of type 2 diabetes in the off-spring than a paternal history, possibly through an effect of maternal hyperglycaemia during pregnancy. This may alter the intrauterine environment, which may in turn affect the risk of diabetes. This is discussed further below.

Type 2 diabetes is a polygenic disorder (see Box 12.3), and it is clear that no single gene explains its inheritance. The advent of modern genetic research tools has led to the identification of several polymorphisms in genes or nearby genes (e.g. in introns) that associate with increased risk of type 2 diabetes. Many of the genes are involved in the control of insulin secretion and action, or appear to be linked to β-cell proliferation (Table 13.3). Other chromosomal loci have been linked with increased risk of diabetes (review Chapter 2 for gene and chromosomal structure).

Environmental factors

The most important environmental risk factors for diabetes are obesity and physical inactivity.

Obesity

The massive explosion in obesity rates worldwide has largely been responsible for the increase in diabetes; it is estimated that up to 80% of all new cases of diabetes can be attributed to obesity. In the UK, the average body mass index (BMI) of a person with type 2 diabetes is 30.0 kg/m², while in the USA, 67% of those with type 2 diabetes have a BMI of greater than 27 kg/m², and 46% have a BMI of greater than 30 kg/m². The risk of developing type 2 diabetes increases across the whole range of BMI, such that the risk in a middle-aged woman whose BMI is greater than 35 kg/m² is 93.2 times greater than in a woman whose BMI is less than 22.5 kg/m² (Figure 13.3). Similar changes are also seen in men.

In addition to total adiposity, the distribution of fat is also important. For any given level of obesity, the more visceral fat an individual has, the greater their risk of developing diabetes. This is reflected clinically by an increased waist circumference.

The importance of obesity is discussed further in Chapter 15.

Physical inactivity

Physical inactivity is also associated with an increased risk of diabetes. People who exercise for around 30 min/day have half the risk of developing diabetes compared to those with a sedentary lifestyle. Although some of the difference can be explained by differences in adiposity, exercise itself accounts for approximately half of the effect.

Intrauterine environment

The intrauterine environment is important for the development of type 2 diabetes. Low birth weight

Table 13.3 Gene and chromosomal loci linked with the development of type 2 diabetes

Specific genes

INSULIN (promoter region)

Peroxisome proliferator-activated receptor γ

KCNJ11 – encoding part of β-cell K+-ATP channel

Insulin receptor substrate 1 (IRS-1)

Adiponectin

Ectonucleotide pyrophosphatase/ phosphodiesterase 1 enzyme (ENPP1)

TCF7L2 and *HHEX* – both encoding transcription factors

SLC30A8 – encoding the zinc transporter ZnT8

CDKAL1 – encoding CDK5 regulatory subunit-associated protein 1

IGF2BP2 – encoding a regulatory protein for IGF-2

Chromosomal regions

Chromosome 1	q21–q25.3
Chromosome 2	q24.1–q31.1
	q35–q37.3
Chromosome 3	q27–q29
Chromosome 6	q23.1–q24.1
Chromosome 8	p23.3–p12
Chromosome 9	q21.11–q21.31
Chromosome 10	q25.1–q26.3
Chromosome 14	q11.2–q21.1
Chromosome 17	p13.3–q11.2
Chromosome 18	p11.32–p11.21
Chromosome 19	p13.3–p13.12
	q13.32–q13.43
Chromosome 20	q11–q13.32
Chromosome 22	q11.1–q12.3

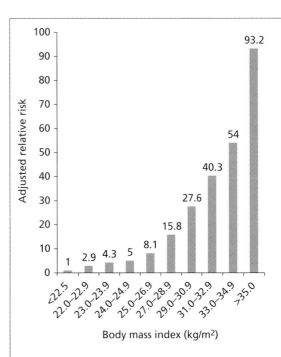

Figure 13.3 Risk of developing diabetes according to body mass index in 114,281 women enrolled in the US Nurses Health Study. Adapted from Colditz GA *et al. Ann Intern Med* 1995;122:481–6.

and thinness at birth are associated with increasing insulin resistance and diabetes in the offspring. In contradiction to this general observation, it appears that babies born to mothers with diabetes are also at increased risk of diabetes, despite the fact that these babies often have a high birth weight. Consequently the relationship between birth weight and subsequent risk of diabetes appears to be J-shaped.

Ageing

The changing world demographics with its ageing population add a further explanation for the increase in diabetes as the prevalence increases with age.

Pathogenesis

Under normal physiological conditions, plasma glucose concentrations are maintained within a narrow range, despite wide fluctuations in supply and demand, through a tightly regulated and dynamic interaction between tissue sensitivity to insulin (especially in the liver) and insulin secretion. In type 2 diabetes, both of these mechanisms break down with impaired insulin secretion through pancreatic β-cell dysfunction and impaired insulin action through insulin resistance (Box 13.1).

> ### Box 13.1 What are insulin sensitivity, insulin responsiveness and insulin resistance?
>
> *Insulin sensitivity* reflects the biological effect of insulin at any given insulin concentration and can be measured in a number of ways to provide a dose response curve
>
> *Insulin responsiveness* refers to the ability of insulin to exert a maximal response.
>
> *Insulin resistance* may be defined as existing when normal insulin concentrations fail to produce a normal biological response.

Insulin resistance

Insulin resistance, defined as the inability of insulin to produce its usual biological effects at physiological concentrations, is a cardinal feature of type 2 diabetes (Box 13.1). It is characterized by an impaired ability of insulin to inhibit hepatic glucose output and to stimulate glucose uptake into skeletal muscle. Insulin also fails to suppress lipolysis in adipose tissue, resulting in increased plasma non-esterified fatty acids (NEFAs) (Box 13.2).

The mechanisms leading to the development of insulin resistance are not fully understood, but may occur at many levels of insulin signalling (Box 13.3; review tyrosine kinase-mediated signalling in Chapter 3; Figure 3.6). It would appear that in type 2 diabetes, most insulin resistance is caused by defects in post-receptor signalling.

β-Cell dysfunction

Insulin resistance does not explain the whole story because people with type 2 diabetes are no more insulin resistant than the most insulin resistant quartile of the general population. Indeed, only ~20% of those with this degree of insulin resistance develop diabetes. Abnormalities in β-cell function are found early in the natural history of type 2 diabetes and in first-degree relatives of people with type 2 diabetes, suggesting that β-cell dysfunction

> ### Box 13.2 Consequences of insulin resistance
>
> *Skeletal muscle*
> - Reduced insulin-mediated glucose uptake
>
> *Adipose tissue*
> - Failure to suppress lipolysis, leading to increased circulating NEFA
>
> *Liver*
> - Reduced ability to inhibit hepatic glucose output
> - Increased NEFAs stimulate gluconeogenesis and glucose production, and triglyceride synthesis
>
> *Vasculature*
> - Impaired endothelial function
> - Increased stiffness of arteries
> - Increased coagulability
>
> *Increased sympathetic tone*
> - Through insulin action on the hypothalamus
>
> *Hyperuricaemia*
> - Insulin reduces renal uric acid clearance and this action is preserved even in the presence of insulin resistance. Consequently, as insulin concentration increases to meet the insulin resistance, uric acid clearance falls to below normal

is an integral component of the pathogenesis of type 2 diabetes.

Normal insulin secretion is biphasic in response to glucose stimulation (review Chapter 11); an acute first phase lasts a few minutes, followed by a sustained second phase. The major β-cell abnormalities in type 2 diabetes are a marked reduction in first-phase insulin secretion and, in established diabetes, an attenuated second phase (Figure 13.4).

By the time of diagnosis, mean β-cell function is already <50%, and it deteriorates further (~4%/year) after diagnosis. Extrapolation from these data suggests that loss of β-cell function begins at least

Box 13.3 Potential mechanisms of insulin resistance (review Figure 3.6)

Absent or reduced number of insulin receptors
- High circulating insulin concentration reduces the number of receptors present on the cell surface (down-regulation)

Abnormal insulin receptor
- Failure of insulin to bind to the insulin receptor
- Failure of insulin binding to activate the insulin receptor:
  - No autophosphorylation
  - No activation of tyrosine kinase
- Evidence for both the above points comes from loss-of-function mutations of the insulin receptor causing diabetes from early life (see Box 3.4)

Post-receptor signalling
- Down-regulation, deficiencies or subtly lowered function from genetic polymorphisms of post-receptor signalling molecules, such as tyrosine phosphorylation of the insulin receptor, insulin receptor substrate (IRS) proteins or phosphatidylinositol-3 (PI-3) kinase

Abnormalities of GLUT-4 translocation and function

Accumulation of skeletal muscle triglyceride
- So-called 'lipotoxicity'

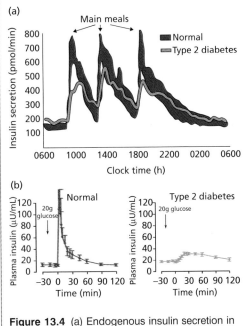

Figure 13.4 (a) Endogenous insulin secretion in type 2 diabetes and under normal conditions throughout a 24-h period. Re-drawn from O'Meara NM *et al. Am J Med* 1990;89:11S–16S. (b) Loss of early-phase insulin release in type 2 diabetes. The first abnormality of insulin secretion seen in type 2 diabetes is loss of the first-phase response. This is compensated for by an exaggerated second-phase response, which can cause hypoglycaemia 3–4 h after a meal. With time, second-phase insulin secretion is also lost. Re-drawn from Ward WK *et al. Diabetes Care* 1984;7:491–502.

a decade prior to the diagnosis. The progressive decline also explains why people with diabetes find it increasingly hard to control their hyperglycaemia with time and require escalations in the number and doses of oral antidiabetes agents, and why eventually they become refractory to oral treatment and require insulin.

The mechanisms underlying β-cell dysfunction appear multifactorial (Table 13.4). As well as genetic factors, a number of environmental factors, includ-

ing obesity, and hyperglycaemia and hyperlipidaemia may all accelerate the decline in β-cell function. Early-life malnutrition seems likely to programme a diminished total β-cell number; one potential mechanism for this is through excessive intrauterine glucocorticoid levels (see Chapter 6).

There has been much discussion about the relative roles of insulin resistance and loss of β-cell function in the natural history of type 2 diabetes, since both components occur early in the disease process. One model for the development of diabetes is as follows (Figure 13.5). As insulin sensitivity falls, β-cell insulin secretion increases to compensate and to maintain glucose concentrations within the normal range. The maximal insulin secretory

Table 13.4 Possible mechanisms of β-cell decline and dysfunction

Innate	Acquired
Genetics	Glucose toxicity
In utero malnutrition	Lipotoxicity
	Obesity
	Hormonal:
	• Inadequate incretin* stimulation
	• Increased glucagon secretion

*Incretins are hormones released by the gut in response to food ingestion. They augment insulin release and include glucagon-like peptide-1 (GLP-1) and glucose-dependent insulinotropic polypeptide (GIP) (see Chapter 10). Drugs that mimic or augment the action of these hormones are used for the treatment of type 2 diabetes.

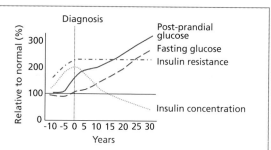

Figure 13.5 Natural history of insulin resistance and insulin secretion in type 2 diabetes. As insulin sensitivity falls, the β-cell compensates by increasing insulin secretion to maintain glucose concentrations in the normal range. Maximal insulin secretion is eventually reached and, beyond that point, insulin secretion declines. Blood glucose concentration rises, initially in the post-prandial period as the individual develops impaired glucose tolerance before the onset of diabetes.

capacity is eventually reached and, beyond that point, insulin secretion declines. As insulin secretion starts to fall, plasma glucose concentrations rise, initially in the post-prandial period, as the individual develops impaired glucose tolerance before the onset of frank diabetes.

This process may, however, be reversible. Although 2–5% of individuals with impaired glucose tolerance will progress to diabetes each year, many revert to normal. Intensive lifestyle intervention at this stage can reduce incident diabetes and so people falling into these categories should be managed actively with advice about their diet and exercise. Bariatric surgery to treat morbid obesity may have a dramatic effect on this process (see Chapter 15). Glucose tolerance often returns to normal following surgery, even in those who require insulin to treat their diabetes. Part of this effect is mediated by the dramatic loss of weight, but changes in glucose metabolism precede weight loss, suggesting a more acute effect, possibly mediated by gut hormones.

Prognosis

Type 2 diabetes is associated with premature mortality, predominantly through cardiovascular disease. Even after adjustment for other cardiovascular risk factors, diabetes is associated with a two- to three-fold increase in the risk of myocardial infarction or stroke. Cardiovascular complications are discussed in greater detail in Chapter 14.

Clinical features

Type 2 diabetes has a gradual and insidious onset, with nearly one-third of cases identified as an incidental finding or following cardiac ischaemic events, e.g. when an asymptomatic individual suffers a myocardial infarction. The diagnosis is often delayed, and some degree of hyperglycaemia may have been present for more than 20 years before the diagnosis is confirmed. In the early 2000s, it was said that there was a 'missing million' in the UK, reflecting the number of people with undiagnosed diabetes (Figure 13.6). With greater awareness of the problem and government incentives to find people with undiagnosed diabetes, this number has fallen to ~800,000, despite overall increasing numbers of people with diabetes. However, the proportion of people with undiagnosed diabetes around the world remains unacceptably high, with varying proportions of undiagnosed cases depending on the provision of local health services. It has been estimated from the 2002 NHANES survey that one-third of the 13.3 million US adults with diabetes were undiagnosed.

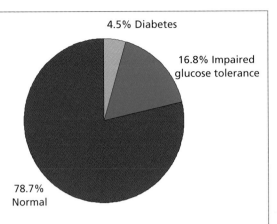

4.5% Diabetes

16.8% Impaired glucose tolerance

78.7% Normal

Figure 13.6 Prevalence of undiagnosed glucose intolerance from the Isle of Ely Diabetes Project. 1122 people aged 40–65 years without known diabetes from one primary care setting underwent a standard 75-g oral glucose tolerance test (review Chapter 11; Box 11.3; Table 11.4) and were classified according to WHO criteria. Williams DR et al. Diabet Med 1995;12:30–5.

Around 50% of people with type 2 diabetes are diagnosed as a result of the typical diabetic symptoms of polyuria, nocturia, thirst, tiredness and blurred vision, although these tend to be less dramatic than in people with type 1 diabetes; a further 16% of people are diagnosed after presenting with an infection.

Hyperosmolar hyperglycaemic state

Hyperosmolar hyperglycaemic state, formerly known as hyperosmolar non-ketotic coma, is a medical emergency and is characterized by hyperglycaemia, dehydration and uraemia without significant ketosis or acidosis. It occurs in middle aged or elderly people with type 2 diabetes and may be the presenting feature in around 25% of individuals. Afro-Caribbean individuals appear to be at a higher risk of developing hyperosmolar hyperglycaemic state (Box 13.4). It is the type 2 diabetes equivalent of diabetic ketoacidosis (DKA) in type 1 diabetes (see Chapter 12); the biochemical differences occur because small quantities of insulin remaining in type 2 diabetes are able to suppress lipolysis and the ensuing acidosis. It occurs less frequently than DKA but has a higher mortality rate (~15%).

Box 13.4 Precipitating causes of hyperosmolar hyperglycaemic state

- Infection
- Myocardial infarction
- Drugs:
  - Diuretics
  - Steroids
  - Omission of oral hypoglycaemic drugs

Hyperosmolar hyperglycaemic state may be complicated by thromboembolism or rhabdomyolysis. The management is similar to the treatment of DKA with fluid and electrolyte replacement and intravenous insulin. Heparin is usually administered because of the high risk of thromboembolic events. Despite the dramatic presentation, following correction of the metabolic abnormalities, many people may only require treatment with lifestyle modification.

Prevention of diabetes

One of the most exciting areas in diabetes at present is the possibility that type 2 diabetes can be prevented or at least delayed by lifestyle and/or pharmacological interventions (Case history 13.1).

Case history 13.1

A 35-year-old woman developed gestational diabetes during her third pregnancy, which required treatment with insulin. She has a strong family history of diabetes and was significantly overweight (BMI 28.2 kg/m²) prior to her pregnancy.

What advice and treatment would you offer her?

Answer, see p. 309

Lifestyle intervention aimed at reducing weight, the amount of fat, in particular saturated fat, in the diet, while increasing the amount of dietary fibre and daily physical activity, has been shown in several countries to reduce new cases of type 2 diabetes by a half over a 3-year period. Public health policies are urgently needed to encourage people to follow this healthy lifestyle and prevent the development of diabetes. Primary prevention strategies should target individuals at especially high risk of developing type 2 diabetes (Box 13.5).

In addition to lifestyle intervention, several drugs have been shown to reduce diabetes (Box 13.6), but at present the place of pharmacological therapy in the prevention of diabetes is not clear. The American Diabetes Association (ADA), however, endorses the use of metformin in younger individuals who are at very high risk of developing diabetes.

Screening for diabetes

The high prevalence of undiagnosed diabetes and the proportion of patients with evidence of complications at diagnosis create a strong imperative for screening (Figure 13.7). Many possible screening methods have been shown to be feasible, acceptable and accurate, but there is still debate about whom to screen.

Universal screening for diabetes is currently impractical because of the burden that would be placed upon primary care, but there is justification for screening of high-risk groups in whom undiagnosed diabetes is common (see Box 13.5).

Although the oral glucose tolerance test is relatively simple and inexpensive and is the gold standard test for diabetes, it is not suitable for routine screening because of the overall cost and inconvenience. A fasting plasma glucose has been endorsed by the WHO, ADA and Diabetes UK as a suitable test for screening. This test is more convenient than the oral glucose tolerance test but lacks sensitivity and may miss a large number of individuals with diabetes (Table 13.5).

Although a random plasma glucose measurement may be unreliable, it does have certain merits. It is easy to perform and has reasonable sensitivity and specificity. As glycated haemoglobin (HbA$_{1c}$) has been endorsed by the WHO and ADA as a diagnostic test for diabetes, this is an alternative easy method of screening and diagnosis in countries

---

Box 13.5 Groups who should be considered for primary prevention programmes and who should be screened for diabetes

- White people aged over 40 years and people from black, Asian and minority ethnic groups aged over 25 years with one or more of the following risk factors:
  - First-degree family history of diabetes and/or
  - Overweight/obese/morbidly obese (BMI* ≥ 25 kg/m^2) and/or
  - Sedentary lifestyle and/or
  - Waist measurement:
    - ≥94 cm (≥37 inches) for white and black men
    - ≥80 cm (≥31.5 inches) for white, black and Asian women
    - ≥90 cm (≥35 inches) for Asian men
- People who have ischaemic heart disease, cerebrovascular disease, peripheral vascular disease or treated hypertension
- Women who have had gestational diabetes
- Women with polycystic ovarian syndrome who have a BMI ≥ 30 kg/m^2
- People known to have impaired glucose tolerance or impaired fasting glycaemia
- People who have severe and enduring mental health problems
- People who have hypertriglyceridemia not caused by alcohol excess or renal disease

*Though more accurate than body weight alone, body fat may be overestimated by BMI in people who are very muscular or underestimated in those who have lost muscle mass.

The more risk factors that a person has, the higher the risk of diabetes; however, just being over 40 years if white or over 25 years if black, Asian or other ethnic origin is not necessarily a risk factor in itself.

Several diabetes risk scores, such as FINDRISK, have been developed to improve the identification of high-risk individuals.

Box 13.6 Measures to reduce the incidence of diabetes

Lifestyle
- ↓ Weight by 5% (ideally to BMI < 25 kg/m²)
- ↓ Fat intake to <30% of energy intake
- ↓ Saturated fat to <10% of energy intake
- ↑ Fibre to >15 g/1000 g
- Take at least 30 min/day of aerobic and muscle strengthening exercise

Pharmacological
- Metformin
- Orlistat (intestinal lipase inhibitor)
- Acarbose (α-glucosidase inhibitor)
- Pioglitazone (thiazolidinedione)
- Blockade of the renin-angiotensin system (conflicting results):
  - ACE inhibitors
  - Angiotensin receptor blockers

These drugs will be considered in greater detail in the section on treatment of diabetes. Randomized clinical trials (RCTs) have shown that the first four drugs can reduce diabetes but with a lesser effect than lifestyle intervention. *Post-hoc* analysis suggested that blockade of the renin-angiotensin system may reduce diabetes but RCTs over the past 5 years have not confirmed this.

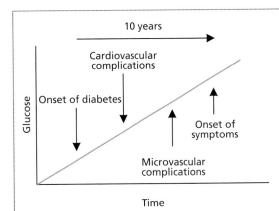

Figure 13.7 The imperative for screening for type 2 diabetes. It is estimated that many patients have diabetes for up to a decade before the onset of symptoms. However, diabetic complications can progress during this period in asymptomatic individuals. For example, approximately 20% of people with newly diagnosed diabetes have retinopathy at presentation and diabetes is frequently diagnosed following myocardial infarction.

where this test is available; the limitations of HbA₁c are shown in Box 12.14.

Screening for diabetes should be undertaken within the community where possible. Many primary healthcare services are overstretched and other settings may be required; e.g. an increasing number of pharmacists in the UK are offering screening using random blood glucose. Individuals with type 2 diabetes who are identified by any screening procedure differ from those who present symptomatically. They are less likely to have established diabetic complications and attitudes to health may differ as the diagnosis is less expected. This has implications for the future management of diabetes.

Table 13.5 Comparison of screening tests for diabetes

Test	Specificity (%)*	Sensitivity (%)**
Fasting plasma glucose	84–99	40–95
Random plasma glucose	92–98	50–69
Glycated haemoglobin (HbA₁c)	79–100	35–98

*Specificity: the probability that the screening test is negative if the person does not have diabetes. This is also known as true negative rate.
**Sensitivity: the probability that the screening test is positive if the person has diabetes. This is also known as the true positive rate.

Management

The aims of managing type 2 diabetes are similar to those of type 1 diabetes. Life-threatening diabetes emergencies, such as hypoglycaemia and hyperosmolar hyperglycaemic state, should be managed effectively and ideally prevented. Symptoms of hyperglycaemia, such as polyuria and polydipsia, need to be addressed. In practice, these two aspects of care occupy only a minority of the work undertaken by diabetes healthcare professionals. The bulk of care is aimed at minimizing the long-term complications through screening and working together with the person with diabetes to support improved glycaemic control and cardiovascular risk factor management.

Target HbA_{1c} levels are ~6.5–7.5% (48–58 mmol/mol), but these must be individualized to prevent iatrogenic side-effects of treatment (further details later in this chapter and in Chapter 14).

Management of type 2 diabetes is a particular challenge when the person has no symptoms; self-care often requires marked lifestyle changes and medications that place a considerable burden on the individual with diabetes. This includes potential side-effects, such as hypoglycaemia. As people with diabetes commonly have limited contact with healthcare professionals, it is paramount that they are involved in planning their diabetes care.

Type 2 diabetes is treated using a step-wise approach, starting with lifestyle modification, which includes dietary changes and an increase in daily physical activity. These remain the cornerstone of management even when treatment escalates to include oral antidiabetes agents, initially alone but subsequently in combination. Later, injectable treatments with either long-acting glucagon-like peptide-1 (GLP-1) receptor agonists or insulin may be added to the treatment regimen.

Diet

The principles of dietary changes to be adopted by a person with type 2 diabetes are identical to those for type 1 diabetes (Box 12.11). In brief, patients should reduce the amount of refined sugar and fat, particularly saturated fat, while increasing the proportion of complex carbohydrate and fibre. Many people with type 2 diabetes are overweight or obese and, therefore, their diet should have a moderate calorie deficit to facilitate weight loss (Case history 13.2). The management of obesity is covered in greater detail in Chapter 15.

Case history 13.2

A 56-year-old office manager presented with thirst, polyuria and tiredness. He admits to drinking large quantities of Coca-Cola. He weighs 90 kg. His fasting blood glucose is 10.0 mmol/L (180 mg/dL) and post-prandial glucose is 25.6 mmol/L (461 mg/dL).

How would you manage this scenario? Would you consider drug therapy at this time?

Answers, see p. 309

Physical activity

People with diabetes should be encouraged to take moderate exercise for at least 30 min/day to improve glycaemic control and reduce cardiovascular risk (Box 13.7). The best exercise is the one that the person enjoys and will still be willing and able to undertake many years after the diagnosis. Both aerobic and strength training are beneficial; however, physical activity is not equivalent to sport and practical advice should be given to help the person with diabetes become more physically active. Examples include using public transport to work, alighting one stop early and walking the extra distance, and using stairs rather than lifts or escalators (Table 15.4). However, take care when advising individuals with peripheral neuropathy to ensure that they wear

---

Box 13.7 Benefits of exercise

- Improved insulin sensitivity even without weight loss
- Reduced blood glucose
- Reduced blood pressure
- Improved lipid profile
- Increased longevity

natural fibres and well-fitting shoes to reduce the risk of foot ulceration.

Oral antidiabetes agents

When diet and exercise fail to maintain normogly-caemia, oral antidiabetes agents are required along-side, but not instead of, lifestyle management. Several antidiabetes agents increase residual insulin secretion and can only be used in type 2 diabetes as they are ineffective in people with established type 1 diabetes where β-cells have been destroyed.

There are currently four main categories of oral agents (Figure 13.8), although new drugs with novel mechanisms of action are being developed:

- Insulin secretagogues:
  - Sulphonylureas
  - Meglitinides
- Insulin sensitizers:
  - Metformin
  - Thiazolidinediones ('glitazones')

- Inhibitors of glucose absorption from the gas-trointestinal tract:
  - Acarbose
- Incretin-based therapies:
  - Dipeptidyl peptidase-4 (DPP-4) inhibitors.

Drugs from different categories can be com-bined if needed as the diabetes progresses.

Insulin secretagogues

Insulin secretagogues, such as sulphonylureas and meglitinides, stimulate insulin release from the pan-creas. Other than generic safety issues, the specific properties of the ideal insulin secretagogue are as follows:

- Rapid restoration of early-phase insulin release to reduce post-prandial glucose excursions
- Plasma insulin should be returned to pre-prandial levels as soon as possible to prevent hypoglycaemia between meals

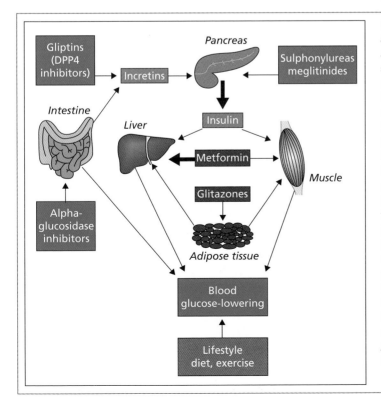

Figure 13.8 Main sites of action for antidiabetes agents. Different antidiabetes drugs target distinct sites as part of their primary mechanism for reducing hyperglycemia. Sulphonylureas and meglitinides stimulate pancreatic insulin release. Biguanides such as metformin primarily suppress hepatic glucose output. α-Glucosidase inhibitors (acarbose) delay digestion and absorption of carbohydrates in the gastrointestinal tract. Thiazolidinediones ('glitazones') decrease insulin resistance in adipose tissue, skeletal muscle and liver. Dipeptidyl peptidase-4 (DPP-4) inhibitors increase the concentration of endogenous incretin hormones. Reproduced from Holt RIG *et al.*, eds. *Textbook of Diabetes: A Clinical Approach*, 4th edn. Oxford: Wiley-Blackwell, 2010, Chapter 29.

• Suitable for use in combination with treatments for insulin resistance.

Sulphonylureas (Table 13.6)

The hypoglycaemic effects of sulphonamide antibiotics were first recognized during a typhoid epidemic in Marseilles, France in 1942. Following this observation, further work led to the development of sulphonylureas to treat diabetes, the first agent being carbutamide in 1955.

Mechani\sm of action

Sulphonylureas act mainly by increasing insulin release from the pancreatic β-cells (see Figure 11.9). Following binding to the sulphonylurea receptor, SUR1, the K^+-ATP channel, KIR6.2, in the cell membrane closes, leading to a rise in intracellular calcium and insulin release (review Chapter 11). The *in vivo* potency of sulphonylureas approximates to their ability to inhibit the K^+-ATP channel *in vitro*. Although there is individual variability, sulphonylureas tend to reduce HbA_{1c} by ~1.5–2.0% (16–22 mmol/mol).

Side-effects

The commonest side-effect of sulphonylureas is weight gain (Box 13.8). When an individual has poorly controlled diabetes, energy expenditure increases through glycosuria and an increase in basal metabolic rate. As glycaemic control improves, energy expenditure decreases with the reduction in glycosuria and basal metabolic rate. Unless the person increases voluntary energy expenditure (by increasing physical activity) or reduces caloric intake, weight gain is inevitable. As such, weight gain may occur with any antidiabetes agent, but appears to be particularly marked with sulphonylureas, thiazolidinediones ('glitazones') and insulin. Weight gain with sulphonylureas and insulin may result from hyperinsulinaemia between meals as increased food intake may be needed to prevent hypoglycaemia.

Associated with this, the second major side-effect of sulphonylureas is hypoglycaemia, which occurs in 0.2 episodes per 1000 patients/year and occurs because the drug prevents the normal physiological reduction in insulin secretion when blood glucose concentration falls. Patients with severe hypoglycaemia on sulphonylureas may need admission to hospital for up to 48 h for observation and glucose support until the drug has cleared from the circulation. Hypoglycaemia is a particular worry in the elderly in whom drug clearance is reduced and the signs of hypoglycaemia may be masked.

Table 13.6 Properties of different sulphonylureas

Drug	Half-life	Duration of action	Route of elimination	Active metabolite
First generation				
Acetohexamide	Medium	Medium	Hepatic	+
Chlorpropamide	Very long	Very long	Hepatic and renal	+
Tolazide	Short	Medium	Hepatic	+
Tolbutamide	Short	Short/medium	Hepatic	
Second generation				
Glibenclamide	Very short	Long	Hepatic	?
Gliclazide	Medium	Medium	Hepatic	
Glipizide	Very short	Short/medium	Hepatic	
Gliquidone	Long	Long	Hepatic	+
Glimepiride	Short	Medium/long	Hepatic	

With the exception of tolbutamide, first generation sulphonylureas are scarcely used today. Glibenclamide, gliclazide and glimepiride are the most commonly used.

Box 13.8 Side-effects of oral antidiabetes agents

Sulphonylureas
• Weight gain
• Hypoglycaemia
• Hyponatraemia
• Alcohol flushing (chlorpropamide)
• Worsening of myocardial ischaemia?
• Acceleration of β-cell loss?

Metiglinides
• Weight gain
• Hypoglycaemia

Metformin
• Gastrointestinal upset
• Lactic acidosis
• Vitamin B_{12} deficiency

Thiazolidinedione
• Weight gain
• Oedema
• Cardiac failure
• Hepatotoxicity (troglitazone)
• Osteoporotic fracture

Acarbose
• Gastrointestinal upset

DPP-4 inhibitors
• Nausea and vomiting

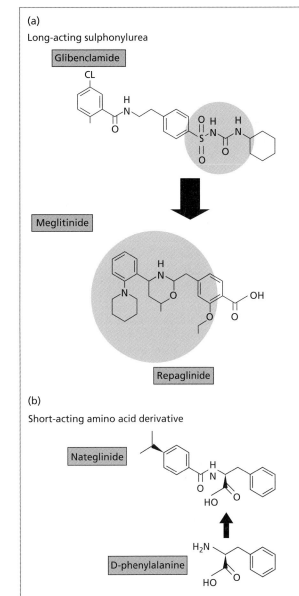

Figure 13.9 Structure of (a) repaglinide and (b) nateglinide. Repaglinide is derived from longer-acting sulphonylureas while nateglinide is derived from the amino acid D-phenylalanine.

Renal failure or intercurrent infection also increase the risk.

Some older sulphonylureas, such as chlorpropamide, are associated with hyponatraemia because they increase the sensitivity of the distal tubule to vasopressin (review Chapter 5), but this is rarely seen with modern sulphonylureas.

There is a concern that sulphonylureas may worsen cardiovascular events in people with type 2 diabetes, although clinical data do not support this. The theoretical reason for concern is that potassium channels exist within the cardiomyocyte, which are the target of the antianginal drug, nicorandil. Nicorandil opens these channels, while sulphonylureas close them. The newer sulphonylureas have lower affinity for the cardiac potassium channels and are more specific for the pancreatic potassium channels at therapeutic concentrations and so the theoretical concern may be lessened.

Compared with other oral antidiabetes agents, the action of sulphonylureas appears less durable (defined as the length of time before treatment needs to be escalated). Accelerated β-cell loss may result from stimulation of an already 'exhausted cell', thereby achieving short-term control at the expense of worsening long-term control.

Meglitinides or post-prandial regulators

There are two drugs in the post-prandial regulator class: nateglinide and repaglinide (Figure 13.9). Repaglinide is the non-sulphonylurea component of glibenclamide, while nateglinide is derived from D-phenylalanine.

Mechanism of action

These drugs also stimulate insulin release by closing the K^+-ATP channel, but bind to a different, but closely related, site on the SUR1 receptor from sulphonylureas. They are designed to restore early-phase post-prandial insulin release without prolonged stimulation during subsequent periods of fasting. However, the effect on glycaemic control with meglitinides is generally less than with other oral antidiabetes drugs. The place of meglitinides in therapeutic options, unlike sulphonylureas, is not yet established.

Side-effects

Hypoglycaemia may occur, but it is usually less severe than with sulphonylureas because of the short duration of action of meglitinides. This makes them potentially useful in older people where hypoglycaemia should be particularly avoided. There is also less weight gain because of a reduced need to snack between meals.

Insulin sensitizers

Insulin sensitizers have no effect on insulin secretion but improve the effectiveness of circulating insulin.

Biguanides

The biguanides are derived from guanidine and the only one currently available is metformin (Figure 13.10). Globally, metformin is the most widely prescribed antidiabetes agent. Although this drug has been available for many years, its mode of action is still not fully understood. Its major actions are:

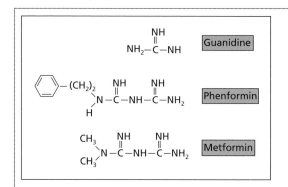

Figure 13.10 Structure of guanidine, phenformin (phenethylbiguanide) and metformin (dimethylbiguanide).

- To increase glucose uptake in skeletal muscle and adipocytes
- To suppress hepatic gluconeogenesis and glycogenolysis
- To reduce glucose absorption from the small intestine (at high concentration).

Metformin appears to work through several intracellular insulin-dependent and insulin-independent mechanisms. Recent work suggests that metformin acts in part by stimulating AMP kinase, an intracellular energy sensor that is usually stimulated during exercise or hypoxia. Stimulation of AMP kinase leads to activation of glucose transporters and facilitates substrate uptake into the cell. New drugs targeting AMP kinase are in development.

Metformin may also suppress appetite and help achieve weight loss, which is useful in patients who are overweight. Metformin may also be used in combination with other oral antidiabetes drugs or insulin and reduces HbA_{1c} by ~1.5–2% (~16–22 mmol/mol).

As well as its effect on glycaemic control, unlike sulphonylureas and insulin, metformin appears to have a cardioprotective effect. The UK Prospective Diabetes Study showed that metformin was associated with reduced cardiovascular mortality and morbidity (Chapter 14). It may also protect against cancer through its insulin-sensitizing action.

Side-effects

The use of metformin is limited by the high prevalence of gastrointestinal side-effects (10–20%), which include anorexia, nausea, abdominal discomfort and diarrhoea. The side-effects can be reduced by starting at low dose and gradually increasing this until the desired therapeutic effect is achieved. A slow-release preparation of metformin appears to be better tolerated.

The most worrying side-effect of metformin is potentially fatal lactic acidosis. Metformin tends to increase lactate production by inhibiting pyruvate metabolism. In situations where lactate clearance is impaired or anaerobic metabolism is increased, such as in shock, lactic acidosis can result. Metformin is therefore contraindicated in renal impairment, cardiac failure and hepatic failure.

Metformin reduces gastrointestinal vitamin B_{12} absorption, but it only rarely causes anaemia. Nevertheless, it is sensible to check haemoglobin annually, particularly for individuals with known or suspected nutritional deficiencies.

Thiazolidinediones or 'glitazones'

Thiazolidinediones have been used clinically since 2000. Pioglitazone and rosiglitazone are the two available, although at the time of writing, rosiglitazone has been withdrawn from Europe and its use

is significantly restricted by the US Food and Drug Administration (Figure 13.11).

Mechanism of action

Thiazolidinediones (TZDs) bind to the peroxisome proliferator-activated receptor gamma (PPAR-γ) (Figure 13.12). This receptor is part of the nuclear hormone receptor superfamily (review Chapter 3 and Figure 3.1). Its natural ligand is unclear, although fatty acids bind PPAR-γ with low affinity. After binding of the TZD, PPAR-γ associates as a heterodimer with the retinoid X receptor (RXR) in the cell nucleus and binds to PPAR-γ response elements in regulatory elements of the insulin target genes (Figure 13.13; Figure 3.20).

PPAR-γ receptors are particularly abundant in adipose tissue, which is the major site of TZD action. TZDs enhance glucose and fatty acid uptake and utilization in adipocytes. They also induce pre-adipocyte differentiation and reduce the secretion of several adipocyte cytokines that inhibit insulin action. Reduced availability of fatty acids to muscle improves insulin sensitivity in myocytes through the Randle cycle (Box 13.9). In addition, TZDs reduce hepatic glucose output (Figure 13.14).

As the effect on plasma glucose is indirect, TZDs may take up to 3 months to reach their

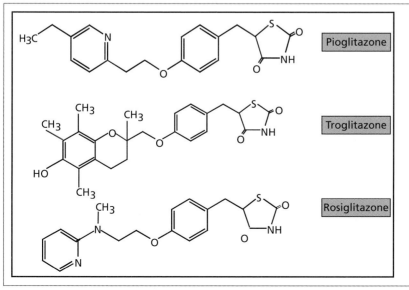

Figure 13.11 Structure of thiazolidinediones. Troglitazone was withdrawn because of hepatotoxicity. Rosiglitazone was withdrawn in Europe because of concerns about cardiovascular safety. Its use is restricted in the USA.

Figure 13.12 Ligand-activated nuclear hormone receptors (review Chapter 3). Thiazolidinediones are ligands for PPARγ receptors. PPAR, peroxisome proliferator-activated receptor; RXR, retinoid X receptor; RAR, retinoic acid receptor α.

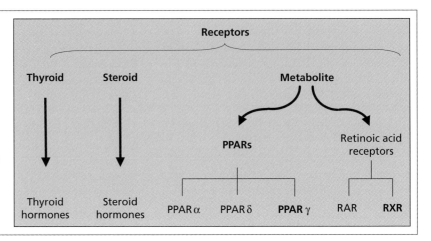

Figure 13.13 Thiazolidinediones: mode of action. After the thiazolidinedione binds to the peroxisome proliferator-activated receptor gamma (PPARγ) receptor, it associates as a heterodimer with the retinoid X receptor (RXR) in the cell nucleus, and binds to PPARγ response elements in the regulatory regions of insulin target genes. LPL, lipoprotein lipase.

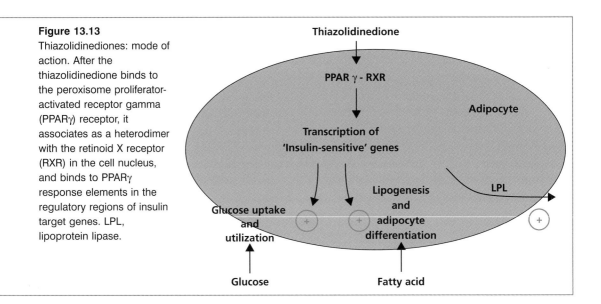

maximal effect [HbA$_{1c}$ reduction of 0.5–1.5% (6–16 mmol/mol)].

In addition to reducing the plasma glucose concentration, pioglitazone improves diabetic dyslipidaemia; plasma triglyceride is decreased while high-density lipoprotein (HDL)–cholesterol concentration increases as a result of increased lipolysis of triglycerides in very low-density lipoprotein (VLDL) –cholesterol. The plasma low-density lipoprotein (LDL)–cholesterol fraction may also become larger and less dense, and therefore less atherogenic. This action may be important in reducing the burden of cardiovascular disease which is discussed in Chapter 14.

The durability of TZDs appears to be greater than that of either sulphonylureas or metformin. They may affect disease progression and several trials have shown that these drugs can slow the progression to diabetes in people with impaired glucose tolerance.

Side-effects

The commonest side-effect associated with TZDs is weight gain, particularly increased fat mass. This

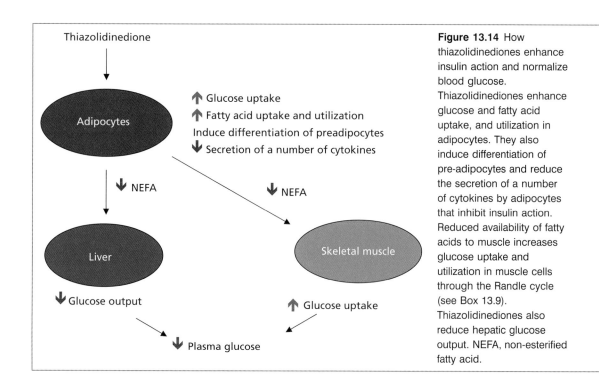

Thiazolidinedione

Adipocytes

↑ Glucose uptake
↑ Fatty acid uptake and utilization
Induce differentiation of preadipocytes
↓ Secretion of a number of cytokines

↓ NEFA   ↓ NEFA

Liver   Skeletal muscle

↓ Glucose output   ↑ Glucose uptake

↓ Plasma glucose

Figure 13.14 How thiazolidinediones enhance insulin action and normalize blood glucose. Thiazolidinediones enhance glucose and fatty acid uptake, and utilization in adipocytes. They also induce differentiation of pre-adipocytes and reduce the secretion of a number of cytokines by adipocytes that inhibit insulin action. Reduced availability of fatty acids to muscle increases glucose uptake and utilization in muscle cells through the Randle cycle (see Box 13.9). Thiazolidinediones also reduce hepatic glucose output. NEFA, non-esterified fatty acid.

appears paradoxical because obesity is associated with increased insulin resistance. However, the TZD-associated fat is distributed preferentially around the hips and thighs, while the metabolically more important 'insulin resistant' intra-abdominal fat is reduced.

TZDs are associated with significant fluid retention and may precipitate overt cardiac failure in those at risk. The fluid retention may also be responsible for some of the weight gain and dilutional anaemia. Rosiglitazone has been withdrawn from use in Europe because of an increased risk of myocardial infarction.

Severe liver toxicity was specific to troglitazone, the earliest marketed TZD, and led to its withdrawal. This does not occur with other TZDs; indeed recent trials have shown that they improve non-alcoholic fatty liver disease.

TZDs also affect bone formation and are associated with increased rates of osteoporotic fracture. Recent epidemiological data have linked pioglitazone with increased rates of bladder cancer.

Box 13.9 What is the Randle cycle?

- Cells are able to utilize either fatty acids or glucose and to switch from one substrate to another depending on the supply
- When fatty acid concentrations fall, the uptake and utilization of glucose increase
- When glucose concentrations fall, the uptake and utilization of fatty acids increase

---

Inhibitors of glucose absorption from the gastrointestinal tract

Guar gum has been used as an additional source of soluble fibre to reduce carbohydrate absorption from a meal. Large quantities are required and the lack of clinical benefit has limited its use.

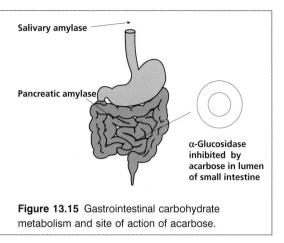

Salivary amylase

Pancreatic amylase

α-Glucosidase inhibited by acarbose in lumen of small intestine

Figure 13.15 Gastrointestinal carbohydrate metabolism and site of action of acarbose.

Acarbose

Acarbose was designed specifically to inhibit α-glucosidase in the brush border of the small intestine and reduce glucose uptake from the gut (Figure 13.15). Carbohydrate digestion is catalyzed by several enzymes that sequentially degrade complex polysaccharides, such as starch, into monosaccharides, such as glucose. Digestion begins with amylases in the saliva and from the pancreas, and is followed in the small intestinal brush border by the digestion of oligosaccharides by β-galactosidases, such as lactase, and various α-glucosidase enzymes that hydrolyze disaccharides.

Acarbose binds with higher affinity than these disaccharides to α-glucosidase, thereby inhibiting dietary carbohydrate breakdown. Digestion and absorption of glucose after a meal is slowed, and consequently the post-prandial peak of blood glucose is reduced, leading to more stable concentrations through the day. Its clinical utility is limited by its lack of efficacy and side-effects. The maximum reduction in HbA$_{1c}$ is approximately half that with metformin or sulphonylureas.

Side-effects

The major side-effects are gastrointestinal and include flatulence, abdominal distension and diarrhoea, as unabsorbed carbohydrate is fermented in the bowel.

Incretin-based therapies

Mechanism of action

Incretin hormones, the most important of which are GLP-1 and glucose-dependent insulinotrophic polypeptide (GIP), are secreted from the intestine in response to eating (Chapter 10). One of their chief actions is to increase glucose-induced insulin secretion by the pancreatic islet β-cells, while suppressing glucagon secretion. In addition, they delay gastric emptying, which may reduce the postprandial rise in plasma glucose. Furthermore, they induce satiety through their actions on the hypothalamus, which has beneficial implications for body weight. There are also animal data suggesting that GLP-1 increases β-cell mass and therefore may potentially affect the disease progression of diabetes.

The incretin response is reduced in people with type 2 diabetes, partly through diminished GLP-1 and GIP secretion, but also through resistance to their actions. To date, therapeutic manipulation of GIP has not proven successful and so the currently available treatments have focussed on GLP-1.

Native GLP-1 is broken down rapidly by the enzyme dipeptidyl peptidase-4 (DPP-4) and so GLP-1 *per se* cannot be used therapeutically. However, inhibitors of DPP-4, which prevent the breakdown of endogenous GLP-1 and GIP, and GLP-1 receptor agonists that are resistant to the actions of DPP-4 have been developed successfully.

DPP-4 inhibitors

Currently, there are four DPP-4 inhibitors in clinical use (sitagliptin, saxagliptin, vildagliptin and linagliptin), although more are in development (e.g. alogliptin). They are oral drugs that are taken once or twice a day and inhibit DPP-4 by >80%, leading to a doubling in the concentration of GLP-1 and GIP. DPP-4 inhibitors reduce HbA$_{1c}$ by 0.6–0.9% (7–10 mmol/mol). Although they can be used as monotherapy, this is not a licensed indication in many countries and so their commonest use is in combination with other oral antidiabetes drugs or with insulin.

Side-effects

DPP-4 inhibitors are well tolerated, with nausea being the commonest side-effect. They are not associated with weight gain and have a low risk for hypoglycaemia. At present there are no long-term safety data for these drugs.

GLP-1 receptor agonists

Currently there are two GLP-1 receptor agonists, exenatide and liraglutide, in clinical use, but other longer acting agents are in development. Unlike DPP-4 inhibitors, these analogues achieve true pharmacological rather than maximum physiological GLP-1 action. This leads to a larger reduction in HbA_{1c} and significant weight loss. All GLP-1 receptor agonists are injectable therapies and yet, despite this, to date they are well tolerated and used by people with diabetes (Case history 13.3).

🔍 Case history 13.3

A 49-year-old man with type 2 diabetes presents with daytime sleepiness and disturbed night-time sleep. His wife complains that he is 'always snoring'. He is currently treated with metformin 850 mg three times daily and gliclazide 160 mg twice daily. His BMI is 36.2 kg/m² and his most recent HbA_{1c} is 10.6% (92 mmol/mol).

What is the likely cause of his sleepiness?

What treatment for his diabetes would you recommend?

Answers, see p. 309

Exenatide

Exenatide is synthetic exendin-4, a molecule that was originally isolated from the saliva of the Gila monster, a lizard living in the Arizonian desert. It has 53% sequence homology with human GLP-1 and is resistant to cleavage by DPP-4. Exenatide is administered by twice-daily subcutaneous injection. It reduces HbA_{1c} by ~1% (11 mmol/mol) and causes a mean weight loss of ~4 kg. Some of the improved glycaemic control is explained by the weight loss, but there is a dissociation between the two as weight loss continues to occur for up to 2 years after the initiation of treatment, while HbA_{1c} usually reaches a nadir after 6 months.

A once-weekly preparation of exenatide has recently been introduced into clinical practice.

Generally exenatide is well tolerated but the main side-effect is nausea and vomiting, which affects up to 50% of people receiving the drug. The incidence of nausea declines with time and can be minimized by judicious meal sizes and timing. Despite this common side effect, only a few people discontinue treatment.

Hypoglycaemia only occurs rarely when used as monotherapy or in combination with metformin, although hypoglycaemia occurs more frequently when combined with either sulphonylureas or insulin. As exenatide is a foreign protein, about 40–50% of people receiving the drug develop antibodies to exenatide; however, the importance of these is unknown as they do not seem to influence the effectiveness of the drug.

Exenatide treatment has been associated with acute pancreatitis. The drug labelling warns about this possibility; however, a direct causal relationship is unclear as the incidence of pancreatitis is increased in people with diabetes *per se*. Nevertheless, exenatide should be avoided in people with an increased of risk of pancreatitis, e.g. those with alcoholism, cholecystolithiasis or hypertriglyceridemia.

Liraglutide

Liraglutide is an analogue of GLP-1 and has 97% amino acid homology to human GLP-1. Liraglutide differs from native GLP-1 by an amino acid substitution (arginine in place of lysine at position 34) and attachment of a fatty acid residue to the lysine at position 26. It has a longer half-life than exenatide and can be administered once daily by subcutaneous injection. Liraglutide is slightly more effective than exenatide, leading to a greater reduction in HbA_{1c}.

The side-effects of liraglutide are similar to exenatide. Overall it is well tolerated. Nausea and vomiting are the commonest side-effects, but the incidence is lower than with exenatide. Hypoglycaemia occurs rarely when combined with either sulphonylureas or insulin. Liraglutide has been associated with pancreatitis but, like exenatide, causation has not been demonstrated.

Which drug and when?

For many years sulphonylureas were the first-line agent for people requiring more than lifestyle modification to treat their diabetes. However, the UK Prospective Diabetes Study published in 1999 showed that metformin improved longevity and reduced cardiovascular mortality, making this agent the first-line treatment for most people (Figure 13.16).

There are differences between national and international guidelines regarding the appropriate time to introduce metformin. The European Association for the Study of Diabetes and ADA consensus statement recommends introducing metformin at diagnosis, while other guidelines, such as the UK National Institute of Health and Clinical Excellence (NICE) guidelines, advocate starting metformin if lifestyle modification fails to achieve adequate glycaemic control (Figure 13.16).

There is considerable debate about the most appropriate second-line agent when metformin no longer maintains adequate glycaemic control. NICE recommends that sulphonylureas, thiazolidinediones, DPP-4 inhibitors and, in some circumstances, liraglutide may all be used as second-line treatments (Case history 13.4). There are advantages and disadvantages of each of these treatments,

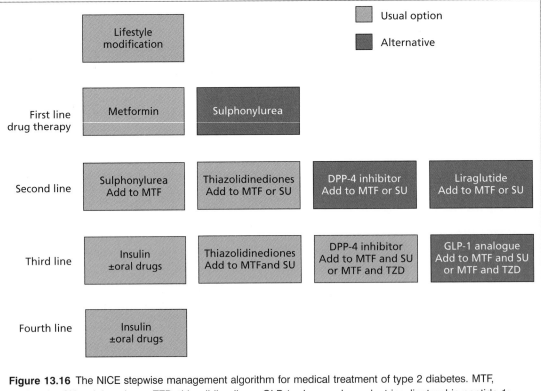

Figure 13.16 The NICE stepwise management algorithm for medical treatment of type 2 diabetes. MTF, metformin; SU, sulphonylurea; TZD, thiazolidinedione; GLP-1, glucose-dependent insulinotrophic peptide 1; DDP-4, dipeptidyl peptidase 4.

Table 13.7 Advantages and disadvantages of second-line antidiabetes agents

	Sulphonylurea	Thiazolinedione	DPP-4 inhibitor	GLP-1 analogue
Advantages	Effective HbA_{1c} reduction	Effective HbA_{1c} reduction with persistent glycaemic control	Well tolerated	Effective HbA_{1c} reduction
	Cheap	No hypoglycaemia	Weight neutral	Weight loss
	Long experience of use	Improves non-alcoholic fatty liver disease	No hypoglycaemia	No hypoglycaemia
Disadvantages	Hypoglycaemia	Slow onset of clinical effect	Less effective HbA_{1c} reduction than other agents	Nausea and vomiting
	Weight gain	Weight gain	Cost	Requires injection
	May hasten β-cell loss	Osteoporotic fracture	Lack of long-term follow-up data	Cost
		Heart failure		Lack of long-term follow-up data
		Bladder cancer?		Pancreatitis?

DPP-4, dipeptidyl peptidase-4; GLP-1, glucagon-like peptide-1; HbA_{1c}, glycated haemoglobin.

Case history 13.4

A 45-year-old woman has had diabetes for 8 years. Her BMI is $28\,kg/m^2$. She has been treated with glimepiride 4 mg/day and has poor diabetic control [HbA_{1c} 11.0% (97 mmol/mol)]. She has background retinopathy and mild renal impairment [serum creatinine 157 μmol/L (1.77 mg/dL)].

What would you do next?

Answer, see p. 309

---

and therefore the choice of agent must be individualized (Table 13.7). Triple therapy is needed when dual therapy no longer controls glycaemia adequately.

Insulin

As type 2 diabetes progresses, many people ultimately require treatment with insulin. In type 2 diabetes, insulin is usually administered as once-daily long-acting insulin, twice-daily mixed insulin or a basal bolus regimen (discussed in Chapter 12). There are advantages and disadvantages with each of these approaches and therefore the insulin regimen must be discussed with the patient (Case history 13.5).

Insulin is frequently used in combination with oral antidiabetes agents, most commonly metformin. Metformin acts as an insulin-sensitizing agent and can reduce the number and severity of hypoglycaemic episodes, and weight gain associated with insulin therapy.

> ### 🔍 Case history 13.5
>
> A 72-year-old woman who lives alone attends the surgery complaining of nocturia, thirst and weight loss. She has had diabetes for 12 years. She has a BMI of 24.8 kg/m². She is currently treated with metformin, tolbutamide and pioglitazone at maximally tolerated doses. Her HbA$_{1c}$ is 10.2% (88 mmol/mol). She is reluctant to start insulin but wants to feel better.
>
> **What are your treatment options?**
> **How would you escalate treatment if your first plan did not solve the problem?**
>
> *Answers, see p. 310*

Emerging antidiabetes agents

There is a continuing need for new and improved antidiabetes agents as current therapies neither reinstate normal glucose homeostasis nor prevent loss of β-cell function nor eliminate the threat of long-term complications. Furthermore, as described above, many current treatments are also accompanied by significant side-effects, including undesirable weight gain and hypoglycaemia. Many new agents are in development and a brief description of some of these drugs is given below.

Sodium–glucose co-transporter 2 inhibitors

Glucose is filtered through the renal glomeruli and almost all of it is re-absorbed in the proximal tubules by the sodium–glucose co-transporter 2 (SGLT2) system. Inhibitors of SGLT2 (termed 'flozins') reduce hyperglycaemia by increasing urinary glucose excretion. Selectivity is needed to prevent co-inhibition of SGLT1, which is responsible for intestinal glucose transport. Clinical trials with SLGT2 inhibitors have shown improvements in glucose control in people with type 2 diabetes. These agents may also have a place as adjunctive therapy in type 1 diabetes. SGLT2 inhibitors do not cause hypoglycaemia and may promote weight loss through an obligate calorie loss in the urine.

The most common adverse effect appears to be an increased incidence of urinary tract and urogenital infection because the increased glucose excretion facilitates bacterial or fungal growth.

Quick release bromocriptine

Bromocriptine is an ergot alkaloid dopamine D$_2$ receptor agonist that has been used extensively in the past to treat hyperprolactinaemia, galactorrhoea (see Chapter 5) and Parkinsonism. However, hypothalamic hypodopaminergic states and disturbed circadian rhythm are also associated with the development of insulin resistance, obesity and diabetes in animal models and humans (see Chapter 5). When administered at daybreak, a new quick-release formulation of bromocriptine appears to act centrally to re-set hypothalamic dopamine circadian rhythms and improve insulin resistance and other metabolic abnormalities.

Clinical studies show that quick-release bromocriptine lowers HbA$_{1c}$ by 0.6–1.2% (7–13 mmol/mol) either as monotherapy or in combination with other antidiabetes medications. Quick-release bromocriptine has recently been approved in the USA for the treatment of type 2 diabetes. Apart from nausea, the drug is well tolerated. The diabetes treatment doses are much lower than those used in Parkinson disease, avoiding the concern over retroperitoneal fibrosis or heart valve abnormalities (see treatment of hyperprolactinaemia in Chapter 5).

Amylin analogues

Amylin is a 37-amino acid peptide co-secreted with insulin. It delays gastric emptying, suppresses postprandial glucagon secretion and increases satiety. Pramlintide is an analogue of amylin that is approved in the USA for use in insulin-treated subjects with either type 1 or type 2 diabetes. It reduces HbA$_{1c}$ by 0.4–0.6% (5–7 mmol/mol) and is associated with a small degree of weight loss (0.8–1.4 kg). It is administered by injection and the main side-effects are nausea (often transient) and hypoglycaemia.

🔑 Key points

- Type 2 diabetes results from the combination of insulin resistance and failure of the pancreatic β-cells
- Type 2 diabetes accounts for approximately 90% of all cases of diabetes in the western world and its prevalence is increasing rapidly
- It is potentially preventable by lifestyle modification
- It has an insidious onset and so patients are frequently asymptomatic for many years

before diagnosis. This provides a strong imperative to screen for the disease
- Treatment is based on lifestyle modification, but pharmacological treatment with oral antidiabetes agents and/or injectable agents may be required
- Hyperosmolar hyperglycaemic state is the most serious complication of type 2 diabetes and is a medical emergency

👤🔍 Answers to case histories

Case history 13.1

This woman is at considerable risk of diabetes in the future. Approximately 50% of woman with gestational diabetes develop diabetes within 10 years of the index pregnancy (i.e. the one in which diabetes occurred). She needs advice and support to help change her lifestyle to minimize risk. This includes both diet and increased physical activity. Drug therapy at this stage is debatable. Although both metformin and orlistat have been shown to reduce the risk of diabetes, the effect size is smaller than lifestyle modification and so the emphasis should be placed on the latter. As diabetes is frequently asymptomatic in its earliest stages, annual screening for diabetes for this woman is important.

Case history 13.2

This man presents with classical diabetic symptoms and has a diagnostic blood test. Given his age and size, type 2 diabetes is most likely, but it is important to be aware that type 1 diabetes or secondary diabetes can occur in this age group. Lifestyle modification, particularly avoidance of sugary drinks, is the most important aspect of this man's treatment, although there may be an

indication to use a sulphonylurea in the short term (<6 weeks) to improve his symptoms while he is adjusting to his new lifestyle. The diet and exercise should also help him to lose weight.

Case history 13.3

This man may well have developed obstructive sleep apnoea as there is a well-established link between obesity, type 2 diabetes and obstructive sleep apnoea. As many as 40% of people with obstructive sleep apnoea have diabetes and almost 90% of obese people with diabetes have obstructive sleep apnoea. Obstructive sleep apnoea is an independent risk factor for cardiovascular disease.

As well as specific treatments for the obstructive sleep apnoea, weight loss is a primary treatment strategy. A GLP-1 receptor agonist would be an ideal treatment for this man as it would improve his glycaemic control and promote weight loss. He should be considered for bariatric surgery.

Case history 13.4

This woman has poor glycaemic control and it is likely that improving this will make her feel better. She is overweight and it is always worth re-emphasizing lifestyle change. She is already on a maximal dose of glimepiride and so a second agent is needed. As she has renal impairment, metformin is contra-indicated and so the treatment options are either a thiazolidinedione or DPP-4 inhibitor. As she is already overweight, avoiding a drug that would promote weight gain would be ideal and so, in the absence of features of non-alcoholic fatty liver disease (which may benefit from treatment with a TZD), a DPP-4 inhibitor would be the treatment of choice.

Case history 13.5

This woman has symptomatic hyperglycaemia and is already taking triple oral therapy. She is not overweight and so the treatment of choice is insulin. However, she is reluctant to start insulin, which is a common phenomenon in people with type 2 diabetes. There is much fear about the use of insulin and these psychological barriers need to be broken down. Education and demonstration of insulin pen devices can help alleviate anxiety associated with starting insulin.

It would be possible for her to commence once-daily long-acting insulin in addition to the oral agents. This is the simplest option and may also be the most acceptable. Most people will require additional treatment, e.g. by adding a single short-acting insulin injection at the main meal (or the meal associated with the greatest post-prandial hyperglycaemia) or with a twice-daily mixed insulin regimen.

CHAPTER 14

Complications of diabetes

Key topics

- Microvascular complications — 312
- Macrovascular disease — 330
- Cancer — 334
- Psychological complications — 334
- How diabetes care can reduce complications — 335
- Diabetes and pregnancy — 336
- Social aspects of diabetes — 339
- Key points — 340
- Answers to case histories — 340

Learning objectives

- To discuss the causes of microvascular and macrovascular complications
- To understand the importance of screening for complications
- To understand the strategies to prevent and treat complications
- To discuss diabetes in pregnancy
- To understand the psychosocial aspects of diabetes

This chapter discusses the microvascular and macrovascular complications of diabetes, diabetes in pregnancy and psychosocial aspects of diabetes

Essential Endocrinology and Diabetes, Sixth Edition. Richard IG Holt, Neil A Hanley.
© 2012 Richard IG Holt and Neil A Hanley. Publlished 2012 by Blackwell Publishing Ltd.

To recap

■ The basic epidemiology and clinical features of type 1 and type 2 diabetes are described in Chapters 12 and 13, respectively, while the diagnostic criteria for diabetes are given in Chapter 11

■ The activation of several intracellular kinases is important in the development of microvascular complications. A detailed description of intracellular signalling is given in Chapter 3

■ HMGCoA reductase inhibitors ('statins') reduce serum total and low-density lipoprotein cholesterol concentration. The synthesis of the hormones from cholesterol is covered in Chapter 2

Cross-reference

■ The risk of developing diabetes complications is strongly linked to poor glycaemic control, which is assessed by measuring glycated haemoglobin (HbA_{1c}). The formation of HbA_{1c} is described in Chapter 11 and its clinical application in Chapter 12.

■ The growth hormone (GH)–insulin-like growth factor (IGF) axis is believed to play a role in the development of microvascular complications. The GH–IGF axis is covered in Chapter 5

■ Bones may be affected by diabetes, either through the effects of renal failure or through foot infection. Bone metabolism is discussed in Chapter 9

■ Many complications could be reduced through prevention of diabetes (see Chapter 13)

Following the introduction of effective treatment with insulin that allowed people to live through the acute metabolic consequences of diabetes, a number of chronic microvascular complications that affect the eyes, kidneys and nerves became apparent. Furthermore, people with diabetes have a higher incidence of macrovascular complications, such as myocardial infarction, stroke and peripheral vascular disease (Figure 14.1). Diabetes is also associated with an increased risk of certain cancers. Pregnancy outcomes for women with diabetes are worse than in the general population. Finally, diabetes is associated with a number of psychosocial sequelae. These complications of diabetes adversely affect the quality of life of people with diabetes and will be considered in turn together with the underlying causes and treatment.

Microvascular complications

Microvascular complications affect over 80% of individuals with diabetes and are present in 20–

50% of patients with newly diagnosed type 2 diabetes (Figure 14.2). With increased screening for type 2 diabetes, the proportion of people with complications at presentation is falling, presumably because of the earlier detection of the disorder and consequently shorter duration of diabetes.

Pathogenesis

The pathogenesis of diabetic microvascular complications is not fully understood and is likely to be multifactorial (Box 14.1). Interestingly, despite long-standing diabetes and its associated hyperglycaemia, some people seem relatively protected against microvascular complications. For instance, the concordance of complications between twins shows the importance of genetic factors in the aetiology of complications: some genotypes may predispose or protect against the generation of microvascular complications.

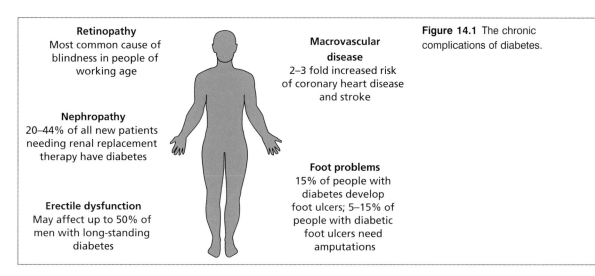

Figure 14.1 The chronic complications of diabetes.

Retinopathy
Most common cause of blindness in people of working age

Macrovascular disease
2–3 fold increased risk of coronary heart disease and stroke

Nephropathy
20–44% of all new patients needing renal replacement therapy have diabetes

Foot problems
15% of people with diabetes develop foot ulcers; 5–15% of people with diabetic foot ulcers need amputations

Erectile dysfunction
May affect up to 50% of men with long-standing diabetes

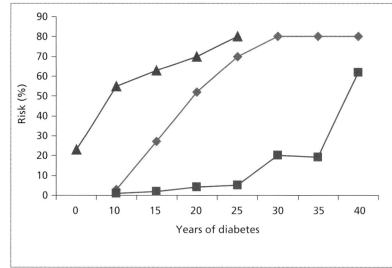

Figure 14.2 Cumulative prevalence of diabetic complications in people with diabetes. Note that at least 20% of people with newly diagnosed type 2 diabetes already have microvascular complications. This reflects the long duration of asymptomatic disease before diagnosis. [Top left line (with triangles)], microvascular complications in people with type 2 diabetes; [middle line with small diamonds], microvascular complications in people with type 1 diabetes; [bottom right line with squares], macrovascular complications in people with type 1 diabetes.

Box 14.1 Why do microvascular complications occur?

- Hyperglycaemia:
  - Development of advanced glycation end-products (AGE)
  - Activation of the sorbitol pathway
  - Activation of several intracellular kinases:
    - Protein kinase C-β
  - Activation of cytokines:
    - Transforming growth factor-β
    - Vascular endothelial growth factor
- Abnormalities in the growth hormone–insulin-like growth factor axis

- Hypertension:
  - Swamping of normal capillary autoregulation
  - Activation of the renin–angiotensin system

Polymorphisms in and around genes in these pathways may correlate to function of the encoded proteins and explain some of the genetic and ethnic differences in predisposition to complications.

Hyperglycaemia

Prolonged exposure to hyperglycaemia undoubtedly predisposes to the generation of microvascular complications. The cell types particularly damaged by hyperglycaemia are those that cannot down-regulate glucose uptake. Furthermore, in either type 1 or type 2 diabetes, improved glycaemic control reduces the incidence of microvascular complications.

Five main underlying mechanisms appear to link hyperglycaemia with the development of microvascular complications (Figure 14.3):

- The formation of advanced glycation end-products (AGEs)
- Altered expression of the receptor for AGE
- Increased flux of glucose through the sorbitol–polyol pathway
- Increased activation of the hexosamine pathway
- Activation of intracellular kinases and cytokines.

Each of these processes is activated by increased mitochondrial production of reactive oxygen species which are induced by hyperglycaemia. The development of microvascular complications is not fully understood and other mechanisms may also be involved.

Formation of advanced glycation end-products

If cellular proteins are exposed to increased glucose over a prolonged period, glucose and its metabolites become attached to the protein through a mechanism that is independent of enzymatic action. Early glycation products are reversible (Box 14.2), but eventually the proteins undergo irreversible changes through cross-linking to form AGEs.

AGEs accumulate in proportion to hyperglycaemia and time. Cells are damaged by three general mechanisms:

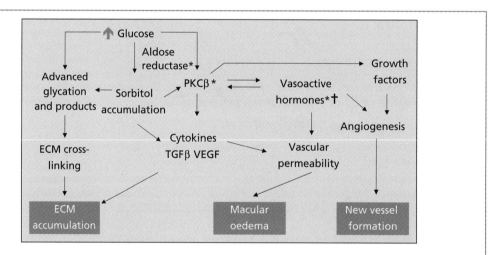

Figure 14.3 Molecular mechanisms that may be important in the generation of microvascular complications. There is no one mechanism that explains the development of microvascular diabetic complications. Hyperglycaemia affects a number of biochemical pathways leading to the accumulation of advanced glycation end-products (AGEs) and sorbitol through the polyol pathway. Hyperglycaemia also activates protein kinase C β (PKCβ). AGE accumulation leads to deposition of material in the extracellular matrix. This impairs the function of the tissue, e.g. the renal glomerulus. Sorbitol and PKCβ activation in turn lead to the secretion of a number of cytokines and growth factors that affect vascular permeability and angiogenesis. *Genetic factors are also important in the development of microvascular complications. Polymorphisms in the aldose reductase enzyme, PKCβ and vasoactive hormones may account for some of the genetic difference. †Hypertension is a strong risk factor for the development of complications. Increased tissue blood flow may affect the function of the vasoactive hormones. ECM, extracellular matrix; TGFβ, transforming growth factor β.

- Glycation directly impairs protein function
- AGEs promote abnormal extracellular matrix accumulation
- AGEs generate reactive oxygen species, which activate nuclear factor κB (NFκB), which in turn activates cellular stress pathways.

Inhibitors of the AGE reaction or antioxidants have largely been unsuccessful at reducing the rate of microvascular complications, possibly because the high quantity of ingested AGEs produced during cooking swamps any effect on reducing cellular formation of AGEs.

Altered expression of AGE receptors

Some of the actions of AGE proteins are mediated through specific receptors that have been identified on a number of different cells, including monocytes, macrophages, glomerular mesangial cells and vascular endothelial cells. These receptors are acti-

---

> ## Box 14.2 Glycated haemoglobin
>
> - Measures the first part of glycation as a measure of glycaemic control (see Chapter 12; Figure 11.5)
> - Non-enzymatic attachment of glucose to the N-terminal of the haemoglobin β-chain

---

vated by pro-inflammatory proteins, which are increased by hyperglycaemia.

Increased flux of glucose through the sorbitol–polyol pathway

In excess, glucose can be metabolized to sorbitol via the polyol pathway, the rate-limiting step of which is catalyzed by aldose reductase (Figure 14.4). This pathway depletes nicotinic acid adenine dinucleotide phosphate (NADPH), leading to decreased formation of reduced glutathione. Reduced glutathione is an important scavenger of reactive oxygen species. Hence, the knock-on consequence of increased flux through the polyol pathway is increased reactive oxygen species, which damage the cell. Other mechanisms have also been proposed to explain the damage to the cells, including sorbitol-induced osmotic stress, and decreased Na^+/K^+-ATPase activity may also have an adverse effect on cellular function.

This polyol pathway can be inhibited by blocking aldose reductase. Clinical trials of aldose reductase inhibitors, however, have been largely disappointing and have not reduced the incidence of microvascular complications. The reason for the lack of efficacy is unclear, but may reflect the multiple and redundant intracellular pathways involved such that blockade of any one pathway may be insufficient to prevent damage.

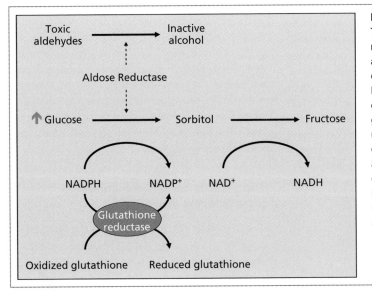

Figure 14.4 Sorbitol–polyol pathway. The normal function of aldose reductase is to metabolize toxic aldehydes generated by reactive oxygen species to inactive alcohols. In the presence of increased glucose concentration, it can also reduce glucose to sorbitol. Both reactions use nicotinic acid adenine dinucleotide phosphate (NADPH) as a co-factor. This can lead to depletion of reduced glutathione, increasing oxidative stress. Sorbitol is oxidized to fructose using NAD^+ as a co-factor.

Increased activation of the hexosamine pathway

When hyperglycaemia is present, glucose metabolism can be shunted into the hexosamine pathway. Excess fructose-6-phosphate is diverted from glycolysis to provide substrates for reactions that utilize UDP-*N*-acetylglucosamine. This activation of the hexosamine pathway then leads to many changes in both protein production, e.g. increased tumour necrosis factor (TNF)-β and plasminogen activator inhibitor (PAI)-I, and in protein function that may contribute to the pathogenesis of diabetic complications.

Activation of intracellular kinases and cytokines

Protein kinase C β (PKCβ) is an intracellular kinase belonging to a family of protein serine–threonine kinases (review Chapter 3). When glucose is metabolized to diacylglycerol, expression of PKCβ is increased. In turn, PKCβ increases production of a number of mitogenic cytokines, such as transforming growth factor β(TGFβ), and vascular endothelial growth factor (VEGF).

Experiments using PKC inhibitors have shown that macular oedema can be reduced in an animal model of retinopathy. Clinical trials in humans are ongoing.

AGEs, hypoxia and PKCβ all increase TGFβ and VEGF production, which in turn increases vascular permeability and angiogenesis, potentially contributing to the macular oedema and new vessel formation seen in diabetic retinopathy. Furthermore, VEGF stimulates angiogenesis and neovascularization. Polymorphisms in and around the genes encoding these cytokines have been associated with an increased risk of retinopathy. The genetic changes themselves may affect protein function, explaining differences amongst individuals in the risk of developing microvascular complications. Recently intravitreal injection of anti-VEGF drugs has been shown to improve diabetic macular oedema.

Haemodynamic theory of diabetic complications

Hypertension is important in the pathogenesis of microvascular complications and may be more important than hyperglycaemia in the progression of microvascular complications once complications are present.

The haemodynamic theory proposes that:

- Through its osmotic effect, hyperglycaemia initiates damage by swamping the normal autoregulatory mechanisms that limit blood flow through a tissue.
- Afterwards, high flow rates that are increased further in patients with hypertension lead to tissue damage; microvascular complications result from chronic abnormalities in blood flow through capillary beds.

This hypothesis is supported by the observation that retinopathy is often less severe in the eye of a patient with an ipsilateral carotid artery stenosis, which restricts downstream blood pressure. This hypothesis is also consistent with the observation that microvascular complications occur in tissues where there is a high capillary blood flow. Aggressive treatment of blood pressure to values of less than 120–130/80 mmHg slows the progression of microvascular complications.

Smoking increases the risk of diabetic complications and this may be mediated through changes in vascular function.

The renin–angiotensin system

Blockade of the renin–angiotensin system with either angiotensin-converting enzyme (ACE) inhibitors or angiotensin receptor blockers slows the progression of microvascular complications to a greater extent than other blood pressure lowering agents, suggesting the renin–angiotensin system may have a role in the generation of microvascular complications. The most convincing evidence is for the treatment of nephropathy but there are studies indicating a benefit for retinopathy.

The growth hormone–insulin-like growth factor axis

The GH–IGF axis (see Chapter 5) has been implicated in the aetiology of microvascular complications for a number of reasons:

- In 1953, a woman with type 1 diabetes was described with background diabetic retinopathy, which regressed after she developed panhypopituitarism from post-partum pituitary necrosis.

- In the 1960s, pituitary ablation was used to treat diabetic retinopathy; its success was related to the degree of GH deficiency.
- People with type 1 diabetes and GH deficiency have decreased incidence and progression of retinopathy.

This area remains somewhat controversial because GH replacement therapy does not increase the incidence of retinopathy in GH-deficient patients with or without diabetes.

In people with diabetes, the GH–IGF axis does not function normally. The reduced portal insulin concentrations that inevitably accompany subcutaneous administration of insulin cause reduced hepatic production of IGF-I. This leads to reduced negative feedback at the anterior pituitary somatotroph and GH hyper-secretion (review Chapter 5). GH concentrations are typically up to two- to three-fold higher in individuals with diabetes compared with healthy subjects. It is possible that correction of the GH hyper-secretion by IGF-I administration could reduce the risk of developing microvascular complications. Similarly, somatostatin analogues or GH receptor antagonists have been shown to produce some reduction of microvascular complications in clinical trials.

Although effective, pituitary ablation was associated with significant morbidity and mortality and was superseded by retinal photocoagulation.

Clinical features

Retinopathy

The most important way that diabetes can affect the eye is the development of retinopathy, which is the commonest cause of blindness in the UK in people under the age of 60 years (Box 14.3; Case history 14.1). Historically, approximately two-thirds of people had sight-threatening retinopathy after 35 years of type 1 diabetes. With improvements in glycaemic and blood pressure control, however, this proportion has fallen. The rate of proliferative retinopathy is lower in type 2 diabetes than in type 1 diabetes, but nevertheless it is esti-

---

> ## Box 14.3 Ways in which diabetes can affect the eye
>
> - Retinopathy
> - Cataract:
>   - Diabetes increases the rate of age-related cataract formation
>   - There is a diabetes-specific cataract that generally affects young people with type 1 diabetes and may progress rapidly
> - Refractory defects:
>   - Hyperglycaemia may alter the osmotic pressure within the lens, leading to temporary refractive defects
> - Glaucoma:
>   - Prevalence is increased in people with diabetes
> - Infection

mated that up to one in three people with type 2 diabetes will develop sight-threatening diabetic retinopathy requiring laser photocoagulation at some time.

> ## 🔍 Case history 14.1
>
> A 24-year-old woman presents with classical symptoms of type 1 diabetes. The diagnosis is confirmed when her blood glucose is measured at 18.2 mmol/L (327 mg/dL). She commences treatment with insulin and re-attends 2 weeks later. She has been experiencing blurred vision and is anxious that she has developed retinopathy and is going to go blind.
>
> **Is it likely that she has developed retinopathy?**
> **What is the cause of the blurred vision?**
> **What reassurance can you give her?**
>
> *Answers, see p. 340*

Retinopathy is also important because it develops in an insidious way and is almost invariably asymptomatic until the patient has a catastrophic intraocular sight-threatening haemorrhage. This is a tragic situation because retinopathy is treatable and with adequate screening, most cases of blindness are preventable.

Natural history

Retinopathy begins with background retinopathy before moving to pre-proliferative retinopathy and finally to proliferative retinopathy (Box 14.4; Figure 14.5). For those without retinopathy, up to 0.6% will progress to proliferative retinopathy over a 4-year period, while for those with background retinopathy, there is a 6.2% risk of progression to proliferative retinopathy within 1 year. However, it is important to recognize that not all people will progress to sight-threatening retinopathy and, indeed, retinopathy may regress.

Screening and diagnosis

As retinopathy is asymptomatic, screening is essential in order to prevent blindness. It is recommended that every patient receives an annual eye test that involves a check of visual acuity and retinal (fundoscopic) examination. Visual acuity should also be checked through a pinhole to assess macula vision.

Traditionally, the retinal examination was performed by a trained physician using an ophthalmoscope through dilated pupils. More recently, this has been replaced where possible by retinal photography as this is more reliable than traditional methods and provides a permanent record for comparison.

As pregnancy can accelerate the progression of retinopathy, pregnant women should be screened in

---

Box 14.4 The different stages of diabetic retinopathy

Background retinopathy
- Dots (micro-aneurysms):
  - A red spot with sharp margins <125 μm (the approximate width of a vein at disc margin)
- Blots (small intraretinal haemorrhages):
  - A red spot with irregular margins and/or uneven density
- Hard exudates:
  - Lipid exudates that often form in a circle around a leaking blood vessel
  - Small white or yellowish-white deposits with sharp margins

Maculopathy
- Background retinopathy that occurs within one disc diameter of the macula
- May cause reduction in visual acuity
- May be associated with macula oedema
- More common in type 2 diabetes

Pre-proliferative retinopathy
- Cotton wool spots:
  - Fluffy white opaque areas that result from retinal ischaemia

- Intraretinal microvascular abnormalities (IRMA):
  - Clusters of irregular branched vessels within the retina that may represent early new vessel formation
- Venous changes:
  - Beading, which appears as segmental dilatations
  - Loops
  - Duplication

Proliferative retinopathy
- New vessel formation:
  - Caused by growth factors that are secreted in response to the retinal ischaemia
  - These are friable and have a high tendency to bleed
  - Haemorrhage from these vessels can lead to temporary or permanent blindness
  - Categorized according to whether they occur at the disc (NVD) or elsewhere (NVE). NVD, new vessels at the disc; NVE, new vessels elsewhere

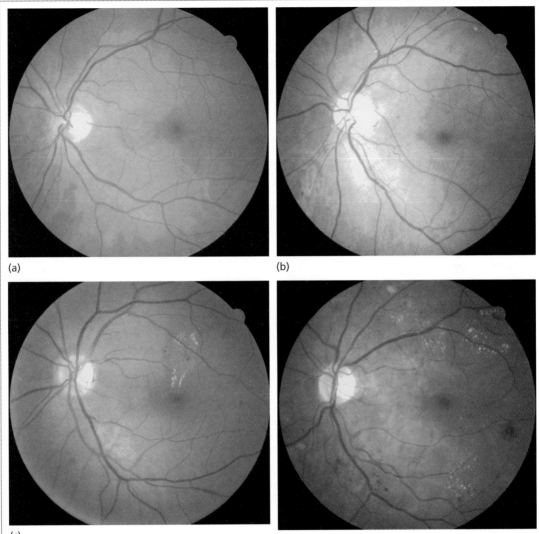

Figure 14.5 Retinal photographs. (a) Normal fundus. (b) Mild background diabetic retinopathy. There are scattered 'dots and blots' and occasional hard exudates in the upper part of the fundus. (c) Diabetic maculopathy. The appearance is similar to (b), but there are lesions within 1 disc diameter of the macula. Note how the hard exudates appear as an ellipse where fat has leaked from a single vessel. (d) Pre-proliferative diabetic retinopathy. The changes are much more extensive and cotton wool spots (areas of retinal ischaemia), venous abnormalities and intraretinal microvascular abnormalities are seen. (e) Proliferative diabetic retinopathy. There are new vessels growing at the disc (NVD; new vessels at the disc). (f) Proliferative diabetic retinopathy. There are new vessels growing close to the macula (NVE: new vessels elsewhere). (g) High-power view of new vessels seen in (f). (h) Fundal photograph showing extensive scarring of the retina following laser treatment of proliferative diabetic retinopathy. Images kindly provided by the Southampton Mobile Retinal Screening Programme.

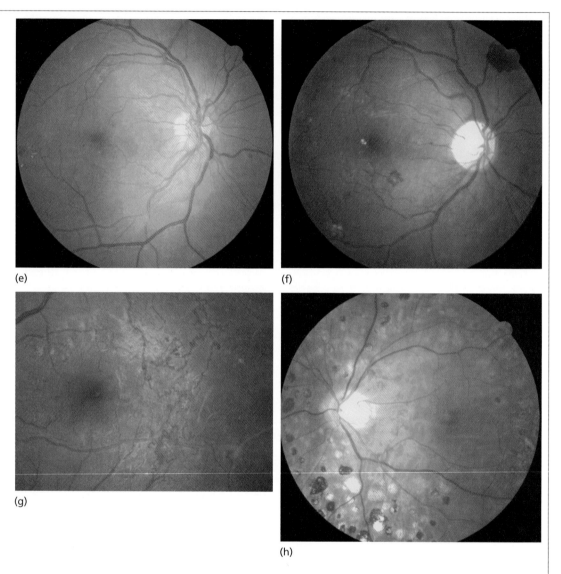

Figure 14.5 (*Continued*)

the first and third trimester and in the second trimester if any retinopathy is present at the outset.

Management

The optimal management of diabetic retinopathy involves close liaison between ophthalmology and diabetes services (Box 14.5).

The development and progression of retinopathy can be prevented or delayed by optimal glycaemic control. The Diabetes and Complication and

Box 14.5 Indications and suggested urgency for referral to an ophthalmologist

- Maculopathy – 1–3 months
- Pre-proliferative – 1 month
- Proliferative – 1–2 weeks
- Sudden loss of vision – same day
- Retinal detachment – same day
- Cataract – non-urgent

Control Trial showed that by lowering glycated haemoglobin (HbA$_{1c}$) by 2% (22 mmol/mol) in people with type 1 diabetes, the incidence of and progression of retinopathy was more than halved. Similarly, in patients with type 2 diabetes, a reduction in HbA$_{1c}$ by ~1% (11 mmol/mol) resulted in a 21% reduction in the incidence and progression of retinopathy. The best results are obtained in patients who also have optimal blood pressure control.

Once a patient has developed pre-proliferative or proliferative retinopathy or maculopathy, further treatment by laser photocoagulation is needed (see Figure 14.5h). Laser treatment is effective in preventing blindness. The principle is that by destroying peripheral parts of the retina, oxygenated blood is preserved for more central regions thus reducing the ischaemic stimulus for new vessel formation. In essence, peripheral vision is sacrificed for central vision. Intravitreal injection of anti-VEGF antibodies has recently been introduced to treat diabetic macular oedema.

Patients may need vitrectomy (removal of the vitreous) if an intravitreal haemorrhage fails to clear.

Regrettably, retinopathy remains the commonest cause of blindness in the UK in people under the age of 60 years. After the onset of blindness, patients should be advised to register as blind and may require additional aids to help them to monitor their diabetes. Less severe visual impairment may prevent the person from driving (see below).

Nephropathy

Diabetic nephropathy is a common cause of established renal failure, accounting for 20–44% of new patients requiring renal replacement therapy. The risk of developing nephropathy is lower in people with type 2 diabetes than in those with type 1 diabetes because of the later onset of type 2 diabetes. However, people with type 2 diabetes requiring renal replacement therapy outnumber those with type 1 diabetes because of the much greater prevalence of type 2 diabetes.

The development of nephropathy is also associated with premature cardiovascular mortality. Cardiovascular disease risk is increased two- to threefold in those with microalbuminuria, the earliest sign of nephropathy, and 10-fold in those with frank proteinuria. Approximately one-third of people with diabetes and proteinuria die from cardiovascular disease before they develop established renal failure. The risk is even higher in those with stage 4 chronic kidney disease.

Natural history

The earliest effect of diabetes on the kidney is increased glomerular filtration rate (GFR). The kidney enlarges through expansion of tubular tissue, but there is no change in serum creatinine or blood pressure. As diabetic nephropathy progresses, there is a progressive increase in urinary albumin excretion and diminished renal function, which results from pathological basement membrane thickening, atrophy and interstitial fibrosis (Table 14.1).

The initial stage of diabetic nephropathy is microalbuminuria, which is defined as a higher than normal albumin excretion that cannot be detected by standard urine dipstick testing (e.g. Albustix), and affects approximately 30–50% of people with diabetes. Protein excretion returns to normal in ~30% of people with microalbuminuria, while only 20–30% of people will progress to frank proteinuria. These latter individuals develop intermittent overt proteinuria before developing persistent overt proteinuria. Occasionally, protein excretion can reach a level that causes nephrotic syndrome. GFR and serum creatinine only become abnormal after the development of frank proteinuria. Hypertension affects virtually all people with persistent proteinuria and some will also develop peripheral oedema.

Screening and diagnosis

Early identification of people with diabetic nephropathy allows intensification of therapy that slows progression of kidney disease and management of the increased risk of other complications, particularly cardiovascular disease.

Annual assessment of urinary albumin excretion and estimated GFR (eGFR) should be undertaken (Box 14.6). Screening for microalbuminuria is most conveniently done by assessing urinary albumin:creatinine ratio, ideally with an early

Table 14.1 Five stages of diabetic nephropathy

	Normal	Micro-albuminuria	Persistent proteinuria	Renal impairment	Stage 4 CKD
Albuminuria (mg/day)	<20	20–300	>300 Up to 15 g/day	>300 Up to 15 g/day	>300 Can fall as renal function declines
GFR (mL/min)	High/normal	High/normal	Normal/decreased	Decreased	Greatly decreased
Serum creatinine (μmol/L)	Normal 60–150	Normal 60–150	High/normal 80–120	High 120–400	Very high >400
BP	Normal	Small increase	Increased	Increased	Increased
Signs	None	None	±Oedema	±Oedema	Uraemic symptoms

GFR, glomerular filtration rate; BP, blood pressure; CKD, chronic kidney disease.

Box 14.6 Estimated glomerular filtration rate (eGFR)

$eGFR = 186 \times ([\text{serum creatinine}/88.4]^{-1.154}) \times \text{age (years)}^{-0.203}$

GFR in mL/min/1.73 m² and creatinine in μmol/L

If the person is female, the result of the formula is multiplied by 0.742

If the person is of black ethnicity the result of the formula is multiplied by 1.21.

---

morning sample (Figure 14.6). As urinary albumin excretion varies considerably from day to day, at least two of three measurements should be abnormal before a diagnosis of microalbuminuria or proteinuria is made.

Management

While optimal glycaemic and blood pressure control are important in the prevention of diabetic nephropathy, there is little evidence that tight glycaemic control influences progression. By contrast, excellent blood pressure control is crucial to slow the progression of nephropathy. Maintaining blood pressure below <125/75 mmHg reduces the annual rate of decline in GFR from 10–12 mL/min/1.73 m² to 3–5 mL/min/1.73 m². The treatment of choice is an inhibitor of the renin–angiotensin system (e.g. an ACE inhibitor or angiotensin type 1 (AT1) receptor antagonist) as these have additional benefits over and above their effect on blood pressure. Other measures include reducing dietary protein intake to 0.7–1.0 g/kg body weight/day as this may slow the deterioration in renal function.

It is important to manage cardiovascular risk factors, such as smoking and lipids, aggressively to reduce the incidence of cardiovascular disease as well as to slow the progression of nephropathy.

It is well recognized that people who are referred as an emergency to a nephrology unit do less well than those whose referral is planned. An early referral to the renal unit allows a structured physical and psychological preparation for renal replacement therapy. It is generally recommended that referral should occur when the serum creatinine approaches 150–200 μmol/L or eGFR falls below 45 mL/min/1.73 m².

Referral to a nephrologist should also be considered if there is increasing proteinuria without diabetic retinopathy because this is a sign of non-diabetic renal damage. Uncontrolled hypertension (Case history 14.2), a rapid decline in renal function and nephritic syndrome are all indications for referral, as are unexplained anaemia and abnormal bone chemistry (serum calcium, phosphate and parathyroid hormone; see Chapter 9).

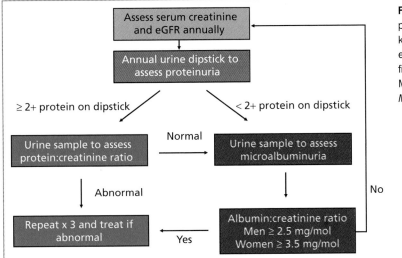

Figure 14.6 A suggested plan for annual screening for kidney disease in diabetes. eGFR, estimated glomerular filtration rate. Adapted from Marshall SM, Flyvbjerg A. *Br Med J* 2006;333:475–480.

Renal replacement therapy can be provided by haemodialysis, continuous ambulatory peritoneal dialysis or renal transplantation. Renal transplantation is considered the treatment of choice for patients younger than 60 years of age as 5-year survival following transplantation is now as good as that in those without diabetes. Patients may also be anaemic secondary to loss of renal erythopoietin. This hormone may need specific replacement.

Neuropathy

Neuropathy affects 20–50% of patients with type 2 diabetes, and its sequelae, such as foot ulceration and amputation, cause considerable morbidity and mortality (Box 14.7). Diabetic neuropathy can be divided into acute and reversible neuropathy and other persistent neuropathies, such as distal symmetrical, and focal and multifocal neuropathies.

Case history 14.2

A 65-year-old man with a 4-year history of type 2 diabetes is referred with uncontrolled hypertension despite treatment with a diuretic and calcium antagonist. He is a heavy smoker. He has proteinuria '+' and an eGFR of 45 mL/min/1.73 m².

His GP reports that there was a sudden deterioration in renal function when he was commenced on ramipril (an ACE inhibitor).

What is the most likely diagnosis?
What clinical features may aid the diagnosis?
What investigations will confirm the diagnosis?
What treatment is available?

Answers, see p. 341

Box 14.7 Classification of diabetic neuropathy

Acute reversible
- Hyperglycaemic neuropathy

Persistent
- Symmetrical:
  - Distal symmetrical neuropathy (peripheral neuropathy)
  - Acute painful neuropathy
- Focal and multifocal:
  - Pressure palsies:
    - Carpal tunnel syndrome (median nerve)
    - Ulnar nerve compression at the elbow
  - Mononeuropathies:
    - Diabetic amyotrophy (femoral nerve)
    - III and VI cranial nerves
    - Truncal
- Autonomic

Hyperglycaemic neuropathy

Hyperglycaemia slows nerve conduction and causes uncomfortable sensory symptoms in those with poor glycaemic control.

Distal symmetrical neuropathy

The commonest neuropathy is distal symmetrical neuropathy, also called 'peripheral neuropathy'. It results from damage to the axon tips of the longest nerves, giving symptoms in a 'glove and stocking' distribution. The longer the nerve, the greater is the risk, explaining why tall stature is a risk factor. Other risk factors include poor glycaemic control, visceral obesity, duration of diabetes, hypertension, age, smoking, hypoinsulinaemia (i.e. patients with β-cell failure) and dyslipidaemia.

Sensory loss is the most obvious component, leading to numbness, but patients may also experience considerable pain or altered sensation. The pain is often described as 'burning' or 'an electrical shock' that may be accompanied by paraesthesiae. Quality of life is reduced as pain interferes with sleep, daily activities and enjoyment. Painful neuropathy is a risk factor for the development of depression.

Pressure palsies

In diabetes, nerves are more susceptible to mechanical injury at sites of compression or entrapment. The commonest is median nerve compression (carpal tunnel syndrome), which causes paraesthesiae and numbness in the lateral three and a half fingers. Most patients respond to surgical decompression.

Mononeuropathies and radiculopathies

People with diabetes are more prone to develop mononeuropathies of the third or sixth cranial nerves or trunk. Damage to nerve roots is also more common. The aetiology of the mononeuropathies and radiculopathies is unclear, but the rapid onset suggests a vasculitic or inflammatory process at least in part.

The commonest radiculopathy is femoral amyotrophy in which there is involvement of the lumbosacral nerve roots, plexus and femoral nerve. Patients present with continuous thigh pain, wasting and weakness of the quadriceps, and sometimes weight loss. The knee-jerk reflex is also lost.

Recovery of the mononeuropathies or radiculopathies is usually spontaneous, but may take many months.

Management of painful diabetic neuropathy

The management of diabetic neuropathy is often difficult (Figure 14.7). It is important to exclude other causes of neuropathy, such as vitamin B_{12} deficiency, alcohol excess and renal dysfunction. Some patients will respond to a cradle or protective film that prevents the affected limb from being touched or rubbed. Simple analgesics, such as paracetamol, aspirin and codeine phosphate, are usually ineffective in the treatment of neuropathy but may provide some relief. Where these measures fail, the antidepressant duloxetine is the first-line treatment. Both serotonin and norepinephrine have been implicated in the mediation of endogenous analgesic mechanisms via inhibitory pain pathways in the brain and spinal cord. Duloxetine is a selective serotonin and norepinephrine reuptake inhibitor thereby modifying pain perception. If this is contra-indicated or is ineffective, amitriptyline is a reasonable alternative. Pregabalin is a further alternative which can be used alone or in addition to duloxetine or amitriptyline.

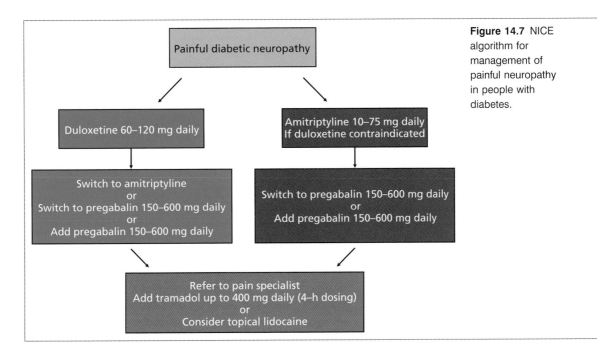

Figure 14.7 NICE algorithm for management of painful neuropathy in people with diabetes.

Painful diabetic neuropathy

Duloxetine 60–120 mg daily

Amitriptyline 10–75 mg daily
If duloxetine contraindicated

Switch to amitriptyline
or
Switch to pregabalin 150–600 mg daily
or
Add pregabalin 150–600 mg daily

Switch to pregabalin 150–600 mg daily
or
Add pregabalin 150–600 mg daily

Refer to pain specialist
Add tramadol up to 400 mg daily (4–h dosing)
or
Consider topical lidocaine

If these measures fail to control the pain, the patient should be referred to a specialist pain clinic and opiate analgesia may be needed. Tramadol is used before considering more potent opiates such as morphine. Topical anaesthetics may also be considered.

Autonomic neuropathy

In people with long-standing diabetes, autonomic neuropathy may develop (Box 14.8). Symptoms are unusual but may be distressing. Management is often challenging and aims to relieve symptoms.

The diabetic foot

Foot problems are a major cause of morbidity in people with diabetes (Case history 14.3). Foot ulceration is common, affecting up to 25% of people with diabetes (Figure 14.8). Diabetes is the commonest cause of non-traumatic lower limb amputation in the developed world and in 85% of cases amputation is preceded by foot ulceration. The rates of non-traumatic lower limb amputation are almost 15 times higher than in people without diabetes. It is estimated that a leg is lost to diabetes somewhere in the world every 30 s. Foot ulceration is the commonest reason for hospitalization and the most expensive complication of diabetes.

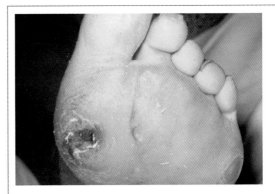

Figure 14.8 Plantar ulcer in a patient with diabetes. Note how dry the skin appears and how the callous has built up around the ulcer. Image kindly provided by Professor Cliff Shearman, University of Southampton.

Major amputations are a tragedy because up to 85% are potentially preventable; however, this requires a coordinated effort by a multidisciplinary team of healthcare professionals. Strategies are aimed at preventing foot ulcers and should be focused on those patients with recognized risk factors for the development of foot problems. These efforts are not only clinically rewarding, but are also cost-effective and can even be cost-saving.

Case history 14.3

A 56-year-old woman develops an infected foot ulcer after a night out at a club. She has had diabetes for 7 years and is treated with metformin 500 mg three times daily and gliclazide 80 mg twice daily. Her HbA_{1c} is 9.0% (75 mmol/mol).

What is your immediate management? What are your long-term plans?

Answers, see p. 341

Box 14.8 Symptoms and signs of autonomic neuropathy

Gastrointestinal
- Gustatory sweating
- Oesophageal dysmotility
- Gastroparesis
- Diabetic diarrhoea

Cardiovascular
- Postural hypotension
- Abnormal cardiovascular reflexes
- Cardiorespiratory arrest
- Neuropathic oedema
- Increased peripheral blood flow

Genitourinary
- Neuropathic bladder
- Erectile dysfunction in men; sexual dysfunction in women

Musculoskeletal
- Charcot arthropathy

Metabolic
- Blunted counter-regulation responses to hypoglycaemia

Eyes
- Abnormal pupillary reflexes

Box 14.9 Cause of diabetic foot ulcers

Neuropathy
- Peripheral neuropathy results in a loss of pain sensation:
  - Patients are unaware of injury to their feet
- Motor neuropathy leads to a characteristic posture of raised arch and clawed toes:
  - Pressure is concentrated on the metatarsal heads and heel
  - Callus forms at these pressure points
  - Haemorrhage or necrosis, which commonly occurs within the callus, can ulcerate
- Autonomic neuropathy:
  - Reduced sweating leads to dry and cracked skin as a portal for infection
- Charcot arthropathy

Peripheral vascular disease
- The reduced blood supply to the feet may compromise both nutrition and oxygen

Infection

Pathogenesis of diabetic foot ulcers

Diabetic foot ulcers are caused by a combination of neuropathy and ischaemia and are frequently complicated by infection (Box 14.9; Figure 14.8). Peripheral vascular disease (PVD) is a major contributor to the pathogenesis of foot ulcers. PVD tends to affect distal vessels and occurs at a younger age in people with diabetes. Although PVD rarely causes ulceration itself, the impaired blood supply compromises the ability to heal minor trauma or infection. Peripheral neuropathy reduces sensation. Consequently infection and trauma may not be perceived by the patient who continues to walk on the injured foot, causing more damage. Autonomic neuropathy in the limbs reduces sweating and alters blood flow, resulting in dry skin that is prone to crack and fissure.

Table 14.2 Principles of good self footcare	
Do	**Don't**
Wash feet daily	Use corn cures
Check feet daily	Use hot water bottles
Seek urgent treatment of problems	Walk barefoot
	Cut or file down corns/callosities
See a chiropodist regularly	Treat foot problems yourself
Wear sensible shoes	
	Wear ill-fitting shoes

Box 14.10 Sites to be tested with monofilament

- Plantar aspect of first toe
- First, third and fifth metatarsal heads
- Plantar surface of heel
- Dorsum of foot

Screening for foot disease

As the treatment of diabetic foot ulcers is difficult, prevention is vital. Patient education, assessment of risk factors and regular examination are vital (Table 14.2).

Screening for foot problems consists of four parts:

- Enquiry about past or present ulceration
- Inspection for abnormalities such as prominent metatarsal heads or clawed toes, hallux valgus, muscle wasting, Charcot deformity, or callus formation
- Testing for neuropathy
- Palpation of foot pulses to detect ischaemia.

There has been considerable discussion about the optimal means of testing for neuropathy. Examination of the feet may reveal distal loss of sensory modalities, such as vibration, touch, pinprick and joint position sense, and temperature. However, formal measurements of vibration sense with a biothesiometer and nerve conduction studies have not been used routinely in clinical practice, creating a lack of clinical standardization. More recently, the introduction of a 10-g monofilaments has allowed reproducible assessments.

The monofilament is applied perpendicular to the foot and buckles at a force of 10 g (Box 14.10). The ability to feel that level of pressure provides protective sensation against foot ulceration. The test is repeated at various sites to detect any area where protective pain sensation is lost.

Lower limb pulses, including dorsalis pedis and the posterior tibial pulse, should be palpated.

Clinical examination can be corroborated by use of Doppler ultrasound, which can also assess the ankle to brachial blood pressure index, a further measure of blood flow to the feet.

Management of diabetic foot ulcers

Diabetes impairs wound healing, which may be exacerbated by sustained pressure on the wound as the neuropathic patient continues to walk on the painless ulcer. Consequently ulcers may be prolonged. Offloading this pressure either by bed rest or total contact casting will facilitate healing of the ulcer. The principle of total contact casting is that pressure is dispersed from the ulcer. The cast is not removable, ensuring compliance. Removable casts that distribute pressure in a similar manner are available, but these are less effective than total contact casting. The casts should be removed weekly to inspect the ulcer, remove callus, and clean and debride the wound as necessary. Ulcers usually heal in 6–12 weeks with this approach, but it is recommended that the cast is worn for a further 4 weeks after healing to allow the repaired tissue to strengthen.

One of the first steps in managing a foot ulcer is to determine whether infection is present or not. Infected ulcers are potentially medical emergencies as inattention can result in massive tissue loss and amputation. The diagnosis of infection is largely clinical as all bacteria colonizing an ulcer are potentially pathogenic. The foot should be inspected for signs of purulent discharge, erythema, local warmth and swelling (Figure 14.9).

The severity of infection should be assessed. Mild infections are relatively superficial and limited; moderate infections involve deeper tissues; while severe infections are accompanied by systematic signs or symptoms of infection or metabolic disturbances.

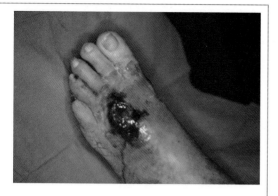

Figure 14.9 Infected diabetic ulcer on the dorsum of the foot. Image kindly provided by Professor Cliff Shearman, University of Southampton.

Swabs should be taken to assess the type and sensitivity of the infecting bacteria. X-rays may help to diagnose osteomyelitis, although this should be assumed if it is possible to probe the ulcer to bone. Magnetic resonance imaging (MRI) or nuclear medicine techniques may also help to confirm the diagnosis.

Antibiotics should only be used where there is evidence of infection to reduce the selection of antibiotic-resistant bacteria. In the case of mild infection, ulcers can usually be treated in an outpatient clinic using oral broad-spectrum antibiotics targeted against the most likely mixture of aerobic and anaerobic bacteria. Treatment can be refined once the results of ulcer swabs are known and bacterial sensitivities determined.

More severe limb-threatening infections require hospitalization and treatment with parenteral antibiotics, while hyperglycaemia is usually treated with intravenous insulin. Early surgical debridement is often indicated. It may be necessary to revascularize ischaemic limbs (Figure 14.10).

As can be appreciated above, the management of diabetic ulcers is challenging and a number of novel approaches have been tried to improve healing (Box 14.11).

Charcot arthropathy

Charcot arthropathy is a rare non-infective complication of severe neuropathy. Diabetes is the commonest cause of Charcot arthropathy in developed

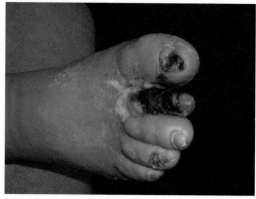

(a)

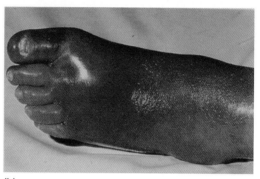

(b)

Figure 14.10 (a) The combination of infection and vascular disease puts the diabetic foot at risk of necrosis, as is seen in the toe of this patient. Image kindly provided by Mr Graham Bowen, Former Chief Podiatrist, Southampton University Hospitals NHS Trust. (b) Moist gangrene. Note the difference in appearance between this figure and Figure 14.10 (a). Image kindly provided by Professor Cliff Shearman, University of Southampton.

countries. Like many other aspects of diabetic foot disease, this complication should be generally preventable. It occurs in a well-perfused foot and can be divided into three phases:

- Acute onset
- Bony destruction
- Radiological consolidation and stabilization

Acute onset

Patients present with an acutely swollen hot foot and about a third are painful (Figure 14.11). The

Box 14.11 Novel adjuvant therapies used in the treatment of diabetic foot ulcers

- Growth factors:
  - E.g. platelet-derived growth factor
- Hyperbaric oxygen
- Negative pressure wound therapy:
  - Utilizes a vacuum device over the wound
  - Decreases tissue oedema
  - Optimizes blood flow
  - Removes pro-inflammatory cytokines
- Bioengineered skin substitutes:
  - Dorsum of foot

Table 14.3 Features that differentiate acute Charcot arthropathy from cellulitis

Charcot arthropathy	Cellulitis
Oedema may resolve with elevation	Typical local and generalized signs of infection may be present More likely if ulcer is present, particularly if discharge is present

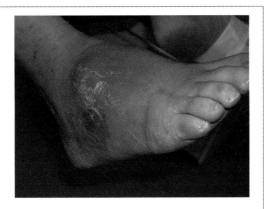

Figure 14.11 Active Charcot arthropathy. Image kindly provided by Mr Graham Bowen, Former Chief Podiatrist, Southampton University Hospitals NHS Trust

initiating event may be an injury, often trivial, that causes bone fracture. Initial X-ray may be normal but a technetium bone scan will detect bony destruction.

It is important to differentiate between Charcot arthropathy and cellulitis (Table 14.3). This can be difficult and so if in doubt, both conditions should be treated. Acute gout and deep vein thrombosis may also masquerade as Charcot arthropathy.

The aim of treating Charcot arthropathy is to prevent or minimize bony destruction. The foot is immobilized in a non-weight bearing cast, which should be checked and replaced regularly. The casting should be continued until the swelling and temperature in the foot has resolved.

Bony destruction

If treatment of the acute stage is delayed, the foot can become deformed as bone is destroyed, often very rapidly over a few weeks. Immobilization is the treatment of choice. Preventing deformity is key as this alters pressure distribution and predisposes the foot to future ulceration, particularly on the plantar surface as part of a 'rocker-bottom' deformity where the alteration in foot architecture generates pressure at the mid-point of the plantar surface rather than the heel and metatarsal heads. (Figure 14.12).

Stabilization

Ultimately the destructive process stabilizes after 6–12 months. Rehabilitation is always necessary after a long period in a cast and reconstructive surgery may be needed.

Genitourinary and sexual problems of diabetes

Male problems

Erectile dysfunction is a major sexual problem among men with diabetes (Case history 14.4). Its prevalence increases with age such that ~60% of men with diabetes over the age of 60 years are affected. The overall prevalence is 35–40%.

In penile erection, nitric oxide relaxes vascular smooth muscle of the corpus cavernosum, expanding the cavernosal space and compressing outflowing venules. This allows blood to flow into, but not

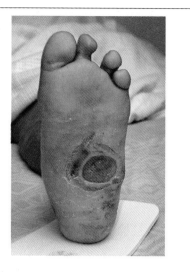

Figure 14.12 Plantar ulcer in a patient with diabetes whose foot has become deformed by a Charcot arthropathy. Note also the amputation. Image kindly provided by Mr Graham Bowen, Former Chief Podiatrist, Southampton University Hospitals NHS Trust.

out of, the penis. Erectile dysfunction in diabetes mainly results from autonomic neuropathy and endothelial dysfunction. Other contributory factors include drugs, psychological issues, and neurological, endocrine and metabolic disorders.

When a man presents with erectile dysfunction, a detailed history is needed to search for reversible causes and to exclude wider sexual dysfunction from androgen deficiency (see Chapter 7). General treatment includes improving glycaemic control, reducing alcohol intake and substituting where possible drugs that may impair erection. First-line pharmacotherapy is with phosphodiesterase type 5 inhibitors, such as sildenafil (Viagra), vardenafil (Levitra) and tadalafil (Cialis). These agents act by inhibiting the breakdown of cyclic GMP, which is a second messenger of nitric oxide (review Chapter 3). As they enhance erections following sexual stimulation, the drugs are taken before intended sexual activity. They are effective in 50–60% of men with diabetes. Phosphodiesterase type 5 inhibitors may cause severe acute hypotension when used concomitantly with nitrates and so this dual use is contra-indicated.

Other treatment options include the use of prostaglandin E, which can be administered by injection into the corpus cavernosum or transurethrally. Apomorphine, a dopamine agonist, has recently been introduced. Vacuum devices allow blood to be drawn into the penis, while a constriction band around the base of the penis prevents blood leaving the penis, facilitating erection. There is also a limited role for surgical insertion of a penile prosthesis.

Case history 14.4

A 55-year-old man with a 10-year history of diabetes presents with impotence. He has no early morning erections. He shaves normally and has a good relationship with his wife. He drinks ½ a bottle of wine daily. In addition to diabetes, he has hypertension for which he takes atenolol and nifedipine, and hypercholesterolaemia for which he takes simvastatin.

What are the possible causes for his erectile dysfunction?
What treatment would you suggest?

Answers, see p. 341

Female problems

Although less well described than in men, women with diabetes may also have sexual problems, including vaginal dryness and impaired sexual arousal. Genitourinary infections, in particular candidiasis, can be problematic and urinary tract infections are frequent in women with poorly controlled diabetes, particularly if there is autonomic neuropathy and bladder distension.

Macrovascular disease

Aetiology

Diabetes confers a two- to four-fold increased risk of myocardial infarction and stroke in men, and up to a 10-fold increased risk in pre-menopausal women, who lose their normal pre-menopausal protection against cardiovascular disease. Mortality following a myocardial infarction is greater in people with diabetes, with cardiovascular disease accounting for 60–75% of all deaths in people with diabetes. Over the last decade, greater emphasis has been placed on managing arterial risk factors.

Pathogenesis

The pathogenesis of atheroma in diabetes is considered to be the same as that in people without diabetes, but it develops earlier and faster, and is more extensive and widespread (Box 14.12). There are also major endothelial abnormalities, including increased endothelial adhesiveness, impaired vasodilatation, enhanced haemostasis and increased permeability.

Hyperglycaemia

There are several mechanisms by which hyperglycaemia and AGEs might contribute to macrovascular disease.

AGEs cross-link vessel wall proteins causing thickening and leakage, and trapping of plasma proteins in the sub-intimal layers. AGEs generate toxic reactive oxygen species that quench the vasodilator nitric oxide and so favour vasoconstriction. AGEs also interact with specific receptors on the endothelium, smooth muscle cells, monocytes and macrophages, causing up-regulation of pro-coagulant and adhesive proteins.

Epidemiological studies have suggested a linear relationship between mean updated HbA_{1c} and the incidence of macrovascular events, but this relationship is weaker than with microvascular events. However, in more recent studies, there appears to be a 'U-shaped' relationship between cardiovascular mortality and HbA_{1c} with a nadir at 7.5–8.0% (58–64 mmol/mol). While there is benefit in treating marked hyperglycaemia (Figure 14.13), trials attempting to normalize glucose from a baseline HbA_{1c} of ~7.5% (58 mmol/mol) showed either no effect or increased overall mortality. Adverse treatment effects may have counter-balanced the beneficial effects of reduced hyperglycaemia; for instance, improving glycaemic control in the type 2 diabetes trials was associated with increased severe hypoglycaemia and weight gain, both of which may increase cardiovascular risk. The duration of follow-up may also be an issue; trials involving people with more marked hyperglycaemia only found improved cardiovascular outcomes 10 years after the end of the trials (Figure 14.13).

It is possible that newer type 2 diabetes treatments associated with weight loss and less hypoglycaemia may be associated with better cardiovascular outcomes. Interestingly, reduced cardiovascular events and mortality rates were seen in people treated with metformin in the UK Prospective Diabetes Study.

Traditional cardiovascular risk factors

Traditional cardiovascular risk factors, such as smoking, hypertension, hyperlipidaemia and obesity, increase the risk of cardiovascular events in people with diabetes. In addition, with the exception of smoking, these factors tend to cluster with higher prevalence in those with diabetes. In the Munster Heart study, for example, 49% of individuals with diabetes had hypertension, 24% had low high-density lipoprotein (HDL)–cholesterol, and 37% had hypertriglyceridaemia, compared with 31%, 16% and 21%, respectively, in people without diabetes.

Diabetes is associated with a dyslipidaemia that is characterized by hypertriglyceridaemia, low

---

Box 14.12 Mechanisms leading to accelerated atherosclerosis in people with diabetes

- Hyperglycaemia:
  - Advanced glycation end-products (AGEs)
- Endothelial dysfunction
- Higher prevalence of traditional risk factors:
  - Hypertension
  - Dyslipidaemia
  - Obesity

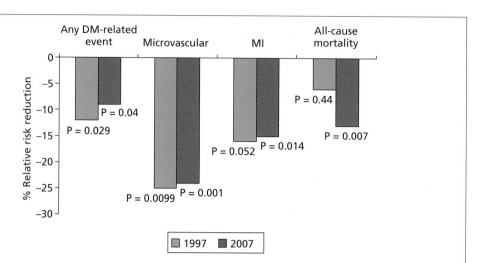

Figure 14.13 Lasting effect of improved glycaemic control on diabetes (DM)-related events, microvascular complications, myocardial infarction and all-cause mortality. The UK Prospective Diabetes Study recruited 5102 individuals with newly diagnosed diabetes and randomized them to intensive or standard glycaemic control. Over the 10-year trial, the glycated haemoglobin (HbA$_{1c}$) was on average 0.9% (10 mmol/mol) lower in the intensive group. At the end of the trial, there was a significant decrease in microvascular events but not macrovascular events or mortality. After the end of the trial, just over 3000 people entered an observational study. After 6 months there was no difference in glycaemic control between the two groups. However, after a further follow-up period of up to 10 years (median 8.5 years), those who had originally had intensive glycaemic control experienced not only significant reductions in microvascular complications but also improved macrovascular complications and decreased mortality. The implication is that early treatment of hyperglycaemia has long-lasting beneficial effects both in terms of microvascular and macrovascular disease, but the benefits for macrovascular disease take a long time to be realized. MI, myocardial infarction. Data adapted from Holman RR *et al. N Engl J Med* 2008;359:1577–89.

HDL–cholesterol concentrations and small dense LDL–cholesterol. These abnormalities of dyslipidaemia are improved, but not reversed completely, by tight glycaemic control. Hypertension is twice as common in people with diabetes and occurs yet more frequently in those who have nephropathy.

This concept of clustering of cardiovascular risk factors is encapsulated in the concept of the metabolic syndrome (Box 14.13). The precise utility of this diagnosis is unclear, but it serves to remind clinicians to think of multiple rather than single risk factors.

Management of cardiovascular disease

Management of cardiovascular complications involves aggressive and systematic attention to each of the risk factors (Case history 14.5).

Case history 14.5

A 67-year-old man with type 2 diabetes for 12 years was treated with gliclazide 160 mg twice daily and pioglitazone 30 mg daily as he was intolerant of metformin. HbA$_{1c}$ was 8.5% (69 mmol/mol). He has a past medical history of myocardial infarction. He has microalbuminuria but no other microvascular complications. His weight is 120 kg, blood pressure 150/100 mmHg, serum total cholesterol 5.1 mmol/L (197 mg/dL), HDL–cholesterol 0.7 mmol/L (27 mg/dL) and triglycerides 2.0 mmol/L (177 mg/dL).

What do you do now?

Answer, see p. 341

Box 14.13 International Diabetes Federation criteria for the metabolic syndrome

- Ethnic specific waist circumference:
  - White European (≥94 cm for men and ≥ 80 cm for women)
  - Chinese and South Asian (≥90 cm for men and ≥ 80 cm for women)

Plus two of the following or treatment of the following:
- Hypertriglyceridaemia (≥1.69 mmol/L or 150 mg/dL)
- HDL–cholesterol:
  - Men <1.04 mmol/L (40 mg/dL)
  - Women <1.29 mmol/L (50 mg/dL)
- Hypertension ≥ 130/85 mmHg
- High fasting glucose ≥ 6.1 mmol/L (≥ 110 mg/dL)

Patients should be advised to quit smoking and blood pressure should be tightly controlled to less than 130–140/70–80 mmHg. There is evidence that the use of ACE inhibitors or angiotensin receptor blockers may confer additional benefit.

HMGCoA reductase inhibitors ('statins'; review synthesis of hormones from cholesterol in Chapter 2, Figure 2.5) reduce the incidence of cardiovascular events as either primary or secondary prevention by ~30% in the general population and in people with diabetes. They should be offered to all people with diabetes with pre-existing cardiovascular disease. Statins should also be considered in those without evidence of cardiovascular disease if other risk factors are present, including age >40 years, the presence of microalbuminuria or proteinuria, and long duration of diabetes. The aim of treatment is to reduce total cholesterol to less than 4.0 mmol/L (~150 mg/dL) and LDL–cholesterol to less than 2.0 mmol/L (~75 mg/dL). The success of statins has largely eclipsed other lipid-lowering therapy, but if they are not tolerated or alone fail to bring the lipid profile to the target, there may be a place for nicotinic acid, omega fish oils and ezetimibe (a drug that inhibits the absorption of cholesterol and thereby disrupts the usual enterohepatic circulation).

Aspirin is not licensed for the primary prevention of vascular events, but has been used extensively for this purpose. Recent studies, however, have suggested that the risk of gastrointestinal haemorrhage outweighs the potential benefit of reduced thromboembolic events, but these may need to be reconsidered in light of the most recent findings that aspirin protects against cancer. Therefore, the balance of benefits and risks of aspirin should be considered carefully for each individual.

Angina in people with diabetes should be managed conventionally. Cardioselective β-blockers may be particularly useful. If symptoms worsen, early consideration should be given to coronary angiography and revascularization. Acute coronary syndrome and myocardial infarction have higher mortality rates among people with diabetes than within the general population, and therefore intensive therapy to revascularize the lesion followed by treatment with low molecular weight heparin, a β-blocker and a platelet inhibitor is needed. Strict blood glucose control at the time of the acute coronary event also improves survival (Case history 14.6).

Case history 14.6

A 60-year-old man without a history of diabetes presents with an uncomplicated acute myocardial infarction. His blood glucose on admission is 11.0 mmol/L (198 mg/dL). His blood pressure is 150/100 mmHg. Serum total cholesterol is 6.0 mmol/L (232 mg/dL), HDL–cholesterol is 1.0 mmol/L (39 mg/dL) and triglycerides are 2.0 mmol/L (177 mg/dL).

What are your immediate plans?

Answer, see p. 342

Coronary revascularization is technically more difficult in people with diabetes because of the diffuse and distal pattern of coronary atheroma. Coronary angioplasty with stenting is the preferred procedure for accessible large-vessel disease. Coronary artery bypass grafting is reserved for

---

> **Box 14.14 Cancers that occur more frequently in people with diabetes**
>
> - Liver
> - Pancreas
> - Colon and rectum
> - Breast
> - Endometrium
> - Bladder

---

difficult or multiple occlusions and for re-stenosis after angioplasty.

Cancer

Diabetes, particularly type 2 diabetes, is associated with an increased prevalence of a number of cancers (Box 14.14), but reduced risk of prostate cancer.

The underlying reason for this association is unclear, but may relate to shared risk factors for the two diseases, such as ageing, obesity, diet and physical inactivity. It has been postulated that hyperinsulinaemia, hyperglycaemia and inflammation seen in diabetes may all increase the risk of cancer.

Recently, there has been debate about the role of antidiabetes treatments in the development of cancer. There is some early evidence to suggest that metformin is associated with a lower risk of cancer, while exogenous insulin, particularly insulin glargine, is associated with an increased cancer risk. However, much more research is needed to clarify this, and at present cancer risk should not be a major factor when choosing diabetes treatments. Nevertheless, it seems appropriate that people with diabetes should be encouraged by their diabetes team to undergo appropriate screening for cancer, as recommended for the general population.

Psychological complications

Diabetes places significant demands on those with the condition. It requires major lifestyle changes, complex and frequently invasive medication regimens, as well as monitoring by invasive blood testing. For many, the disorder is a continual presence every day. The knowledge of the condition and its long-term complications may affect self-esteem and can adversely affect quality of life.

The diagnosis of diabetes may provoke a grief reaction and multidisciplinary support is needed during this period. Engagement is required to help the person with diabetes come to terms with their diagnosis and take control; too often, people feel that their diabetes or healthcare team take control of them. For some, acceptance of the diagnosis and its demands may take a long time. Therefore, emotional and psychological support and techniques are required long term as well as at diagnosis.

All members of the diabetes team should be trained to recognize and address basic psychological issues. While much support may be gained through healthcare professionals, it is important to recognize that other sources of support exist, including friends and family, patient support groups and national charities, such as Diabetes UK and the American Diabetes Association.

Overall quality of life for those with diabetes is similar to that of people with other chronic conditions, such as arthritis. However, poor health-related quality of life is associated with biomedical complications, being female, physical inactivity, low income and recurrent hypoglycaemia. Interventions to reduce psychological distress include individual psychotherapy or counselling, and group therapy.

Despite the imperative to support the psychological needs of those with diabetes, the lack of psychological support for those with diabetes is well recognized, with few diabetes services having adequate access to specialist psychological support.

Depression

The prevalence of depression is increased two- to three-fold among people with diabetes, particularly amongst those taking insulin or those with diabetic complications. As well as the effects on mental well-being, depression adversely affects diabetes care. People with depression and diabetes are less likely to exercise, eat healthily, monitor glucose and take medication as prescribed. Their glycaemic control is worse, the incidence of both microvascular and macrovascular complications is increased, life-expectancy is shortened and health costs are increased.

> ### Box 14.15 Simple screening questions that can be used to identify people with depression
>
> - During the past month, have you been bothered by having little interest or pleasure in doing things?
> - During the past month, have you been bothered by feeling down, depressed or hopeless?
> - If the answer to either is 'yes', ask if the patient wants help with this problem.
> - If the answer to this is also 'yes', then it is reasonable to make a formal assessment and offer treatment.

Healthcare professionals need to be aware of the effects of diabetes on mental well-being. Several short questionnaires have been developed to identify those with depression and clinicians should consider these during the consultation (Box 14.15). While it is well established that treatment of depression is effective at ameliorating depressive symptoms, it has only recently been shown that both psychological and pharmacological therapies are also effective in improving diabetes outcomes.

Psychological therapies, such as cognitive behavioural therapy, are particularly effective, possibly because they provide the individual with coping strategies to manage their diabetes more effectively.

Children show remarkable psychological resilience to the diagnosis of diabetes, but nevertheless about one-third report some psychological distress shortly after diagnosis. This 'adjustment disorder' is characterized by symptoms of depression, anxiety, social withdrawal and sleep disturbances. A similar adjustment reaction is often seen in parents, particularly mothers, of newly diagnosed children.

The relationship between diabetes and mental illness is complex. While depression was traditionally viewed as an understandable reaction to the diagnosis of a life-long condition with considerable treatment demands and complications, other biological aspects of diabetes, such as hyperglycaemia itself, may contribute to the development of depression. Furthermore, depression and other mental illnesses, including schizophrenia and bipolar illness, are associated with an increased risk of developing of diabetes.

Cognitive dysfunction

Type 1 diabetes has a modest effect on cognitive function. Measures of intelligence, psychomotor speed and academic achievement are the most affected, with children showing greater deficits than people who are diagnosed with diabetes during adulthood. These changes occur early in the natural history of diabetes, within 2–3 years after diagnosis. It was previously thought that hypoglycaemia was the main cause of the dysfunction but it appears that it only affects cognition if it is profound and protracted. By contrast, chronic hyperglycaemia may be important in the aetiology of this problem.

Older adults with type 2 diabetes have memory deficits. Chronic hyperglycaemia and the presence of other complications, in particular retinopathy and peripheral neuropathy, predict this problem.

How diabetes care can reduce complications

High-quality diabetes care is essential for all people with diabetes in order to achieve the best possible health outcomes. The growing numbers of people with diabetes has meant that traditional specialist care services are oversubscribed and new models of care are being developed. No single person or setting can provide all that is required in diabetes care. Consequently both primary and secondary sectors are needed to ensure delivery of the appropriately structured and integrated care that is the hallmark of a high-quality diabetes service.

People with diabetes should be seen as individuals with a condition that has medical, personal and social consequences, rather than passive recipients of healthcare. The person living with diabetes will spend the vast majority of their time managing their own diabetes and only an estimated 1% of their time in contact with healthcare professionals. Therefore, empowering the individual with the responsibility of managing diabetes is critical. Contact with the diabetes healthcare team requires well-defined, clear aims and objectives delivering maximum benefit from the consultation, and providing the individual with the necessary skills and coping strategies to manage their diabetes.

The multidisciplinary diabetes team involves dieticians, podiatrists, pharmacists, opticians (or equivalent) and psychologists, as well as doctors and nurses. Diabetes specialist nurses play a crucial role, with important duties in clinical care, counselling and advice, and education to both people with diabetes and other healthcare professionals.

Care must be structured and systematic to ensure that patients receive appropriate advice and management on the different aspects of care (Box 14.16). It is important that complications are considered and should be sought at least annually.

Diabetes and pregnancy

Diabetes is the commonest chronic medical problem in pregnant women, affecting 2–5% of all pregnancies in the UK. Gestational diabetes (GDM) is diabetes that is diagnosed for the first time in pregnancy (see Chapter 11). Among other pregnancies complicated by diabetes are women with pre-existing type 1 diabetes and an increasing number of women with pre-existing type 2 diabetes, a combined consequence of an increasing prevalence of type 2 diabetes and women delaying pregnancy until they are older.

Effect of diabetes on pregnancy

Diabetes can affect pregnancy from conception to birth and may have life-long consequences for the offspring. Women with diabetes may find it harder to conceive and are at increased risk of miscarriage. Hyperglycaemia is teratogenic during the first trimester. There is a six- to 10-fold increased risk of all congenital malformation with heart and central nervous system congenital abnormalities being the commonest. However, the caudal regression syndrome (sacral agenesis) is the most specific for diabetes, being 200 times commoner in diabetic than normal pregnancies.

During the second and third trimesters, maternal hyperglycaemia leads to accelerated fetal growth and macrosomia (defined as a baby whose weight is above the 95th centile for gestation age). This

---

Box 14.16 Issues to consider during the diabetes consultation

Lifestyle
- Smoking
- Driving and its legality [Driver and Vehicle Licensing Agency (DVLA) in the UK (www.dvla.gov.uk)]
- Weight and diet (including alcohol)
- Physical activity
- Review social situation (e.g. carers)
- Pregnancy and pre-pregnancy advice

Macrovascular screening
- Medication review
- Lipids
- Blood pressure
- Aspirin
- Angina
- Claudication:
  - Consider referral for intervention if deterioration of symptoms
- Transient ischaemic attacks/ cerebrovascular accident

Glycaemia
- HbA_{1c}
- Hypoglycaemia
- Oral medication
- Insulin:
  - Injection sites
  - Technical problems

Microvascular screening
- Retinal photography (but including other aspects of eyecare)
- Microalbuminuria
- Feet
- Erectile dysfunction

Education
- Assess need for formal education
- Promote patient charities, e.g. Diabetes UK, American Diabetes Association

Mental well-being
- Diabetes-related distress
- Depression

increases the risk of an operative or traumatic birth, which may result in brachial plexus injury. Despite their size, a baby born to a mother with diabetes behaves like a premature baby in many ways; the risk of respiratory distress, jaundice and hypoglycaemia are all increased. In the later stages of pregnancy, pre-eclampsia and preterm labour are also commoner in women with diabetes. The risk of stillbirth and perinatal death is three- to five-fold higher than in the general population.

In adulthood, offspring of mothers with diabetes have a greater risk of obesity and diabetes themselves.

Tight control of blood glucose will reduce all pregnancy-related complications of diabetes, but even in the best centres, the outcomes for women with diabetes and their pregnancies remain worse than for the general population.

Effect of pregnancy on diabetes

Pregnancy induces a state of insulin resistance that is maximal in the second and third trimesters. Largely caused by placental hormones, this encourages nutrient transfer to the growing fetus. The increase in insulin resistance affects diabetes management with insulin requirements typically going up by 50–100% in the second half of pregnancy.

By contrast, the insulin requirement may fall in the first trimester, risking increased frequency and severity of hypoglycaemia and hypoglycaemia unawareness.

Pregnancy may accelerate diabetic retinopathy and nephropathy, in part because of rapid tightening of glycaemic control and in part because of the pregnancy itself.

Management of the diabetic pregnancy

Pre-existing diabetes

The outcome of a diabetic pregnancy is heavily dependent on the optimization of glycaemic control from the outset of pregnancy and so management begins well before the woman considers pregnancy. Planning is the key to a successful and healthy pregnancy. Treatment and care should take account of the woman's needs and preferences to allow her to

make informed decisions. This can only happen if she is educated about the risks of diabetes in pregnancy and plans the pregnancy. Therefore, pre-conception advice, education and planning should begin once a woman reaches childbearing age in adolescence.

Pre-conception care

Pre-conception care is critical for good outcomes. Many centres run specific pre-conception clinics to allow these issues to be discussed more fully. It is important to check for microvascular and macrovascular complications. Potentially harmful drugs should be discontinued and other medical therapy reviewed. The insulin regimen should be adjusted to optimize glycaemic control without inducing hypoglycaemia. Women with pre-existing diabetes have a higher risk of neural tube defects (spina bifida and anencephaly), and so a higher dose of folic acid (5 mg) is recommended while trying to conceive to prevent this. Once a positive pregnancy test is obtained, fetal neurogenesis has already begun.

Antenatal care

Once the pregnancy is confirmed, women should attend a specialized joint antenatal diabetes clinic. Regular contact with the diabetes team is important to facilitate suitable adjustment to the insulin regimen as insulin requirements change. The women should be supplied with concentrated glucose solution and glucagon injections because of the increased risk of hypoglycaemia and 'hypo' unawareness. Their partners should be instructed how to use the glucagon. It is important to screen for retinopathy regularly during the pregnancy.

Diabetic ketoacidosis is frequently lethal to the fetus and so women should be educated about the early identification of this and provided with the means to test for urinary or blood ketones. If diabetic ketoacidosis occurs, the woman should be admitted and the ketoacidosis treated as an emergency.

A detailed ultrasound scan for fetal anomalies, including a four-chamber view of the fetal heart and outflow tracts, should be offered at 18–20 weeks. Growth scans and other tests of fetal well-being should also be performed during the third trimester.

Birth

Most babies born to mothers with diabetes are delivered before term because of the higher risk of stillbirth. For many women this will involve induction of labour or elective caesarean section. During labour it is important that glycaemic control is maintained and this is usually achieved by an intravenous insulin and glucose infusion.

Postnatal care

Following birth, the insulin requirement drops quickly and most women will return to their pre-conception doses. Where possible, the baby should remain with the mother. As the baby is at increased risk of hypoglycaemia, early feeding should be encouraged with breast-feeding being the preferred option. Maternal glucose should be monitored as breast-feeding may increase the risk of hypoglycaemia. Neonatal glucose should also be assessed regularly until it is clear that the pre-feeding glucose levels are being maintained in the normal range.

Gestational diabetes

GDM is defined as diabetes occurring for the first time in pregnancy. Its importance was first recognized around 40 years ago when it became apparent that women with GDM were more likely to develop diabetes in later life. More recently, the dangers of maternal hyperglycaemia to the fetus have been fully appreciated. It occurs in at-risk women because their pancreatic β-cells are unable to secrete sufficient insulin to meet the increased insulin requirements of pregnancy (Box 14.17). The risk factors for GDM are the same as for type 2 diabetes and so, GDM can be regarded as the early unmasking of a metabolic abnormality brought on by the demands of pregnancy. In a few cases, GDM may unmask pre-clinical type 1 diabetes.

There is a lack of international agreement regarding diagnosis of GDM, in terms of the amount of glucose to be used (75 or 100 g) during the oral glucose tolerance test (OGTT), diagnostic cut-off values and number of abnormal values required to make the diagnosis (Table 14.4). The discrepancies in the diagnostic criteria have arisen largely because of the absence of high-quality evidence regarding the effects of milder degrees of hyperglycaemia on the fetus and the benefits of treating this. The International Association of Diabetes and Pregnancy Study Groups (IADPSG) has recently published a consensus document recommending that the diagnostic criteria for GDM should be changed, with the hope of achieving international harmonization. While their recommendations are based on sound epidemiological findings, they have not been backed up by high-quality randomized controlled trials and further research is needed to assess the clinical benefit and cost-effectiveness of the changes.

The management of GDM begins with lifestyle modification. Although the diet should provide sufficient calories and nutrients to meet the needs of the pregnancy, micronutrient-rich foods such as fruit, vegetables and low-fat dairy products rather than energy-dense high-fat foods will help control maternal glycaemia. The woman should be encouraged to include at least 30 min/day of physical activity in her daily routine.

When this is insufficient to control the glucose, pharmacotherapy is required. Although insulin is the most commonly used means of maintaining glucose control, certain oral hypoglycaemic agents, metformin and glibenclamide (glyburide), may be used safely in pregnancy.

Approximately 50% of women with GDM will develop diabetes (mostly but not exclusively type 2) within 10 years of the pregnancy. They should be targeted for lifestyle intervention to reduce their risk and should be screened regularly for diabetes (see Chapter 13).

> **Box 14.17 Major risk factors for gestational diabetes**
>
> - BMI above 30 kg/m²
> - Previous macrosomic baby weighing 4.5 kg or above
> - Previous gestational diabetes
> - First-degree relative with diabetes
> - Family origin with a high prevalence of diabetes:
>   - South Asian, black Caribbean and Middle Eastern

Table 14.4 Comparison of diagnostic criteria for gestational diabetes

Association	Glucose load (g)	Number of high readings needed	Fasting glucose	1 h glucose	2 h glucose
IADPSG	75	≥1	5.1 mmol/L (90 mg/dL)	10.0 mmol/L (180 mg/dL)	8.5 mmol/L (153 mg/dL)
WHO	75	≥1	7.0 mmol/L (126 mg/dL)		7.8 mmol/L (140 mg/dL)
Former ADA*	100	≥2	5.3 mmol/L (95 mg/dL)	10.0 mmol/L (180 mg/dL)	8.6 mmol/L (155 mg/dL)
ADIPS	75	≥1	5.5 mmol/L (100 mg/dL)		8.0 mmol/L (144 mg/dL)
CDA	75	≥2	5.3 mmol/L (95 mg/dL)	10.6 mmol/L (190 mg/dL)	8.9 mmol/L (160 mg/dL)
EASD	75	≥1	6.0 mmol/L (108 mg/dL)		9.0 mmol/L (162 mg/dL)
NZSSD	75	≥1	5.5 mmol/L (100 mg/dL)		9.0 mmol/L (162 mg/dL)

*The ADA has now adopted the IADPSG diagnostic criteria.
IADPSG, International Association of Diabetes and Pregnancy Study Groups; WHO, World Health Organization; ADA, American Diabetes Association; ADIPS, Australasian Diabetes in Pregnancy Society; CDA, Canadian Diabetes Association; EASD, European Association for the Study of Diabetes; NZSSD, New Zealand Society for the Study of Diabetes.

Social aspects of diabetes

Diabetes affects many aspects of the daily lives of people with the condition.

Driving

The main issues for drivers with diabetes are hypoglycaemia and visual impairment from either retinopathy or cataract. Disability from leg amputation or neuropathy may also affect the ability to drive safely.

Drivers with diabetes must take precautions to avoid hypoglycaemia while driving as this may impair motor skills and judgement (Box 14.18). Although people with diabetes are not involved in more accidents than the rest of the population, hypoglycaemia is the commonest cause of accidents in this group. Impaired awareness of hypoglycaemia is a relative contra-indication to driving and these

> **Box 14.18 Advice to reduce the risk of a road traffic accident**
>
> - Check blood glucose before driving and regularly on long journeys:
>   - Testing kit should be available within the vehicle
> - Take frequent rests with snacks and meals
> - Ensure that there is fast and longer-acting carbohydrate in the vehicle in case of hypoglycaemia
> - Do not drive if hypoglycaemia occurs:
>   - Stop the car if driving
>   - Turn off the engine and remove the keys from the ignition
>   - Leave the driver's seat
> - Do not drive for at least 45 min after the glucose has returned to normal following an episode of hypoglycaemia

individuals need extra blood glucose testing prior to and during breaks in driving.

In most countries, the licence of a driver with diabetes is legally restricted in duration and is subject to medical review to assess fitness to drive. In most countries, drivers with diabetes are therefore required to inform the relevant authorities of their diagnosis.

Employment

Certain employment opportunities are restricted where hypoglycaemia may pose a risk to the worker with diabetes or others. This includes work in the Armed Forces, civil aviation or emergency services. Commercial driving (e.g. of public transport or goods vehicles) or work in dangerous areas such as offshore or overhead working is restricted. While some restriction is justifiable, it is important to recognize that diabetes is not a bar to most occupations and people with diabetes should not be discriminated against on the grounds of disability.

Key points

- Diabetes is associated with a number of long-term complications
- These can be divided into microvascular and macrovascular
- Microvascular complications include:
  - Retinopathy
  - Nephropathy
  - Neuropathy
- The aetiology of microvascular complications is not fully understood, but improved glycaemic control and blood pressure can slow progression
- The burden of myocardial infarction, stroke and peripheral vascular disease is increased in people with diabetes
- The cause of macrovascular disease is multifactorial and so a systematic review of all cardiovascular risk factors is needed
- Diabetes is associated with a number of psychological sequelae including diabetes-related distress and depression
- Pregnancy outcomes in diabetes are worse than in the general population, but may be improved by assiduous glycaemic control
- A systematic approach to the management of diabetes is needed with a multidisciplinary team.
- Diabetes has a number of social implications for driving and employment

Answers to case histories

Case history 14.1

It is highly unlikely that she has developed diabetic retinopathy as this is rarely seen in the first 5 years after diagnosis in people with type 1 diabetes. In contrast, 20% of people with type 2 diabetes have retinopathy at diagnosis. Retinopathy is frequently asymptomatic in its earliest stages.

The most likely explanation for the blurred vision is a change in osmotic pressure in the eye as a result of correction of the hyperglycaemia. Prior to treatment glucose equilibrates between the eye and blood. When the glucose is lowered in the blood, this sets up an osmotic gradient between the eye and the blood. Water flows down the osmotic gradient. This leads to swelling of the eye and in particular the lens, resulting in a refractory defect.

With time, the glucose concentration in the eye falls and the refractory defect corrects itself.

From a clinical perspective, it is important to warn patients about this phenomenon to prevent their understandable anxiety and also to advise them not to replace their glasses during this period as their eye prescription will undoubtedly change as the glucose comes under control.

Case history 14.2

The combination of uncontrolled hypertension, smoking and proteinuria coupled with deterioration in renal function in response to ACE inhibition suggests renal artery stenosis. This is commoner in people with type 2 diabetes and is a differential diagnosis in someone with proteinuria. Clinical features may include an abdominal bruit and evidence of peripheral vascular disease (absent peripheral pulses). Conventional angiography is the investigation of choice in many centres, but spiral computed tomography and magnetic resonance angiography have begun to replace conventional angiography. Isotope renography can provide an estimate of renal function but is of limited value when there is bilateral disease or renal function is seriously impaired. Treatment must be tailored to the individual; it may be possible to control the hypertension with additional antihypertensive agents, but angioplasty may improve renal function as well as reduce blood pressure.

Case history 14.3

An infected foot ulcer in a patient with diabetes is potentially a medical emergency. Left untreated it can develop into a limb-threatening condition within a few days. Treatment will include debridement of the ulcer, culture of swabs and broad-spectrum antibiotics. Pressure must be taken off the foot and so bedrest should be advised.

It is important to obtain good glycaemic control to improve healing and resolution of the infection. Depending on the severity of the infection, she may need insulin acutely. Her presentation provides a good

opportunity to assess her feet for neuropathy and peripheral vascular disease. Advice and education about foot care and appropriate shoes should be given.

Case history 14.4

There are a number of reasons why this man may have developed erectile dysfunction. It is likely that the cause is organic because of the lack of early morning erections. Furthermore, he has a good relationship with his wife. Diabetes-induced autonomic neuropathy and endothelial dysfunction are likely to be major contributors, while his antihypertensive medication, simvastatin and excessive alcohol intake may also worsen the erectile dysfunction.

It is important to institute simple measures such as advice to reduce his alcohol consumption. It may be possible to switch some of the antihypertensives to drugs that are less associated with erectile dysfunction. However, this must be balanced against the need for cardioprotective drug treatment. The drug of choice for this man would be a phosphodiesterase type 5 inhibitor, such as sildenafil.

Case history 14.5

This man is at high risk of further cardiovascular events and all risk factors should be targeted. His total cholesterol is above the ideal and so introducing a statin is the most important step. His HDL–cholesterol is low and nicotinic acid or fish oils may be indicated if dyslipidaemia is not corrected by the statin. His blood pressure is above ideal and needs aggressive treatment. Although the blood pressure target is more important than the agent used, it is likely that an ACE inhibitor or angiotensin receptor blocker should be included as he has microalbuminuria. He is overweight and efforts should be made to help bring down his weight through lifestyle modification. His glycaemic control is not ideal and the use of a GLP-1 analogue is likely to be of benefit as this will improve his weight as well as the hyperglycaemia. Aspirin is indicated for secondary prevention of cardiovascular events.

Case history 14.6

His myocardial infarction should be managed in the usual way with coronary revascularization, analgesia, low molecular weight heparin, β-blockers, aspirin, clopidogrel and oxygen. Although a formal diagnosis of diabetes cannot be made at this stage, it is important to manage his blood glucose aggressively. This is most easily achieved with intravenous insulin.

CHAPTER 15
Obesity

Key topics

- What is obesity? — 344
- Control of body weight — 347
- Prevention — 353
- Management — 353
- Key points — 358
- Answers to case histories — 358

Learning objectives

- To understand the importance of obesity, including its links with diabetes
- To understand the normal mechanisms that control eating behaviour
- To understand the pathogenesis of obesity and the public health measures needed to reduce the prevalence of obesity
- To know the treatment options for obesity

This chapter examines the epidemic of obesity. To reduce the health burden of obesity, it is important to define it, understand its causes and complications, and establish realistic weight management programmes

To recap

- Obesity may result from gain or loss of function mutations; the importance of genetic mutations in endocrine disease is described in Chapter 2
- Body weight is highly regulated through classical endocrine feedback mechanisms, the principles of which are covered in Chapter 1

Essential Endocrinology and Diabetes, Sixth Edition. Richard IG Holt, Neil A Hanley.
© 2012 Richard IG Holt and Neil A Hanley. Publlished 2012 by Blackwell Publishing Ltd.

Cross-reference

■ Obesity is a strong risk factor for type 2 diabetes. The relationship between these two conditions is described in Chapter 13

■ Appetite is regulated by the hypothalamus, which is described in Chapter 5

■ One short-term regulator of appetite is gastrointestinal endocrine function. Various gastrointestinal hormones are described in Chapter 10, while analogues of glucagon-like peptide 1 (GLP-1) are discussed in Chapter 13

The global prevalence of obesity has increased dramatically over the last 30 years. It is associated with a range of medical and psychological complications and is one of the most important public health problems of our time. Despite this, the trend of obesity continues to increase, indicating that current preventative measures are failing. Although there is a high degree of heritability for obesity, the rapid rise in prevalence suggests that environmental factors, such as altered diet and decreased energy expenditure, are more important factors in the development of today's epidemic.

Body weight is tightly regulated; even small mismatches of less than 100 kcal between daily energy intake and expenditure may result in massive obesity in the long term.

Management of the individual with obesity is challenging. There is much pessimism regarding weight reduction programmes and it has been said that 'most obese people do not enter treatment, most who do fail to lose weight and most who lose weight re-gain it'.

What is obesity?

Normal weight and degrees of either overweight or underweight are classified by the World Health Organization (WHO) using body mass index (BMI) (Box 15.1). The classification is based on data from white Europeans, and for individuals of other ethnicities, in particular people from South Asia, the upper limit of normal BMI needs to be reduced.

Box 15.1 How to calculate body mass index?

Body mass index is calculated according to the formula:

Weight in kilograms/(height in metres)^2

Box 15.2 The WHO definitions of underweight, overweight and obesity

- Underweight – BMI < 18.5 kg/m^2
- Normal weight – BMI 18.5–25 kg/m^2
- Overweight – BMI > 25 kg/m^2
- Obese – BMI > 30 kg/m^2
- Morbidly obese – BMI > 40 kg/m^2

The definitions of obesity and being overweight are based on actuarial data that show that mortality has a J-shaped relation to BMI, with mortality being lowest within the BMI range of 20–25 kg/m^2, but increasing at BMIs below and particularly above this range (Box 15.2). The effect of low BMI on mortality may have been over-estimated because of potential confounders. Smoking and intercurrent illness may cause weight loss *per se*, while leading to increased mortality (Figure 15.1).

Why worry about weight excess?

'Thou seest that I have more flesh than another man and therefore more frailty...'

(King Henry IV Part 1 Act III, Scene III)

It is estimated that obesity reduces life-expectancy by around 9 years and accounts for 30,000 deaths in the UK per annum. Overweight and obesity are also associated with significant morbidity via a number of metabolic and cardiovascular complications, musculoskeletal disease and several cancers (Table 15.1). Obesity is costly both in terms of the direct medical treatment costs caring for its complications and indirect costs through lost productivity.

Obesity increases the risk of diabetes, dyslipidaemia and insulin resistance by more than three-

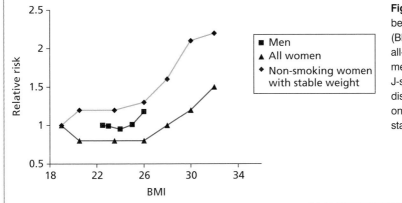

Figure 15.1 Relationship between body mass index (BMI) and relative risk of all-cause mortality in American men and women. Note how the J-shaped relationship disappears in women when only non-smoking women with stable weight are considered.

Table 15.1 Health risks of obesity		
Relative risk >3	**Relative risk 2–3**	**Relative risk 1–2**
Diabetes	Cardiovascular disease	Cancers – post-menopausal breast, endometrial, colon
Gallbladder disease	Hypertension	Reproductive hormone abnormalities – polycystic ovarian syndrome, impaired fertility, fetal defects
Dyslipidaemia	Osteoarthritis	Back pain
Insulin resistance	Hyperuricaemia	↑ Anaesthetic risk
Breathlessness	Gout	
Sleep apnoea		

fold, while increasing that of coronary heart disease and hypertension two- to three-fold. It is estimated that up to 80% of all new cases of diabetes can be attributed to obesity. The risk of developing type 2 diabetes increases across the normal range (see Chapter 13); however, the risk of diabetes in a middle-aged woman with a BMI of greater than $35\,\text{kg/m}^2$ is 93.2 times greater than in a woman whose BMI is less than $22.5\,\text{kg/m}^2$.

There is compelling evidence that our society discriminates against 'fat people' and this is damaging to the psychological well-being of obese individuals. Obese women are likely to have left school earlier, are less likely to be married and have higher rates of household poverty than women who are not overweight. These findings are independent of baseline socioeconomic status and are not seen in people with other chronic conditions such as asthma or musculoskeletal disorders.

The limitations of body mass index

As the health risks associated with obesity relate to the excess storage of body fat and in particular visceral fat, certain individuals will be misclassified by BMI. For any given BMI, women have a higher percentage of body fat than men (Box 15.3). This can lead to the anomalous situation where a lean but heavily muscled young male bodybuilder may have a higher BMI than a middle-aged obese

---

Box 15.3 Percentage body fat in men and women

In adult men of average weight, the expected percentage body fat is 15–20%

In women of average weight, the expected percentage body fat is 25–30%

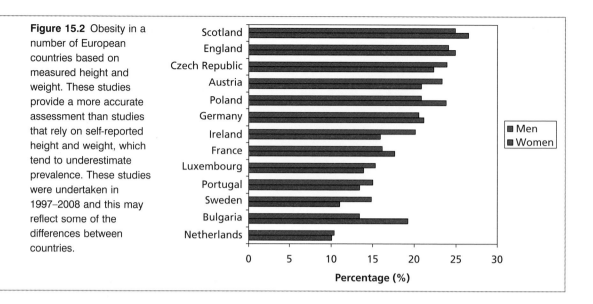

Figure 15.2 Obesity in a number of European countries based on measured height and weight. These studies provide a more accurate assessment than studies that rely on self-reported height and weight, which tend to underestimate prevalence. These studies were undertaken in 1997–2008 and this may reflect some of the differences between countries.

woman. Nevertheless, across populations BMI correlates well with percentage body fat, making it an easy measure of obesity.

Body fat may be preferentially located in the abdomen (central obesity) or surrounding the hips and thighs (peripheral obesity). Central obesity more accurately predicts adverse health risk; for the same BMI, the more visceral fat, the greater the risk of developing cardiovascular and metabolic complications of obesity. This may explain some ethnic differences in complication risks. Asians tend to have greater central fat distribution than white Europeans and carry a higher risk of obesity complications for any given BMI. There are also gender differences in body fat distribution, with most women developing peripheral obesity while men develop central adiposity.

Waist measurement can be used to identify those at high risk of developing metabolic complications of obesity. Waist measurements in excess of 100–102 cm in men and 88–90 cm in women are independent predictors of metabolic dysfunction. However, again, suitable adjustments are needed in people from non-white ethnic backgrounds.

Obesity trends

An estimated 300 million people around the world are obese and conservative estimates suggest that

obesity levels will continue to rise in the early 21st century. The WHO MONICA project followed obesity trends in 21 countries among randomly selected middle-aged participants from the early 1980s to the late 1990s. Mean BMI as well as the prevalence of overweight and obesity increased in virtually every western European country studied (Figure 15.2), as well as in Australia, the USA and China.

Within the UK, the prevalence of obesity in adults has almost trebled since 1980; in 2008, 24% of men and 25% of women were obese. The prevalence of obesity among children is lower, but the rate of increase is similar to that in adults. Obesity rates are higher in low social classes and in some ethnic minority groups.

The Centers for Disease Control's Behavioral Risk Factor Surveillance System provides dramatic evidence of the continuing rise in the prevalence of obesity in the USA. Each year, state health departments use standard procedures to collect data through a series of monthly telephone interviews with US adults. In 1991, four states had a prevalence of obesity between 15% and 19% and no state had a prevalence above 20%. In 2010, no state had a prevalence of obesity less than 20%. Thirty-six states had a prevalence of 25% or more; 12 of which had a prevalence of 30% or more. As these data rely on self-reported height and weight, it is possible that they underestimate the true prevalence of obesity.

The causes of obesity

The causes of obesity are multifactorial and range from purely genetic conditions, such as monogenic leptin deficiency, to entirely environmental conditions, as seen in sumo wrestlers. However, obesity can only occur when energy intake remains greater than energy expenditure for a long period of time. Thus, if energy intake increases and/or energy expenditure decreases, an individual will gain weight. Both energy intake and expenditure are affected by internal homeostatic mechanisms as well as external environmental factors.

Given the diversity of factors affecting energy balance, it is remarkable how well body weight is regulated. Most healthy adults are able to maintain their body weight to within a few kilograms over 40 or more years in spite of having eaten in excess of 20 tonnes of food. A rise of a few kilograms represents a gain of around 10,000–20,000 kcal stored as fat. As the average energy consumption in western societies is approximately 0.75–1 million calories per year (2000–2500 kcal/day), such weight gain represents an energy mismatch between intake and expenditure of much less than 1%.

Even in individuals who become obese, the mismatch between energy intake and energy expenditure is extremely small. Daniel Lambert earned a living in Leicestershire, UK, during the 18th century by exhibiting himself as a natural curiosity having reached the weight of 700 pounds (320 kg). It is estimated that when he died at the age of 39 years, he weighed 52 stone 11 pounds (336 kg), of which approximately 230 kg would have been fat, containing approximately 2 million kilocalories. Assuming that there was progressive weight gain throughout his life, the excess consumption would have been only approximately 140 kcal/day; this number of calories is contained in an apple.

In order to understand the causes of obesity we need to examine the mechanisms that regulate normal body weight.

Control of body weight

There are two main mechanisms regulating appetite and body weight: a short-term control that prevents over-eating at meals and a longer term system that regulates body weight and energy stores, largely in fat. These mechanisms involve the hypothalamus (see Chapter 5). The ventromedial hypothalamus acts as a satiety centre and stimulation of this area removes the drive to feed (anorexia), while lesions lead to over-eating (Figure 15.3; see Table 5.1). By contrast, the lateral hypothalamus acts as a hunger (and thirst) centre. It is tonically active but is inhibited transiently by the satiety centre in the postprandial period. Destruction of the lateral hypothalamus causes anorexia and cachexia.

Appetite is stimulated by the activation of neurones containing neuropeptide Y (NPY) or Agouti-related protein (AGRP). It is suppressed by neurones containing α-melanocyte stimulating hormone (α-MSH) or cocaine and amphetamine-regulated transcript peptide (CART). α-MSH is derived from the protein precursor pro-opiomelanocortin (POMC) that also gives rise to adrenocorticotrophic hormone (ACTH) in the anterior pituitary (see Figure 5.11 and associated text). Several other neurotransmitters, such as orexins and brain-derived neurotrophic factor (BDNF), also have a role in regulating appetite.

There is considerable redundancy in the mechanisms stimulating appetite; loss of function of either the *AGRP* or *NPY* gene or both genes together is not associated with any obvious change in energy metabolism or food intake. By contrast, loss-of-function mutations in either *POMC* affecting α-MSH or in the gene encoding the receptor through which α-MSH signals, the *melanocortin 4 receptor* (*MC4R*), disrupt satiety and are monogenic causes of early-onset severe obesity.

Signals from the gastrointestinal tract

Several gastrointestinal hormones (see Chapter 10; Table 10.1) and neuronal signals from the afferent vagus nerve provide short-term information about hunger and satiety by responding to gastrointestinal mechanical distension, macronutrients, pH and tonicity. Ghrelin, whose secretion by the stomach increases before meals, is the only hormone to

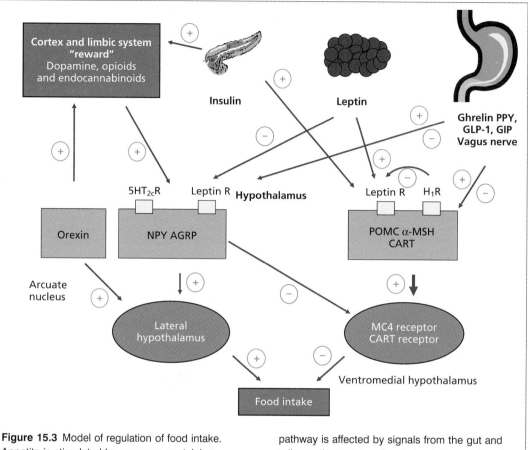

Figure 15.3 Model of regulation of food intake. Appetite is stimulated by neurones containing neuropeptide Y (NPY) and Agouti-related protein (AGRP) in the lateral hypothalamic area. Food intake is inhibited by α-melanocyte stimulating hormone (α-MSH) and cocaine and amphetamine-regulated transcript peptide (CART). Regulation of this final pathway is affected by signals from the gut and adipose tissue, as well as being influenced by the hedonistic control of food intake. PPY, peptide YY$_{3-36}$; GLP-1, glucagon-like peptide 1; GIP, glucose-dependent insulinotrophic hormone; POMC, pro-opiomelanocortin; MC4, melanocortin 4.

stimulate hunger, while cholecystokinin, glucagon-like peptide 1 (GLP-1) and peptide YY$_{3-36}$ (PPY) all reduce appetite.

Long-term control of fat mass – the role of leptin

The adipose tissue hormone, leptin, acts in the brain as a satiety hormone and as a negative regulator of fat mass. It is transported actively across the blood–brain barrier to reach the hypothalamus, where it binds to leptin receptors located on the surface of NPY-containing neurones. Loss-of-function mutations in the genes encoding either leptin or its receptor cause severe obesity from over-eating in both mouse models and rare human patients. Where leptin is absent or non-functional but its receptor is intact, replacing the hormone by injection restores normal BMI to individuals with early-onset severe obesity (Figure 15.4). Under normal circumstances, leptin increases with increasing fat mass to suppress appetite and increase basal metabolic rate, and *vice versa* (a classical negative feedback mechanism; see Figure 1.4).

These findings led to the hope that subtle abnormalities in leptin action underpin common obesity (e.g. polymorphisms in the leptin signalling pathway). However, in most situations, as predicted

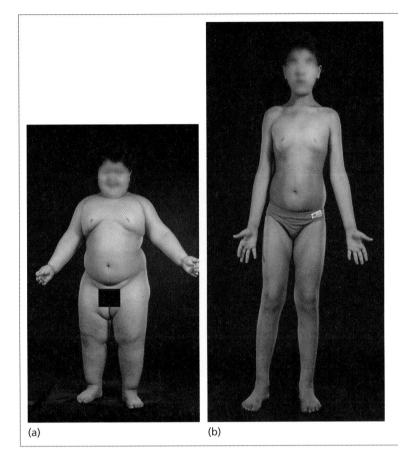

Figure 15.4 Effects of recombinant human leptin treatment in a patient with congenital leptin deficiency. (a) Before, showing a 3-year-old boy weighing 42 kg, and (b) after treatment, showing the boy now 7 years old and weighing 72 kg. Reproduced from Farooqi IS. *Eur J Clin Invest* 2011;41:451–455, with permission.

(a)   (b)

physiologically, leptin is already increased in obesity and treatment with further leptin does not lead to a decrease in body weight.

Other mechanisms involved in eating behaviour

As well as eating for homeostasis, many of us also eat for pleasure as part of our normal social lives. These hedonistic aspects of eating are controlled by a separate but complementary mechanism to the hypothalamic control of appetite. Subtle differences in this system lead to less inhibited eating patterns. For instance, altered food choices are seen in overweight people.

Several hormones and neurotransmitters are involved in this aspect of eating behaviour, including dopamine and central opioid activity. Endogenous endocannabinoids stimulate food intake through activation of cannabinoid-1 (CB1) receptors in the lateral hypothalamus. Blockade of CB1

receptors causes a reduction in food intake and subsequent weight loss. This mechanism was targeted by rimonabant, a drug used to treat obesity and its associated metabolic abnormalities. The drug was withdrawn, however, because of an increased risk of depression.

Genetic factors

Why one person is better adapted than another to withstand small mismatches in intake and expenditure is an important question, and probably has a genetic basis. Much of the variance in BMI within a population is explained by genetic factors; twin studies have produced the most consistent and highest heritability estimates for BMI, suggesting that as much as 60–90% of variance in BMI is explained by genetics.

Over the last decade, several human genes have been identified in addition to those encoding leptin and α-MSH in which loss-of-function mutations

Table 15.2 Genetic causes of and associations with obesity

Genetic syndromes that feature obesity	Monogenic causes of obesity	Polymorphisms linked to obesity
Prader Willi	Leptin deficiency	*FTO* gene
Laurence Moon Biedl	Leptin receptor deficiency	Melanocortin 4 receptor
Bardet Biedl	Pro-opiomelanocortin deficiency	
Biemond syndrome II	Melanocortin 4 receptor deficiency	
Alström	Prohormone convertase 1 deficiency*	
Carbohydrate-deficient glycoprotein syndrome type 1 Short stature obesity	Neurotrophin receptor TrkB	
Albright hereditary osteodystrophy		
Borjeson–Forssman–Lehmann syndrome		
Fragile-X syndrome		
Germinal cell aplasia Sertoli cell-only syndrome		
Simpson dysmorphia		

*The importance of prohormone convertase 1 in POMC and insulin processing is discussed further in Chapters 5 and 11 respectively.

have caused severe early-onset obesity; most disrupt the normal appetite control mechanisms (Table 15.2). Although they only affect a minority of people, these monogenic causes of obesity are important because they help to identify the critical pathways regulating human energy balance and provide clues to where new therapies might be directed in future.

The possibility of other obesity-susceptibility alleles occurring at relatively higher frequencies was raised by the discovery that polymorphisms in the *fat mass and obesity-associated* (*FTO*) gene and *MC4R* gene associate with increased weight and predispose to obesity.

Environmental changes

Despite the important contribution of genetics to the development of obesity, the current obesity epidemic cannot be explained by genetics alone given the rapid change over the last 30 years. It is likely that changes in the environment interacting with a susceptible genotype have led to the marked increase in obesity prevalence.

Dietary intake

Food and drink provide our entire energy intake and so changes in eating patterns have a profound influence on body weight. In the last 50 years, there have been dramatic changes in the availability and types of food that may have contributed to the obesity epidemic.

Total energy intake

The National Food Survey in the UK provides the longest running continuous survey of household consumption in the world. This has shown that over the last 50 years food consumption within the home has decreased. At first sight these data appear to be paradoxical until it is remembered that as much as 50% of all food is now consumed outside the home; the prevalence of obesity increases in people who live near fast-food restaurants. It is difficult to assess total energy intake but it would appear that while energy intake remained relatively stable during the first 80 years of the 20th century, over the last 30 years, intake has increased by 10–15% or ~300 kcal/day, which is more than enough to account for the 50 kcal/day net (100 kcal gross) required to produce a 1 kg weight gain each year. There are several reasons to explain this increase and these are described below.

Cost of food

Since the Second World War, in Europe and elsewhere more food is produced than is required. This has led to intense competition and incentives to bulk buy such as 'two for the price of one' offers or better value 'jumbo' packs. What we eat is influenced by the cost of food and in real terms, the cost of food has fallen. The relative costs of certain food types have also changed; in absolute terms the price of fruit and vegetables, fish and dairy products has increased much more than high energy density foods containing fat and refined sugar. This is one reason why the type of foods being consumed has changed.

Portion size

Portion sizes have increased dramatically in the last 40 years. This is apparent in a number of settings but particularly in fast-food outlets (Table 15.3).

Types of food

The National Food Survey indicated that there have been changes in the types of food that we are eating, with a shift from carbohydrate to fat consumption. This is important because most individuals regulate their meals size according to weight or volume rather than caloric intake. Fat contains approximately 9 kcal/g while carbohydrate and protein contain 4 kcal/g. Short-term metabolic studies show that when the dietary fat content increases, individuals continue to eat the same quantity of food and consequently move into positive energy balance.

There is some evidence from cross-sectional and longitudinal studies that the proportion of energy consumed as fat is linked to an increase in the prevalence of obesity. More recently, however, particularly in the UK and USA, there has been a decline in the proportion of energy consumed as fat, while the prevalence of obesity continues to rise. This may reflect the relatively long lag phase in the development of obesity and it may be many years before this recent dietary change affects the prevalence of obesity.

The water content of a meal is important. If water is added to food, the energy density falls and total calorie intake is reduced. Drinking water at meal times is also important as there is an inverse relationship between water intake and total energy intake and subsequent obesity. Since the 1970s, there has been a shift from consumption of water to sugary carbonated drinks. These beverages contain corn starch and considerable energy. When these soft drinks are consumed, there is little adjustment to decrease energy intake from other sources and so overall calorie consumption increases.

Physical activity

We have evolved to undertake vigorous physical activity and therefore it should be unsurprising that inactivity is associated with ill-health. Total energy

Table 15.3 Examples of how the size of commercially available portions has increased over the last 50 years

Retailer	Then		Now	
Burger King burger	2.8 oz (79 g) 202 kcal	1954	4.3 oz (122 g) 310 kcal	2004
MacDonald's French fries	2.4 oz (68 g) 210 kcal	1955	7 oz (198 g) 610 kcal	2004
Cinema popcorn	720 ml 174 kcal	1950	5040 mL 1700 kcal	2004

Table 15.4 Examples of light, moderate and vigorous physical activity			
	Light **EE (<3.0 x BMR)**	**Moderate** **EE (3.0–6.0 x BMR)**	**Vigorous** **EE (>6.0 x BMR)**
Walking	Slowly	Briskly	Fast or jogging
Cycling	Slowly	Steadily or up slopes	>10 mph or up hills
Swimming	Slowly	Moderate exertion	Fast or treading water
Gym work	Stretching exercises	Sit-ups	Stair ergometer, ski machine
Housework	Vacuum cleaning	Heavier cleaning	Moving furniture
Gardening	Weeding	Mowing the lawn with a power mower, sweeping, raking	Hand mowing or digging

EE, energy expenditure; BMR, basal metabolic rate.

expenditure is the sum of our basal metabolic rate, dietary-induced thermogenesis, adaptive thermogenesis, such as shivering, and physical activity. Of these, physical activity offers the greatest scope for an individual to increase their energy expenditure. Physical activity can be defined as any bodily movement produced by skeletal muscle that results in energy expenditure, and can be subdivided into different components such as exercise or sport. Activity can be also divided according to its intensity and duration (Table 15.4). Low-intensity activities may include walking or housework, while more intense activities may include running or cycling faster than 10 mph or uphill. Sedentary behaviour, such as television viewing, is also significant when considering weight gain as it constrains the opportunity to be active and therefore reduces energy expenditure.

Physical inactivity is a major determinant of the current obesity epidemic. Several studies have shown that physically active people have lower levels of body fat and weigh less than inactive people. There are also strong relationships between indicators of inactivity, such as television viewing and car ownership, with population trends in obesity. In one study from the USA, 11–12% of children who watched television for less than 2 h/day were overweight compared with 20–30% who watched it for more than 5 h/day.

Unfortunately, epidemiological studies have shown that we are becoming progressively less active. The Allied Dunbar National Fitness Survey undertaken in 1995 indicated that 29% of men and 28% of women were classed as sedentary, while only 16% of men and 5% of women possibly partici-

pated in regular vigorous activity. Inactivity increases with age but social class differences are not strong because occupational activity is often balanced with leisure time activity. In the USA, 60% of adults are not regularly active and 25% reported no significant activity at all. Similarly, children are also becoming increasingly inactive.

Technological advances have also reduced our physical activity. Increasing car use across society has reduced physical activity undertaken travelling to and from work. Household appliances are estimated to have reduced our energy expenditure by around 500 kcal/day. Instead, we have tended to compartmentalize exercise into 30–40 min gym sessions two or three times a week rather than focusing on increasing our energy expenditure throughout the day.

Psychological factors

There is much to be learnt from studying the eating behaviours of people who gain weight. Overweight individuals select more energy dense food, display enhanced hunger traits with less satiety, and eat larger and more frequent meals. Their eating behaviour is also less inhibited. Individuals who tend to gain weight have a greater readiness to eat and will eat opportunistically. There are differences in the timing of eating; obese individuals tend to eat more in the afternoon and less in the morning, and some may even eat throughout the night. In contrast, enjoyment from food is less important in those who do not gain weight, and health rather than taste becomes a more important factor when choosing food (Case history 15.1).

Case history 15.1

A 25-year-old female secretary attends to ask for help with her weight (BMI 27.4 kg/m²). She has read many magazines about 'slimmer of the year' and has tried a commercial weight programme. She buys most of her food as ready prepared meals at the supermarket. She eats her lunch sitting at her desk with her work colleagues and eats her supper at home in front of the TV. She snacks on biscuits while at work.

What advice can you offer her?

Answer, see p. 358

The prevalence of obesity is increased in people with severe mental illness. While this partly reflects the illness and the environment in which the individual lives, antipsychotics are associated with significant weight gain (Case history 15.2).

Case history 15.2

A 28-year-old man with schizophrenia speaks to his community psychiatric nurse about his concerns that he has gained 10 kg in weight since starting treatment with clozapine. As they are chatting, it becomes apparent that he is eating throughout the day, including at night, and his diet includes a high proportion of fat and sugary carbonated drinks. He usually spends his days watching TV.

What advice can the psychiatric nurse offer?
Are there any medications that may help?

Answers, see p. 358

Time spent sleeping is inversely proportional to body weight. It is unclear why short sleepers weigh more as sleeping is associated with physical inactivity. It may relate to the seasonal and diurnal changes in hypothalamic control of food intake and nutrient storage.

Prevention

Despite the apparent simplicity of the solution to preventing obesity, there is little evidence to show that health education programmes within the general population are effective. Education alone is insufficient and behaviour modification is also needed. Healthcare professionals need to take obesity seriously and must collectively support obesity prevention strategies to avoid undermining of healthy lifestyle advice.

Public health and governmental responses are also needed to reduce the obesity epidemic. This could include legislation or a more 'ecological' approach in which there is a coordinated strategy to influence the individual by education and behaviour change, and the 'obesogenic' environment through economic, physical and socio-cultural pressures.

Management

The major aim of a weight management programme is to improve health by reducing morbidity and mortality associated with obesity, rather than simply normalizing weight and adiposity. A relatively modest 10% weight loss is associated with a major reduction in death and metabolic complications of obesity (Table 15.5).

Table 15.5 Benefits associated with 10% weight loss

Death	↓ 20–25% in premature mortality
Diabetes	↓ 50% in type 2 diabetes ↓ 30–50% in blood glucose
Lipids	↓ 10% in total cholesterol ↓ 30% in triglycerides
Blood pressure (BP)	↓ 10 mmHg in systolic BP ↓ 20 mmHg in diastolic BP

Patient selection

Unfortunately, the scale of the problem means that healthcare resources cannot treat all patients with obesity and therefore it is important to select patients who are likely to benefit most.

Characteristics of patients likely to lose weight during a weight management programme are:

- High initial body mass
- High central obesity
- High energy intake
- Those who have achieved initial weight loss.

Early weight loss probably reflects the patient's ability to follow the weight management programme. Patients need to be well motivated to undertake the lifestyle changes. High self-esteem and the acceptance of the need to change also predict weight loss. This is particularly challenging in those with mental illness where obesity may well affect the mental state of the patient.

It is important to set appropriate goals to prevent disappointment and frustration during the programme. A 10% weight loss is an appropriate goal because it is achievable, results in significant health benefits and can be maintained. However, in one study, when patients were asked how much weight they would like to lose, only 1% said that they would be happy with a weight loss of less than 10% while 63% expected to lose more than 20% of weight. The natural history of body weight throughout a lifetime is gradual increase and therefore, the first aim of a weight management programme is to prevent further weight gain before progressing to weight loss (Figure 15.5). Congratulating patients

on maintaining weight can improve self-esteem and promote long-term adherence to the programme.

Patients should also be aware of the long-term challenge of weight loss. In the same way that weight gain occurs over many years, a lifelong change to lifestyle is needed to reduce weight. Patients should be encouraged not to think of 'short-term fixes'. The basal metabolic rate makes up a significant portion of our total energy expenditure. If energy intake falls below the basal metabolic rate, the control mechanisms described earlier in the chapter are activated to try to maintain weight. The patient will feel lethargic, tired and listless, and will be unable to maintain this approach for any length of time. Too great a calorie deficit will therefore lead to failure. On the other hand, if a calorie deficit of around 500 kcal is advocated, the patient will lose around 1 kg of weight/week, an amount that is sustainable over the long term.

Dietary strategies

There is a huge popular literature about diets that will aid weight loss. Most of these diets fail to appreciate that nutrition is a 'demand-led' process and that any diet should meet the basic bodily requirements. There is a need to include both fats and carbohydrates as energy supplies and any diet that excludes either of these components will create a mismatch between supply and demand. Diets need to be sustainable over the long-term and most diets that exclude many different food types, such as the 'Atkins' or 'Ornish' diets, usually cannot be maintained for more than several months (Box 15.4). It is important, however, to recognize that individuals respond differently to different interventions and any dietary recommendations should be discussed on this basis.

The first aim of dietary advice therefore must be to ensure that the individual eats sufficient food to meet their metabolic needs (Figure 15.6). Patients should be advised to avoid extreme eating restraints and dieting. In order to reduce calorie consumption, two dietary changes should be considered: the types of food should be changed and portion sizes reduced. A systematic review of all dietary interventions lasting longer than 1 year found that there is little evidence to support the use

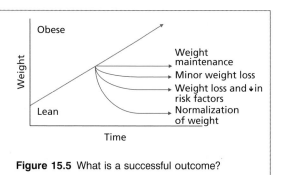

Figure 15.5 What is a successful outcome?

Box 15.4 Eating and activity objectives in weight management programmes

Eating objectives
- Regain control (rehabilitation):
  - Avoid extreme eating restraint/dieting
  - Eat sufficient food to ensure metabolic control and adequate intake of nutrients
  - Re-establish 'normal' eating behaviour and attitudes towards food
  - Appreciate scale of challenge
- Modest reduction in energy intake (~500 kcal/day)
  - Eat well but with lower fat, refined sugar and alcohol intake
  - Maintain sufficient energy (>BMR) and nutrients to satisfy minimal requirements

Activity objectives
- Decrease amount of time sitting and supine
- Aim for low-intensity activity – not what is characteristically termed exercise
- Factor in the total time spent active; it does not have to be a single bout of continuous activity sufficiently vigorous to cause breathlessness or heavy perspiration, i.e. 10 times for 3 min each is as good as once for 30 min
- Activity must fit in with daily life and functional capabilities of individual
- Activity should be pleasurable

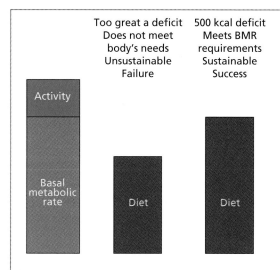

Figure 15.6 Rationale of a 500-kcal deficit diet.

of diets apart from low-fat diets for weight reduction. *Ad libitum* low-fat diets for up to 36 months resulted in modest weight losses of around 3.5 kg. The consumption of low energy dense foods and sweeteners may also reduce meal energy intake. Short-term studies, however, have suggested that weight loss on low-carbohydrate diets is comparable with fat-restricted diets with higher carbohydrate content. Low-carbohydrate diets may have benefits for those with type 2 diabetes as they appear to have a beneficial effect on glycaemic control, hypertriglyceridaemia, and high-density lipoprotein (HDL)–cholesterol in some patients.

Portion size is extremely important. One way of achieving this is to use a smaller plate as the same volume of food will appear more than on a larger plate and therefore will promote reduced food intake.

It is important to re-establish 'normal' eating behaviour and attitudes towards food. Many people eat for reasons that have nothing to do with hunger. For example, people might eat from boredom, to cope with sadness or to be sociable. Encouraging healthy eating patterns can lead to a reduced energy intake. It is important that while food is consumed, the individual's attention is focused on the food. If the attention is divided, such as by simultaneously working at a computer, the reward gained from eating is reduced and therefore people tend to eat more. It is important that food does not become associated with other activities, such as watching television, because this will lead to less healthy eating behaviours. Patients should be advised to eat only at a dining room or kitchen table at mealtimes. Cravings for food are often short lived and therefore, a useful strategy can be to distract the patient with an alternative activity such as a 5-min walk when a craving occurs.

The value of commercial weight loss programmes has not been fully established, but it appears that they may lead to greater weight loss than an individual's attempts on their own. The peer support derived from others attending the group helps maintain motivation.

Physical activity

Physical activity plays an important part in a weight management programme (Box 15.4). While high energy expenditure can outstrip energy intake and therefore promotes weight loss in its own right, exercise particularly has a role in the prevention of weight re-gain when combined with dietary interventions. It is important that patients decrease the amount of time that they spend sitting or occupied in sedentary activities. Low intensity activity is also of great importance; for example, an 80-year-old person with agitated Alzheimer disease will expend more calories per day than a professional athlete because the patient with Alzheimer disease is walking for nearly 24 h every day. The total time spent active is important and exercise does not need to be undertaken in a single period. Patients need to think about ways of incorporating more physical activity in their everyday lives. This can be achieved in many ways:

- Use the stairs rather than lifts
- Alight the bus one stop early and walk
- Park at the far end of the supermarket car park rather than right next to the door.

Physical activity needs to fit in with daily life and the functional capabilities of the individual. Ideally, the activities should be pleasurable as the most appropriate type of exercise to undertake is the one that will still be pursued a decade later.

Drugs

Pharmacological treatment of obesity has a chequered history and many physicians still regard these drugs with suspicion and scepticism. Indeed, in the last few years two drugs used to treat obesity (rimonabant and sibutramine) have been with-

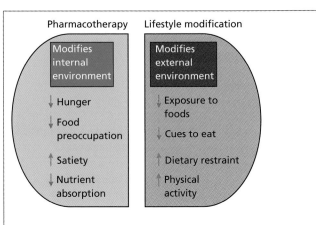

Figure 15.7 Additive effects of diet and drugs.

drawn. The only drug currently available is orlistat and, when used in combination with lifestyle and behavioural modification programmes, is a useful adjunct in the management of obesity (Figure 15.7).

Orlistat inhibits pancreatic and gastric lipases, thereby reducing hydrolysis of ingested triglyceride. It produces a dose-dependent reduction in dietary fat absorption that is near maximal at the currently available dose of 120 mg three times a day. In clinical trials lasting up to 4 years, it leads to modest weight loss of up to 10%. This weight loss is associated with a reduction in other cardiovascular risk factors, including waist circumference, blood pressure, dyslipidaemia and hyperglycaemia. In people with impaired glucose tolerance, it reduces the risk of incident diabetes by 37% over and above the effect of lifestyle intervention alone. In people with pre-existing diabetes, many are able to reduce or discontinue their oral hypoglycaemic medication.

The main limiting factor for the use of orlistat is the development of gastrointestinal side-effects secondary to fat malabsorption. These include loose or liquid stools, faecal urgency and anal discharge, and can be associated with fat-soluble vitamin deficiency and malabsorption. As the consumption of a high-fat diet will inevitably lead to severe gastrointestinal side-effects, it is important that the prescription of orlistat is accompanied by behavioural and dietary advice. In some people, orlistat can be highly effective, but it is salutary to note that only around 1% of those prescribed the drug are still taking it 2 years later.

Several other drugs have been considered for use in the management of obesity, including pseudoephedrine, ephedra, sertraline, yohimbine, amphetamine or its derivatives, bupropion, benzocaine, threachlorocitric acid and bromocriptine. There is currently a paucity of data about their effectiveness and they were not recommended in a recent Cochrane systematic database review.

Of the drugs that are currently being developed for the management of obesity, GLP-1 receptor agonists deserve a special mention (see Chapter 13). Trials of liraglutide at higher doses than are used to treat diabetes are on-going. The first short trial over 20 weeks demonstrated a mean 7.2-kg weight reduction in people receiving 3 mg of liraglutide compared with 2.8 kg with placebo and 4.1 kg with orlistat.

Bariatric surgery

Bariatric surgery is currently the only long-term cure for obesity. There are two main types of surgery; malabsorption techniques bypass part of the stomach and small intestine, while restrictive surgery leads to reduced dietary intake by reducing the size of the stomach and therefore improves satiety. Some operations utilize a combination of both. In some situations, apronectomy is also needed to remove redundant abdomen skin and this may contribute to further weight loss.

The best evidence for the long-term effects of bariatric surgery for obesity comes from the Swedish Obese Subjects Study in which the weight loss after 2 years was typically between 30 and 40 kg. After 10 years, the weight losses stabilized at 25% in those with bypass operations and 14–16% in those with restrictive operations.

Quality of life improves dramatically following surgery and this is associated with major improvements in the metabolic sequelae of obesity. Gastric bypass surgery is associated with a 99–100% pre-vention of diabetes in people with impaired glucose tolerance and a 50–80% clinical resolution of diagnosed early type 2 diabetes. The improvement in glycaemic control occurs shortly after surgery, before the weight loss, suggesting that mechanisms other than weight loss are involved. In the long term, obesity surgery decreases mortality. In the Swedish Obese Subjects Study, deaths were reduced by a quarter in those who had had surgery.

At present, obesity surgery is only recommended for those with morbid obesity (Case history 15.3). Each patient requires an extensive preoperative assessment, which includes a psychological assessment, as surgery will not treat an eating disorder and may lead to worsening of the mental state if patients are dependent on food.

Case history 15.3

A 49-year-old woman with a 10-year history of type 2 diabetes attends her GP surgery for her diabetes review. She has been treated with pre-mixed insulin with increasing doses for 2 years, currently 170 units three times a day. She is intolerant of metformin. She has reduced mobility because of markedly swollen legs as a result of venous insufficiency and two ulcers around her ankles. Her BMI is 48.7 kg/m^2. Her HbA$_{1c}$ is 13.4% (123 mmol/mol).

When the GP starts to discuss her weight, she becomes distressed and says that she has tried to lose weight all her life. She has spent lots of money on commercial weight programmes and has tried several medications in the past. She does not know what else she can try.

What treatment options are available?

Answer, see p. 359

New less invasive techniques are being developed as alternatives to surgery, including gastrointestinal barriers. Gastrointestinal barriers are impervious liners that prevent the duodenum and upper jejunum coming into contact with partly digested food, thereby mimicking the foregut bypass surgery without altering the patient's anatomy. Pancreatic and biliary secretions pass along the outside of the devices and then mix with partly digested food in the upper jejunum. These liners can be inserted by an endoscope and left *in situ* for 6 months. Trials of their effectiveness are currently on-going.

🔑 Key points

- The prevalence of obesity has increased dramatically over the last two decades and shows no sign of slowing
- Obesity is associated with significant morbidity and premature mortality
- Societal changes leading to a sedentary lifestyle and altered food consumption mean that there is a mismatch between energy intake and expenditure
- The management of the individual with obesity is challenging and should include lifestyle modification for all, pharmacotherapy for some and surgery for a few

🔍 Answers to case histories

Case history 15.1

It is important to take a full dietary and exercise history, although she has given you clues that she has unhealthy eating behaviours. Her expectations may be unrealistic if she wants to win 'slimmer of the year' and she needs to know what is achievable. It would be better for her to eat away from her desk at lunch – partly to increase her activity levels and partly because eating at her desk may become associated with feelings of relaxation. She is snacking on biscuits, which might be a coping behaviour for a stressful job. Lower calorie snacks could be suggested, but snacking should be discouraged if possible. Cravings do not last long and so it might be worth suggesting she gets up and does something else for a few minutes when she has the urge to eat. It is likely that eating by the television will increase her calorie intake and will lead to eating outside meal times. Encourage her to eat at a table where she can devote all her attention to the food. She has a sedentary job and should be encouraged to become more physically active.

Case history 15.2

People with schizophrenia have a two- to three-fold increased prevalence of obesity compared with the general population. The underlying cause is multi-factorial but it seems that clozapine, a second-generation antipsychotic, has contributed to his problem. This is important because weight gain can lead to discontinuation of the psychiatric treatment and possible psychiatric relapse. Treatment of the mental illness, however, is important if the man is to make lifestyle changes to reduce his weight.

It would have been better to institute weight management when the treatment was initiated. People who have long-term problems with antipsychotic weight gain usually experience some weight gain within the first 2–3 weeks of treatment. It is important to weigh people receiving antipsychotics weekly during the early phase of treatment to identify those who are developing weight gain.

Contrary to expectation, lifestyle modification programmes are possible in people with severe mental illness and are at least as successful as in the general population. Longer term support may be needed, but simple lifestyle messages can lead to significant weight loss or prevention of weight gain. Many patients have never received basic health education.

Where lifestyle modification is not possible, there is preliminary evidence to suggest that metformin is beneficial in reducing weight gain or promoting weight gain. It also has the additional benefit in reducing the risk of diabetes. The latter is important as this person is at increased risk of diabetes and is consuming a large quantity of sugary drinks.

Case history 15.3

This woman has morbid obesity and has tried all conventional means of losing weight. She is markedly insulin resistant. Despite large doses of insulin, she has poor glycaemic control. She also has

venous ulceration, again a result of her obesity.

Bariatric surgery would be an option for her. With a bypass operation she may lose 20–30% of her body weight. This will lead to improvements in her glycaemic control and she may be able to stop insulin. The strongest predictor of whether insulin can be stopped post surgery is the duration of diabetes. She needs to be aware that surgery will change her eating patterns for the rest of her life. It is important to exclude medical causes of obesity, such as Cushing syndrome, but these are unlikely given the duration of her obesity.

Another option that could be used instead of or prior to surgery is a GLP-1 receptor agonist as this may improve her glycaemic control and promote weight loss. The combination of GLP-1 receptor agonist and insulin is not licensed in some countries.

The weight loss will also improve her venous ulceration and facilitate healing of the ulcer.

Although surgery is expensive, when considered alongside the cost of daily dressings and insulin, it is likely that the operation would be cost-saving within a short period of time.

Index

Page numbers in bold refer to tables. Page numbers in italic refer to figures. Page numbers suffixed with 'b' refer to boxes.

acarbose *297*, 299b, 304
acetohexamide **298**
acetylation of DNA 17
acetyl CoA carboxylase 252, *254*
acid labile subunit 74
acidosis
    diabetic ketoacidosis 279, **280**
    parathyroid hormone 196
acromegaly 75, 77–80, **81**, 97, 201
ACTH *see* adrenocorticotrophic
        hormone
Addison disease 13, 108–11, 124,
        177, 231, 283
Addisonian crisis 111
adenosine-3',5'-cyclic
        monophosphate 37, *38*
adenylate cyclase 35, 37
adjustment disorder, diabetes in
        children 335
adrenal cortex **10**, 100–19
    ACTH on 87
    insufficiency 88, 108–11, 231
        pigmentation 88, 124
    tumours 116–18
adrenalectomy 114
    Conn syndrome 116
adrenal gland, incidentaloma 60–1,
        117, 125–6
adrenaline (epinephrine) **53**,
        119–22
adrenal medulla **10**, 119–23
adrenal vein sampling 116, 125
adrenarche 102b, 138
adrenocorticotrophic hormone
        (ACTH) **53**, 86–8, 102–5
    on aldosterone synthesis 107
    Cushing syndrome 113–14

stimulation test 231
    synthetic ACTH test 88, 110,
        124
adrenoreceptors 120
adult respiratory distress syndrome,
        diabetic ketoacidosis 282
advanced glycation end-products
        (AGEs) 314–15
    cardiovascular disease 331
    receptors 315
age
    GH and IGF-I secretion 75–6
    male sexuality 138
    osteoporosis 206
AGEs *see* advanced glycation
        end-products
Agouti-related protein 347
AIRE gene 212
Albright hereditary osteodystrophy
        40b, 199
albumin
    calcium and 191, 211–12
    see also microalbuminuria
aldose reductase inhibitors 315
aldosterone 101, 106–7, *108*
    excess (Conn syndrome) 115–16,
        125
    insufficiency, congenital adrenal
        hyperplasia 117–18
    reference ranges **53**
alendronate 207
alkalosis, respiratory 211
allergy, insulin 270
alopecia *see* male-pattern balding
α-cells 219, 244, *248*
α-melanocyte stimulating hormone
        347

α subunits *see* Gα protein subunits
Amadori reaction *246*
amenorrhoea 83, 151–7, 164
American Diabetes Association,
        classification of diabetes
        238–40
amino acids
    derivatives 8–9, 20–4
    growth hormone test **78**
amiodarone 182, 184b, 189
AMP kinase 300
amputations, diabetes 325
amylin analogues 308
anabolic actions
    growth hormone 74–6
    insulin 250, *251*
    insulin-like growth factor I 75
anabolic drugs
    osteoporosis 207–8
anaemia
    hypothyroidism 187
    metformin 300–1
analgesics, diabetic neuropathy
        324–5
anaplastic carcinoma of thyroid 186
androgens 134–6
    adrenal *see* sex steroid precursors
    deficiency 132
    hirsutism 157
    polycystic ovarian syndrome 154
androstenedione **53**
aneuploidy 56
angina, diabetes 333
angiotensins 107, *108*
    see also renin–angiotensin–
        aldosterone axis
antacids, hypercalcaemia 200

---

antenatal care, diabetes 337
antibiotics, diabetic foot 328
antidepressants, diabetic neuropathy 324
antidiabetes agents *see* oral antidiabetes agents
antidiuretic hormone *see* vasopressin
anti-inflammatory agents, glucocorticoids as 106
anti-Müllerian hormone **53**, 130
antipsychotics, obesity 358–9
antiresorptive drugs, osteoporosis 207
antithyroid drugs 171b, 180, 188, 189
    fetus 181
aorta, Turner syndrome **154**
apparent mineralocorticoid excess 41
appetite control 347–50
arachidonic acid *43*
arginine vasopressin *see* vasopressin
aromatase inhibitors 229
array comparative genomic hybridization 57
arteries to thyroid 168
aspirin 333
atheroma, diabetes 331–2
ATP-sensitive K⁺ channel 218
atrial natriuretic peptide 38
autocrine cells *4*
autoimmune diseases 124, 175b, 231
    type 1 diabetes 258, 259–60
autoimmune polyendocrine syndrome type 1 198, 211
autoimmune thyroiditis 175
    see also Graves disease
autonomic neuropathy, diabetes 325, 326
autonomic symptoms, hypoglycaemia 276

baldness, male-pattern 157, 163–4
bariatric surgery 357–8, 359
    diabetes prevention 293
Beckwith–Wiedemann syndrome 20b

β-blockers, hyperthyroidism 181, 188
β-cells 244, *248*
    type 2 diabetes 290–2
bicarbonate, diabetic ketoacidosis **280**, 281, 282
big IGF-II 217
biguanides *297*, 300–1
binding proteins 24
biphasic release of insulin 244, *249*, 290, *291*
birth weight, diabetes 288
bisphosphonates 202, 207
blindness, diabetic retinopathy 321
blood pressure
    aldosterone on 107
    control, diabetes 322, 333
    cortisol action 106
blood specimens 49
    hypercalcaemia 202
    hypoglycaemia 217
blood supply
    islets of Langerhans *248*
    thyroid 168
body mass index 344
    diabetes 288, *289*
    limitations 345–6
bone 202–10
    cortisol action 106
    diabetic foot 328, 329
    growth hormone excess 77–8
    insulin-like growth factor I 75
    parathyroid hormone on 196–7
bone mineral density 205–6, 207
bread, calcium 192
breast
    cancer 229–30
        prolactin and 86
    oxytocin on 96
    pregnancy 151
    thelarche 151
breast-feeding, diabetes 338
bromocriptine 86, 308
bruit, Graves disease 188

cabergoline 86
calcification, ectopic 201

calcitonin **195**, 197, 207
calcitriol *see* 1, 25-dihydroxyvitamin D
calcium 191–203
    albumin and 191, 211–12
    exocytosis and 20
    negative feedback on vitamin D 193, *195*
    parathyroid hormone and 196
    screening 226
    in second messenger pathways 37–8, *42*
calcium-sensing receptor (CaSR) 196
    activation 203
    inactivation 200
calibration ofimmunoassays 49
cAMP (cyclic adenosine monophosphate) 37, *38*
cAMP response element binding protein (CREB) 37
cancer *see* malignant disease; neoplasia syndromes; *specific organs and tissues*
candidiasis, autoimmune polyendocrine syndrome type 1 211
cannabinoid-1 receptors 349
capillary blood glucose monitoring 272–3
carbimazole 188, 189
    fetus 181
carbohydrates
    counting 271–2
    digestion 304
carbon dioxide tension, vasopressin action 92
carcinoid syndrome 221–3
carcinoid tumours 221–2, 232
cardiac failure, acromegaly 78
cardiomyocytes, K⁺ channels 299
cardiovascular complications
    diabetes *313*, 330–4, 341–2
        glucose levels 243
        glycated haemoglobin *vs 245*
        mortality 264
        nephropathy 321
        sulphonylureas 299

Carney complex 227
carpal tunnel syndrome 324
cascades of enzymes 20–2
CaSR *see* calcium-sensing receptor
casts (plaster) 327
catabolism 106
catecholamines 119–22, 126
   sample collection 49b
   thyroid hormones and 173
catheterization (urinary), diabetic
     ketoacidosis 281
cavernous sinus, cranial nerves **71**
CBG (cortisol-binding globulin)
   101–2, 112
C-cells 167
   hyperplasia 226
cell-surface receptors 28–31
cellulitis, Charcot arthropathy and
   329
central obesity 346
cerebral oedema, diabetic
     ketoacidosis 282
Charcot arthropathy 328–9
chemicals, diabetes triggers 262b
chemotherapy, testicular tumours
   141
children, diabetes 258–9
   adjustment disorder 335
   ketoacidosis 280
chlorpropamide **298**
   hyponatraemia 299
cholecalciferol (vitamin D$_3$) 192–3,
   210
cholecystokinin **216**, 221
cholesterol
   hormones from 23, 103
   reduction of levels 333
   synthesis *24*, 252
   vitamin D synthesis from 192–3,
     194
chromaffin cells 119, *120*
chromogranin(s) 119
chromogranin A **53**
chromosomes 15, *16*
   abnormalities 20b
   G-banding 56
   karyotypes 56
   sex determination 128–30

cinacalcet 203
circadian rhythm 13b, 73, 104, 110
   see also diurnal variation
clozapine 358
codons 18
co-enzyme A 23
cognitive impairment
   diabetes 335
   hypoglycaemia 276
collagen 204b
colloid, thyroid 168, 171
colorectal carcinoma, growth
     hormone excess 80
competitive-binding assays 51
complete gonadal dysgenesis 130,
   131, 132
computed tomography 59–60
congenital adrenal hyperplasia 13,
   117–18, *119*, 126, 133,
   162–3
congenital hyperinsulinism 218
congenital malformations
   maternal diabetes 336–7
   see also teratogenesis
Conn syndrome 115–16, 125
continuous subcutaneous insulin
     infusion 269, *270*
contrast media (radiographic),
     thyroid inhibition by 175
control mechanisms 9–13
co-repressors, thyroid hormone
     receptors and 41
coronary arteries, surgery 333–4
corpus luteum 143–4
corticotrophin-releasing hormone
   87, 102–5
cortisol **53**, 101–6
   excess (Cushing syndrome) 88,
     111–15, 124–5
   fetus 106, 150–1
   growth hormone release 77
   target cell conversion 41
cortisol-binding globulin (CBG)
   101–2, 112
cortisone 105
Cortrosyn 110
C-peptide 214–17, 244, *247*
   hypoglycaemia 217

cranial diabetes insipidus 94, **95**
cranial nerves, cavernous sinus **71**
craniopharyngioma 70, 140
cravings for food 355
creatinine, estimated GFR 322b
CREB (cAMP response element
     binding protein) 37
cretinism 170b
crystalloids 281
Cushing disease 88, 114
Cushing syndrome 88, 111–15,
   124–5
cycles *see* rhythms
cyclic adenosine monophosphate
   (cAMP) 37, *38*
cyclo-oxygenases *43*
CYP21A2, congenital adrenal
     hyperplasia 117, 118
cyproterone acetate 229
cytochrome P450 enzymes 23–4
   congenital adrenal hyperplasia
     117
   steroidogenesis 103, **104**
   see also 1α-hydroxylase
cytokine receptors 34
cytosolic guanylate cyclase 38

DAX1 gene 15, 42
DCCT-aligned HbA$_{1c}$ 273
dehydration, diabetes 263
   ketoacidosis 278, 281
dehydroepiandrosterone (DHEA)
   101, 107
   fetus 150, *151*
   polycystic ovarian syndrome
     154
δ-cells 219, 244, *248*
depression, diabetes 334–5
De Quervain's subacute thyroiditis
   176
desmopressin 94, **95**
DEXA (dual energy X-ray
     absorptiometry) 201–2,
   205–6, 207
dexamethasone 151
   suppression tests 113, 114, 232
DHEA *see* dehydroepiandrosterone
diabetes insipidus 93–4, **95**, 97–8

diabetes mellitus
 aetiology
  type 1 260–3
  type 2 287
 bariatric surgery 357, 359
 care strategy 335–6
  pregnancy 337–8
 classification 236, 238–41, **265**
 complications 311–42
  cancer 334
  epidemiology *313*
  psychological 334–5
  see also cardiovascular
   complications; ketoacidosis;
   microvascular complications
 diagnosis 241–3, *244*, 256, 264,
  265
 environmental factors 262–3,
  288–9
 epidemiology 236–7, **238, 239,**
  255
  type 1 258–9
  type 2 286–7
 historical aspects 5, 238,
  239–40b
 ketoacidosis 263, 277–82, 284
  pregnancy 337
 management
  type 1 264–74
  type 2 296–308
 neonates 218, 246
 obesity 288, *289*, 309, 344–5
 orlistat 356
 pathogenesis
  type 1 259–60
  type 2 289–92
 pregnancy 150, 336–9
  gestational diabetes 309, 338,
   339
  screening for retinopathy
   318–20
 prevention 293–4, 295b
 prognosis
  type 1 263–4
  type 2 292
 screening *see under* screening
 social aspects 339–40
 type 1 257–84

 type 2 285–310
 undiagnosed 292, *293*
 see also maturity-onset diabetes of
  the young
diacylglycerol 37–40, *42*
DIDMOAD syndrome **95**
diet
 calcium intake 192
 diabetes 271–2, 293–4, 295b,
  296
 for obesity 354–6
 trends 350–1
 vitamin D 192
 on zona glomerulosa 107
DiGeorge syndrome 56, 198
5α-dihydrotestosterone 130
1,25-dihydroxyvitamin D (calcitriol)
  193,
  194
 for hypocalcaemia 199
24,25-dihydroxyvitamin D 193
dipeptidyl peptidase 4 (DPP-4),
  inhibitors 221, *297*, 299b,
  304, **307**
diplopia, pituitary tumours and 69
distal symmetrical neuropathy 324
diurnal variation
 insulin secretion *266*
 loss in Cushing syndrome 113
 testosterone 136
 see also circadian rhythm
DNA 15, 17, 20b
DNA repair genes 224b
dopamine agonists 80
 for prolactinomas 85
dopamine receptor antagonists, on
  prolactin 85
DPP-4 *see* dipeptidyl peptidase 4
drinks, obesity and 351
driving, diabetes 339–40
dual energy X-ray absorptiometry
  (DEXA) 201–2, 205–6,
  207
duloxetine, diabetic neuropathy 324
duodenum, hormones **11**
duplication of chromosomes 15
dynamic testing 52, 56b
 hypoadrenalism 110

eating behaviour 349, 350–1, 352,
  355, 358
ectopic ACTH secretion 114, 232
ectopic calcification 201
ectopic hormone syndromes
  227–8
education, diabetes 270–1
eflornithine 158
eicosanoids 38–40, *43*
embryogenesis 143
embryology
 adrenal cortex 100, *101*
 adrenal medulla 119
 parathyroid glands 196
 pituitary 66–7
 reproductive organs 128–34
 thyroid 166–8
embryonal carcinoma 141b
emergencies
 diabetes 274–82
 hypercalcaemia 202
 hyperosmolar hyperglycaemic
  state 293
employment, diabetes and 340
endocannabinoids 349
Endocrine Postulates (Doisy) 9b
endocrine system 4
endometriosis 158
endometrium
 cancer 230
 menstrual cycle 145–7
endopeptidases 20
energy balance 347
enteroendocrine cells 220
enzymes 20–2
 assays 52
 mineralocorticoid receptors and
  106–7
 steroidogenesis *103*, **104**
epidermal growth factor receptor
  blockers 229–30
epigenetics 17, 20b
epinephrine **53**, 119–22
eplerenone 116
ε-cells 244
erectile dysfunction, diabetes *313*,
  329–30, 341
ergocalciferol (vitamin D₂) 192–3

erythropoietin receptors (EPO receptors) 34
estimated glomerular filtration rate 322b
ethnicity
    diabetes 287
    obesity 346
exenatide 304–5
exercise
    diabetes 272, 288, 293–4, 295b, 296–7
    obesity and 351–2, 356
exocytosis 20
exophthalmos (proptosis) 181–2, *183*
extracellular domains, cell-surface receptors *29*
ezetimibe 333

falls 207
familial benign hypercalcaemia 200–1, 212
familial endocrine neoplasia 223–7
familial isolated hyperparathyroidism 226
familial male precocious puberty *39*
familial phaeochromocytoma syndromes 227
familial risk of diabetes 262, 287–8
fast-food outlets 350, 351
fasting
    glucose levels
        diabetes diagnosis 241, *244*, 294
        regulation *251*
        see also impaired fasting glycaemia
    growth hormone regulation 77
    insulin secretion 244
    sample collection and 49b
fat (dietary) 351
fatty acids
    insulin on metabolism 252, **253**
    non-esterified 278–9
    Randle cycle 303b
    release, catecholamines 120–1
    see also free fatty acids

feedback see negative feedback; positive feedback
feminization, adrenocortical 116
femoral amyotrophy 324
fertility
    management 153
        polycystic ovarian syndrome 157
    sub-fertility 159–62, 164
fertilization 148
fetus
    adrenal androgens 107
    antithyroid drugs 181
    cortisol 106, 150–1
    hyperthyroidism 181
    iodine deficiency 170b
    maternal diabetes 336–7
    steroid hormone synthesis 150, *151*
FFA see free fatty acids
fibroids 158
finasteride 229
fine-needle aspiration cytology, thyroid nodules 185
flozins 308
fludrocortisone 110
fluid retention, thiazolidinediones 302
fluid therapy, diabetic ketoacidosis **280**, 281
fluorescence *in situ* hybridization 56–7
follicles
    ovary 142–3
    thyroid 167, 168
follicle-stimulating hormone 89–90
    hypogonadism 139–40
    menopause 149
    molecule 8
    on ovary 144, 145, *146*
    reference ranges **53**
    synthesis *21*
    testis regulation 136–7, 138
follicular carcinoma of thyroid 186
follicular phase of menstrual cycle **149**
food trends 350, 351, 355

foot ulcers, diabetes *313*, 325–9, 341
fractures 212
    osteoporosis 206
free fatty acids (FFA)
    cortisol on metabolism 105
    growth hormone and 77
fructosamine 273–4

galactorrhoea 158, 163
Gα protein subunits 36, 38b, **39**
gas chromatography 52
gastrin **53**, **215**, 220
gastrinomas 219b, 220, 231
gastrointestinal barriers 358
gastrointestinal hormone-secreting tumours 219b
gastrointestinal tract 220–3
    acarbose 304
    appetite control 347–8
    metformin on 300
G-banding of chromosomes 56
G-cells 220
gender differences, obesity 345, 346
genes 15
    diabetes 261, 288, **289**
    obesity 347, 349–50
    sequencing 57
    transcription 16–17
    translation 18
    tumours and 223–4, *225*
genome-wide microarray technology 57
genomic imprinting 17
genomics 57
genotypes 57
germ cells
    embryology 130
    oogenesis 142
germ cell tumours of testis 141
germline mutations, catecholamine-secreting tumours 122–3
gestational age 147
gestational diabetes 309, 338, **339**
ghrelin 77, **215**, 220, 347–8
gigantism 77–80
glibenclamide **298**
gliclazide **298**

glimepiride **298**

glipizide **298**

gliquidone **298**

glitazones (thiazolidinediones) *297*, 299b, 301–3, **307**

glomerular filtration rate, estimated 322b

glucagon **215**, 219, 254
  for hypoglycaemia 276–7
  reference ranges **53**

glucagon-like peptide 1 (GLP-1) **216**, 221
  receptor agonists 304–5, **307**, 357, 359

glucagonomas 219

glucocorticoids
  growth hormone release 77
  therapeutic uses 106, 118–19
  see also cortisol

gluconeogenesis 252

glucose
  cortisol on metabolism 105
  diabetes
    diagnosis 241–3, *244*
    effect of exercise 272b
    ketoacidosis management 281
    monitoring 272–3, 283
    screening 294, **295**
  digestion 303–4
  GH and IGF-I on homeostasis 74
  insulin on metabolism 250–2, *253*
  insulin stimulation 244–6
  reference ranges **53–4**
  release, catecholamines 120
  renal threshold 263
  tolerance test *see* oral glucose tolerance test
  see also hyperglycaemia

glucose-dependent insulinotropic peptide **216**, 221

glucose transporters (GLUT) 31, 251–2

glucosidase inhibitors *297*

glutathione, reduced 315

glycated haemoglobin (HbA$_{1c}$) 315b
  Amadori reaction *246*

diabetes complications *245*, 331, *332*

diabetes control 273

diabetes diagnosis 243

diabetic retinopathy 321
  limitations 274b
  reference ranges **54**
  screening 294–5
  target levels 296

glycogen, metabolism 252

glycolysis 252

goitre *170*, 175
  Graves disease *176*
  multinodular 184–5, 189

goitrogens 170

gonadotrophin-releasing hormone (GnRH) 89, 137
  analogues 229
  test 140, 153
  treatment with 73

gonadotrophins 89–90, 136–7, 138
  amenorrhoea 153
  molecules 8
  pulsatility 148
  see also follicle-stimulating hormone; luteinizing hormone

gonads
  complete dysgenesis 130, 131, 132
  embryology 128–30

G-protein–coupled receptors 30, 34–40

G-proteins 35
  subunits 35
  see also Gα protein subunits

Gqα subunit 37–8

Graafian follicles 143

granules (secretory) 20

Graves disease 178–82
  goitre *176*

Graves orbitopathy 181–2, *183*, 188–9

growth
  cortisol action 106
  insufficiency *82*

growth factor receptor-bound protein type 2 (Grb2 protein) 31

growth hormone 73–83
  deficiency 80–3
    hypoglycaemia 217
  excess (acromegaly) 75, 77–80, **81**, 97, 201
  immunoassay 49–50
  reference ranges **54**
  regulation 76–7
  replacement therapy 82–3
  resistance syndromes 37
  signal transduction 34, *35*, 76

growth hormone–IGF-1 axis 76
  diabetic complications 316

growth hormone-releasing hormone (GHRH) 76

guanylate cyclase, cytosolic 38

guar gum 303

guidelines, diabetes type 2 management 306

gynaecomastia 142

haemodynamic theory, diabetic complications 316

half-life of growth hormone 76

Hashimoto thyroiditis 175

hCG *see* human chorionic gonadotrophin

headache, pituitary tumours 70

heart
  Turner syndrome **154**
  cabergoline 86
  carcinoid syndrome 223b
  see also cardiovascular complications

heart failure, acromegaly 78

heat-shock proteins, steroid hormone receptors and 41

hemianopia 68, 96

hepatocyte nuclear family, transcription factors 43

HER2 antagonists 229–30

hermaphroditism 130–4

heterozygosity 57

hexosamine pathway 316

high-dose dexamethasone
  suppression test **113**, 114
hirsutism 157–8
  polycystic ovarian syndrome
    155
historical aspects 4–5, 6b, **7–8**
  diabetes 5, 238, 239–40b
  insulin *267*
HLA haplotypes, diabetes 261
HMGCoA reductase inhibitors 23,
  333
home testing, Cushing syndrome
  113
HONK *see* hyperosmolar
  hyperglycaemic state
hormone(s) 5–6
  historical aspects 4–5
hormone replacement therapy 153,
  158, 207
hormone response elements
  steroid hormone receptors 41
hormone-secreting tumours
  gastrointestinal 219b
hormone-sensitive lipase *278*
hormone-sensitive tumours
  228–30
human chorionic gonadotrophin
  (hCG) 141, 145, 149–50
  delayed puberty and 159
  molecule 8
  synthesis *21*
  as tumour marker 230
human leukocyte antigens (HLA)
  262b
  haplotypes, diabetes 261
human menopausal gonadotrophins
  141
hydrocortisone 110, 114, 124, 231
hydroxyapatite 203
5-hydroxyindoleacetic acid 222
1α-hydroxylase 193–5
  magnesium deficiency on 198
24-hydroxylase 193
hydroxymethylglutaryl co-enzyme A
  23
hydroxymethylglutaryl co-enzyme A
  reductase inhibitors 23, 333
17-hydroxyprogesterone **53**

11β-hydroxysteroid dehydrogenase
  105
  type 2 41
25-hydroxyvitamin D 193
hygiene hypothesis 263
hyperadrenalism 111–19
hypercalcaemia 200–3, 211–12
hyperemesis gravidarum,
    hyperthyroidism
  178
hyperglycaemia 278
  cardiovascular complications 331,
    332
  microvascular complications
    313b, 314–16
  neuropathy 324
  teratogenesis 336–7
  see also hyperosmolar
    hyperglycaemic state
hyperinsulinism, congenital 218
hyperkalaemia
  diabetic ketoacidosis 279
  neonates 118
hyperosmolar hyperglycaemic state
  293
hyperparathyroidism 200, 201–3,
  210
  familial isolated 226
  MEN-1 224
  screening 226
hyperprolactinaemia 83–6, 97
hypertension
  Conn syndrome 115
  diabetes 313b, 316, 341
    nephropathy 322
  phaeochromocytoma 122
hyperthyroidism 178–85, 188
  thyroid function tests 174
  treated thyroid nodules 185
hypertriglyceridaemia, diabetes
  331–2
hyperventilation 211
hypoadrenalism 108–11, 231
  secondary 111
hypocalcaemia 198–9, 211
hypoglycaemia 217–18, 231,
  274–7, 283–4
  antenatal care 337

driving and 339–40
sulphonylureas 217, 298
hypogonadism
  female 153
  male 138–41, 163
  secondary 90
hypogonadotrophic hypogonadism
  90
hypokalaemia
  causes 116b
  Conn syndrome 115
hyponatraemia 93, 108–9
  chlorpropamide 299
hypoparathyroidism 198, 199, 211
hypophosphataemic rickets 210
hypophyseal portal vessels *68*
hypopituitarism 90–1
hypoprolactinaemia 86
hypospadias 132
hypothalamic–anterior pituitary
    hormone axes 72–3
  adrenal cortex 102–5
  ovary 144, *147*
  testis 136–7
hypothalamus 66, 67, *68*, 70–2
  amenorrhoea 153
  growth hormone regulation 76–7
  hormones **10**, 72
  nuclei **69**
  weight regulation 347
hypothyroidism 175–8, 187–8
  cretinism 170b
  hypothalamic–anterior pituitary
    hormone axis 72–3
  iodide deficiency 170
  Pendred syndrome 171
  pituitary 174
  secondary 178
  thyroid function tests 174, 177–8
hypovolaemia, diabetes 263

IGF-I *see* insulin-like growth factor I
IGF-binding proteins 74
immunoassays 49–51
impaired fasting glycaemia 241, 243
impaired glucose tolerance 241, 243
incidentalomas, adrenal 60–1, 117,
  125–6

incretins 221
    antidiabetes agents and 304–6
infections, diabetes 262b
    foot 327–8, 341
    ketoacidosis 277
inferior petrosal sinus sampling 114
infertility (sub-fertility) 159–62,
    164
inflammation, cortisol action 106
infradian rhythm 13b
inhibin 137, 139–40
inhibition 11, 12
injections of insulin 268–70
    after diabetic ketoacidosis 282
inositol triphosphate (IP₃) 37–8
insulin 214–19, 243–54
    action 246–54
    analogues 267, 282
    diabetes management 265–70,
        283
        type 2 diabetes 307, 309–10
    diabetic ketoacidosis **280**
        management 281–2
    effects of GH and IGF-I 74
    fetus 150
    formulations 266–7
    molecule 8, *11*
    reference ranges **54**
    resistance
        cortisol promoting 105, 106b
        diabetes 289–90, 291b
        polycystic ovarian syndrome
            155
        pregnancy 337
        syndromes 34b
    responsiveness 290b
    secretagogues 297
    secretion 244–6, *247, 249,* **249**
        type 2 diabetes 290, *291, 292*
    sensitivity 290b
    sensitizers 300–1
    signal transduction 31–3, 34b,
        248, *250,* 291b
    synthesis *21,* 214–17, 244, *247*
    tolerance test **78,** 88
insulin-like 3 130
insulin-like growth factor I (IGF-I)
        34, 35b, 74

anabolic actions 75
    diabetic complications 316
    gene defects 37b
    reference ranges **54**
    signal transduction 76
insulin-like growth factor-II,
        alternative 217
insulinomas 217–18, 219b
insulin promoter factor 1 43
insulin receptor 31, 248, 291b
insulin responsive substrates 248
insulin zinc suspensions 267
intermediate metabolism, insulin on
        249–54
internal carotid artery, pituitary
        tumours enveloping 69
intersex 131–3
intrinsic TK receptors 31
in vitro fertilization 164
iodide
    deficiency 170
    thyroid inhibition 175
    uptake 168, *169*
iodination of thyroglobulin 170
iodine-131 180–1
islets of Langerhans **10,** 214–20,
        244, *248*
IVF (*in vitro* fertilization) 164

Janus kinase family 34, *36*
jejunum, hormones **11**
juxtaglomerular apparatus 107, *109*

Kallman syndrome 90, 139
karyotypes 56
K-cells 221
ketoacidosis 263, 277–82, 284
    pregnancy 337
ketone bodies 278–9
    monitoring 281
kidney
    aldosterone on 107
    cortisol action 106
    nephrons *109*
    proximity to adrenal 100
    vasopressin action 92
Klinefelter syndrome 15, 133,
        163

lactation 151
    cortisol action 106
    prolactin 83
lactic acidosis 301
Laron syndrome 37
laser photocoagulation, diabetic
        retinopathy 321
late-onset male hypogonadism 138
L-cells 221
leprechaunism 34b
leptin 348–9
Leydig cell tumours 141
life-expectancy, diabetes 264
lipids
    cortisol on 105
    diabetes 331–2, 341–2
    growth hormone and FFA
        on 77
    insulin on metabolism 252, **253**
    pioglitazone on 302
lipoatrophy 270
lipohypertrophy 270
lipolysis, diabetic ketoacidosis 278
liquid chromatography 52
liraglutide 305, 357
lithium 175
liver
    hormone **11**
    insulin on 250
    thiazolidinediones 302–3
loss of heterozygosity 57
low-dose dexamethasone suppression
        test 113
low-fat diets 355
lung
    cancer 232
    cortisol on development 106,
        150–1
luteal phase of menstrual cycle 145,
        149
luteinizing hormone 89–90
    hypogonadism 139, 140
    menopause 146
    molecule 8
    on ovary 144, 145, *147*
    reference ranges **54**
    synthesis *21*
    on testis 136–7, 138

macroadenomas, pituitary 67
macrocytosis 124
macroprolactin 84
macrosomia 336
macrovascular complications *see*
      cardiovascular complications
magnesium deficiency 198
magnetic resonance imaging 59–60
malabsorption, orlistat 356
male-pattern balding 157, 163–4
malignant disease
      diabetes 334
      hypercalcaemia 200, 201b
      see also neoplasia syndromes;
            specific organs and tissues
malnutrition-related diabetes 240
MAPK pathway *33, 36*
mass spectrometry 51–2
maternal diabetes 288, 336–7
maternal history, diabetes 288
maturity-onset diabetes of the young
      256
      mutations 43, 240, **241**, 246
      type 1 diabetes *vs* 264
McCune–Albright syndrome *40,*
      227
medullary thyroid carcinoma 57,
      186, 226
      familial 227
meglitinides 297, 300
meiosis 15, *16, 17*
melanocortin receptors 87, 347
melatonin 73
MEN-1 (multiple endocrine
      neoplasia) 224–6
MEN-2 (multiple endocrine
      neoplasia) **225**, 226, 232
menopause 146
      gonadotrophins 89
      hormone replacement therapy
            158
      osteoporosis 206
menstrual cycle 142, 144–5, **149**
      sub-fertility 161
mesonephric ducts 130
metabolic acidosis
      diabetic ketoacidosis 279, **280**
      parathyroid hormone 196

metabolic syndrome 332, 333b
metabolism, effects of GH and
      IGF-I 74–6
metacarpals,
            pseudohypoparathyroidism
            198
meta-iodobenzylguanidine,
      radiolabelled 61
metanephrine
      reference ranges **54**
      screening 226
metastases
      adrenal cortex 116
      carcinoid tumours 232
      endometrial cancer 230
metformin 299b, 300–1, 306
      cardiovascular complications and
            331
      insulin with 307
methylation of DNA 17, 20b
microadenomas, pituitary 67
microalbuminuria 321–2
microarray technology 57
microheterogeneity 52
microvascular complications of
            diabetes 312–30
      clinical features 317–30
      glucose levels and 243
      glycated haemoglobin *vs 245*
      pathogenesis 312–17
midwifery, diabetes 338
milk, goitrogens 170
mineralocorticoid receptors 106–7
      cortisol inactivation 41
mineralocorticoids
      Conn syndrome 115–16, 125
      see also aldosterone
mitogen-activated protein kinase
            pathway *33, 36*
mitosis 15, *16*
mitotane 117
mixed insulin 268
monofilaments, sensory testing 327
monogenic disorders 259
      obesity 349–50
      renal tubules 116b
mononeuropathies, diabetes 324
morning sample collection 49b

mortality
      body mass index 344
      diabetes 237, 263–4
mosaicism 56
motilin **216**, 221
mRNA 17, 18
      insulin on 252
Müllerian ducts 130
multinodular goitre 184–5, 189
multiple endocrine neoplasia
            syndromes 122–3, 200,
            224–7, 232
muscle, cortisol action 105–6
mutations 18, 20b
      catecholamine-secreting tumours
            122–3
      diabetes 240, **241**
      diagnosis 57
      see also specific genes
myocardial infarction, diabetes
            330–1, 333, 342
myxoedema coma 177b

nateglinide 300
National Institute of Health
            and Clinical Excellence,
            diabetes type 2 management
            306
necrolytic migratory erythema 219
needles, insulin injection 268–9
negative feedback 11, *12,* 72–3, *74*
      calcium on vitamin D 193, *195*
      parathyroid hormone 196
      testosterone 137
negative pressure wound therapy
            329b
Nelson syndrome 88
neonate
      congenital adrenal hyperplasia
            118, *119*
      diabetes 218, 246
      hypocalcaemia 198
      hypoglycaemia 218
      sexual development 138
neoplasia syndromes 223b
      carcinoid syndrome 221–3
      familial endocrine neoplasia
            223–7

multiple endocrine neoplasia
syndromes 122–3, 200,
224–7, 232
nephrogenic diabetes insipidus 94,
95
nephrologists, referral for diabetic
nephropathy 322
nephrons *109*
nephropathy, diabetic *313*,
321–3
neural crest 119
neuroendocrine cells *4*
neurofibromatosis type 1 227
neurogenin-3 214
neuroglycopaenic symptoms 276
neurohypophysis *see* pituitary,
posterior
neuropathy, diabetes 323–5
foot ulcers 326, 327
neuropeptide Y 347
neutrophils, glucocorticoids and
106
nicotinamide adenine dinucleotide
phosphate 252
nitrates, phosphodiesterase type 5
inhibitors and 330
Nobel prize winners **7–8**
nodules, thyroid 184–5
non-esterified fatty acids 278–9
non-functioning adenomas, pituitary
67–70, 88, 90
norepinephrine 119–22
reference ranges **54**
normetanephrine
reference ranges **54**
screening 226
nuclear medicine 60–1
hyperthyroidism 180
nuclear receptors 40–2, *44*, *45*, *46*
thiazolidinediones on 301, *302*
nucleosides 15b
nucleotides 15b

obesity 343–59
cortisol promoting 105
diabetes 288, *289*, 309,
344–5
environmental factors 350–2

prohormone convertase 1/3
deficiency 87
trends 346–7
obstructive sleep apnoea 309
octreotide 221
oedema, growth hormone 76
oestradiol 144, 145
reference ranges **54–5**
from testosterone 136
oestrogen receptors, breast cancer
229
oestrogens 144–146, *146*, **149**
feto-placental unit 150, *151*
on growth hormone release 77
menopause 146
replacement therapy 153
oncogenes *225*
see also proto-oncogenes
oogenesis 142
ophthalmologists, referral for
diabetic retinopathy 320
ophthalmopathy (Graves) 181–2,
183, 188–9
ophthalmoplegia 68
opiates, diabetic neuropathy
324–5
optic chiasm compression 67, 70,
71
oral antidiabetes agents 297–308
pregnancy 338
oral glucose tolerance test (OGTT)
241, 242, 243b
growth hormone status 77, **78**
orlistat 356–7
orphan nuclear receptors 40, 41–2
osmolality, vasopressin action 92
osmotic effects, diabetes 263,
340–1
osteoblasts 204
parathyroid hormone on 196–7
osteoclasts 204
osteodystrophy, renal 200
osteoid 203
osteomalacia 208, 210
osteomyelitis, diabetic foot 328
osteopaenia 207
osteoporosis 205–8, 212
ovarian reserve 146

ovary 142–6
cancer 230
embryology 128–30
hirsutism 157
hormones **11**
premature failure 153
see also polycystic ovarian
syndrome
ovulation 142–3, 144–5
induction 162
oxygen tension, vasopressin action
92
oxytocin 94–6
molecule 8

pain,
diabetic neuropathy 324–5
retro-orbital 188–9
pancreas **10**, 214–20
pancreas duodenal homeobox factor
1 43
pancreatic polypeptide **215**, 220
reference ranges **55**
pancreatitis, exenatide 305
papillary cell cancer of thyroid
185–6
paracrine cells *4*
paraesthesia 211
paragangliomas 121, 122, **123**,
227
parathyroid glands 166, 196
insufficiency 198, 199, 210
selective excision 202
venous sampling 202
see also hyperparathyroidism
parathyroid hormone **195**, 196–7
hypercalcaemia 202
reference ranges **55**
resistance syndromes 198–9
venous sampling 202
see also teriparatide
parathyroid hormone-related peptide
197
parturition 151
diabetes 338
pathognomonic (term) 265b
PCSK1 (prohormone convertase
1/3) 87, 221, 244

pegvisomant *35*, 80
pelvic inflammatory disease 164
pen devices, insulin 268–9, *270*
Pendred syndrome 171
peptide hormones 8
  sample collection 49b
  storage and secretion 20
  synthesis 19–20
perchlorate 168
performance-enhancing drugs,
     hypogonadism 139
perinatal factors, diabetes 262b
periodicity *see* rhythms
peripheral neuropathy 324
peripheral vascular disease, diabetic
     foot 326
pernicious anaemia 175b
peroxisome proliferator-activated
     receptor gamma 301, *302*
pertechnetate, technetium isotope
     168
phaeochromocytoma 121–3, 126,
     232
  familial syndromes 227
  MEN-2, screening 226
  nuclear medicine 61
phenotypes 57
phenoxybenzamine 122
phenylethanolamine *N*-methyl
     transferase 119
PHEX gene 192
phosphate 192
  parathyroid hormone on 197
  on vitamin D synthesis *195*
phosphatidylinositol (PI) *35, 38, 42*
phosphatidylinositol-3-kinase 31
phosphodiesterases 37
phosphodiesterase type 5 inhibitors
     330
phospholipase C 35, *42*
phosphorylation of proteins, signal
     transduction 30, 31–3
physical activity *see* exercise
phytic acid 192
PI3 kinase pathway *33, 36*
pigmentation, adrenocortical
     insufficiency 88, 124
pioglitazone 301

PIT1 mutations 43
pituitary 66–7, *68*
  ablation for retinopathy 317
  anterior 66–7
    amenorrhoea 153
    cell types **73**
    hormones **10**, 73–91
    see also hypothalamic–anterior
      pituitary hormone axes
  hypothyroidism 174
  infarction 91
  insufficiency 90–1
  magnetic resonance imaging *60*
  posterior 66–7
    hormones **10**, 91–6
  tumours 67–70, 96–7
    acromegaly 78
    Cushing disease 88
    hyperprolactinaemia 85
    non-functioning adenomas
      67–70, 88, 90
    radiotherapy 70, 71
    TSHomas 89
    visual field defects 67–8, *71*,
      96
    see also Cushing disease
pituitary-specific transcription factor
     1 43
placenta, steroid hormone synthesis
     150, *151*
placental lactogen 151
poly-A tail 17
polycystic ovarian syndrome
     (PCOS) 154–7, 163
  sub-fertility 161–2
polycythaemia, testosterone
     replacement therapy 140–1
polydipsia 94, **95**, 98
polymerase chain reaction 57, *58*
polyol pathway *314*, 315
POMC *see* pro-opiomelanocortin
portal vein (hepatic), insulin 250
portal vessels (hypophyseal) *68*
portion sizes, food 351, 355
positive feedback 12, *74*
  oxytocin 96
  prolactin 83
postnatal care, diabetes 338

post-prandial regulators
     (meglitinides) 297–8, 300
post-translational modification of
     peptides 19–20, *21*
potassium, diabetic ketoacidosis
     279, **280**, 281
potassium channels
  ATP-sensitive 218
  cardiomyocytes 299
  inward rectifying channel type 6.2
    246, 298
PPAR-γ (peroxisome proliferator-
     activated receptor gamma)
     301
pramlintide 308
pre-conception care, diabetes 337
pregabalin 324
pregnancy 147–51
  diabetes 150, 336–9
    gestational diabetes 309, 338,
      339
    screening for retinopathy
      318–20
  Graves disease 178, 181
  prolactin 83
  prolactinomas 86
  sex hormones **149**
  thyroid-stimulating hormone
    174
premature ovarian failure 153
pre-prohormones 19
pressure palsies, diabetic neuropathy
     324
pretibial myxoedema *183*, 188
progestagens, endometrial cancer
     230
progesterone **149**
  endometrial cancer prevention
    230
  measurement 145
  menopause 158
  polycystic ovarian syndrome 157
  reference ranges **55**
  synthesis 144
progestins 229
prohormone convertase 1/3 (PC1/3)
     87, 221, 244
prohormones 8, 19–20, *21*

proinsulin *247*
prolactin 83–6, *137*, 151
    reference ranges **55**
    signal transduction 34
prolactinomas 84, 85, 163
    pregnancy 86
promoters, gene transcription 16
pro-opiomelanocortin 86, *87*
    mutations and appetite 347
propranolol, hyperthyroidism 181,
        188
proptosis 181–2, *183*
propylthiouracil, fetus 181
prostaglandin(s) *43*
prostaglandin E 330
prostate
    cancer 228–9
    testosterone replacement therapy
        141
protamine insulin 267
protein(s)
    insulin on metabolism 252–3
    phosphorylation, signal
        transduction 30, 31–3
protein binding 24
    androgens 136
    calcium 191
    cAMP response element binding
        protein 37
    competitive-binding assays 51
    cortisol-binding globulin 101–2,
        112
    IGF-binding proteins 74
    thyroid hormones 172
    see also sex hormone-binding
        globulin
protein kinase A 37
protein kinase C (PKC) 38–40
protein kinase C β *314*, 316
proton pump inhibitors 220
proto-oncogenes 223–4
    RET 57, 226, 232
provocative tests 52
pseudo-Cushing syndrome 113
pseudohypoparathyroidism 198–9
psychogenic polydipsia 94, **95**, 98
psychological complications of
        diabetes 334–5

psychological factors, obesity
        352–3
    eating behaviour 355
puberty
    delayed 90, 159, 164
    failure 133
    female 146
    male 138
    precocious 159, **160**
        central 89–90
        familial male *39*
        sex steroid precursor action *vs*
            107
pubic hair, female 146
pulsatility
    gonadotrophins, female 146
    growth hormone release 76
    hypothalamic hormone release 73
pumps (insulin infusion) 269, *270*
pyramidal lobe of thyroid 167

quality of life, diabetes 334

radiculopathies, diabetes 324
radiocontrast dyes, thyroid
        inhibition by
        175
radioiodine 180–1
radionuclide imaging *see* nuclear
        medicine
radiotherapy
    acromegaly 80, **81**
    hypopituitarism from 91
    pituitary tumours 70, 71
Randle cycle 303b
Rathke's pouch 66–7
receptors 27–47
    see also nuclear receptors
recombinant insulin 267
recombination, chromosomes *16*
5α-reductase (SRD5A2) 135–6
    inhibitors 157–8, 229
reduced glutathione 315
reference ranges 52, **53–5**
regulation (control mechanisms)
        9–13
remodelling of bone 204–5
renal artery stenosis 341

renal failure
    hyperparathyroidism 200
    hypocalcaemia 198
renal replacement therapy 323
renal threshold, glucose 263
renal tubules, monogenic defects
        116b
renal units, referral for diabetic
        nephropathy 322
renin 107, 110
    Conn syndrome 116
    reference ranges **55**
renin–angiotensin–aldosterone axis
        108
    Conn syndrome 115
    diabetic complications 316
repaglinide 300
reproductive endocrinology 127–64
    female 142–58
    male 134–42
resistance syndromes
    G-protein–coupled receptors 40b
    growth hormone 37
    insulin 34b
    nuclear receptors 41
    parathyroid hormone 198–9
    thyroid hormone 89
respiratory alkalosis 211
retinoid X receptor 301, *302*
retinopathy, diabetic *313*,
        317–21
    glycated haemoglobin *vs 245*
RET proto-oncogene 57, 226, 232
retro-orbital pain 188–9
reverse T$_3$ and T$_4$ *169*
reversibility of hormone–receptor
        interactions *30*
rhythms 13
    see also circadian rhythm
ribosomes 18
rickets 208–10
Riedel thyroiditis 175
rimonobant 349
RNA polymerase 17
rosiglitazone 303

salt wasting congenital adrenal
        hyperplasia 117–18

sample collection 49b
  hypercalcaemia 202
  hypoglycaemia 217
sandwich assays 50–1
sarcoidosis, hypercalcaemia 200–1
satiety centre 347
saturability of hormone receptors *30*
schizophrenia, obesity 358–9
scintigraphy *see* nuclear medicine
screening
  diabetes 294–5
    depression 335
    foot disease 327
    nephropathy 321–2
    retinopathy 318–20
  MEN-1 224–6
  MEN-2 226
SDHB, SDHD genes 227
second messengers 30, 34, 37–40
secretin **216**, 221
secretory vesicles 20
selective oestrogen receptor modulators 207
selenodeiodinases 172
  propranolol on 181
self-antigens, diabetes 262
semen analysis 134, 140
seminiferous tubules 134, *135*
seminoma 141b
sensory testing, diabetic neuropathy 327
septo-optic dysplasia 90
sequencing of genes 57
serotonin **216**, *222*
Sertoli cells 134, *135*
  see also inhibin
sex chromosomes 15
sex determination, embryonic 128–30
sex development, disorders of 130–4
sex hormone-binding globulin 136, 139
  polycystic ovarian syndrome 154
  reference ranges **55**
sex steroid precursors 107
  tumours secreting 116

sexual differentiation *129*, 130, *131*, *132*
sexual dysfunction, diabetes *313*, 329–30, 341
SH2 domains 31
SH3 domains 31
Sheehan syndrome 91
short stature *82*
short Synacthen test 110
sick euthyroid syndrome 174
signal transduction 30–1
  growth hormone 34, *35*, 76
  insulin 31–3, 34b, 248, *250*, 291b
  prolactin 34
  second messengers 30, 34, 37–40
sildenafil 330
single nucleotide polymorphism arrays 57
skin
  cortisol action 105
  pigmentation, adrenocortical insufficiency 88, 124
sleep time, weight *vs* 353
social aspects
  diabetes 339–40
  obesity 345
sodium, homeostasis
  aldosterone on 107
  cortisol action 106
  GH on 76
sodium–glucose co-transporter 2 inhibitors 308
soluble insulin 266–7
somatostatin **215**, 219
  analogues 80, **81**, 221
    hypoglycaemia 218
  reference ranges **55**
somatostatinomas 219
sorbitol *314*, 315
space-occupying lesions, pituitary tumours as 67–70, 96
specimens *see* sample collection
spermatogenesis 134
spermatozoa, function 147
spironolactone 116
  for hirsutism 158
SRY gene, translocation 133

stalk disconnection syndrome 85
START domain containing 3 23
STAT family proteins 34, *36*
static testing 52
statins 23, 333
steroid acute regulatory protein 23
steroid hormones 9
  nomenclature 23
  receptors 41, *46*
  storage 23–4
  synthesis *19*, 23, *25*, 103
    enzymes **104**
    fetus 150, *151*
    ovary 144
  see also specific hormones
steroidogenic factor-1 17, 42
stimulus-response testing *see* dynamic testing
stomach, hormone **10**
stress 87–8
  on gonadotrophin-releasing hormone *137*
  hypogonadism 90
stroke, diabetes 330
strontium ranelate 208
sub-fertility 159–62, 164
sulphonylureas 297–9, **307**
  hypoglycaemia 217, 298
  mechanism 246
superfamilies, hormone receptors 29b
suppression tests 52
  dexamethasone 113, 114, 232
surfactant (lung)
  cortisol on development 106, 150–1
Synacthen (tetracosactide) 110
syndrome of inappropriate ADH 93, 97
  Addison disease *vs* 109
synthetic ACTH test 88, 110, 124
syringes, insulin *270*

T$_3$ (tri-iodothyronine) 168, *169*
  metabolism 172–3
  protein binding 172
  reference ranges **55**
  see also thyroid, hormones

T₃-toxicosis 184
T₄ (thyroxine) 168, *169*
   competitive-binding assay 51
   metabolism 172–3
   protein binding 172
   reference ranges **55**
   replacement therapy 177, 187
      antithyroid drugs with 180
   see also thyroid, hormones
tadalafil 330
tamoxifen
   breast cancer 229
   endometrial cancer metastases
      230
Tanner stages of puberty *138*
target cell hormone conversion 41,
   45
'TATA' boxes 16
technetium isotope, pertechnetate
   168
television, obesity and 352
teratogenesis
   hyperglycaemia 336–7
   see also congenital malformations
teriparatide 208
testis 134
   embryology 128–30
   hormone **11**
   tumours 141, 230
   undescended 132
testosterone 135
   diurnal variation 136
   hirsutism 157
   hypogonadism 139
   negative feedback 137
   polycystic ovarian syndrome 154
   reference ranges **55**
   replacement therapy 140–1
testotoxicosis *39*
tetracosactide 110
thelarche 151
thiazide diuretics, hypercalcaemia
   200
thiazolidinediones *297*, 299b,
   301–3, **307**
thirst regulation 71–2
thromboembolism
   diabetic ketoacidosis 282

hyperosmolar hyperglycaemic
   state 293
thyroglobulin 168–71
   iodination 170
   reference ranges **55**
   resorption 171–2
thyroglossal cysts, positions *166*
thyroid 165–89
   anatomy 168
   cancer 57, 185–6, 189
      see also medullary thyroid
         carcinoma
   dyshormonogenesis 175
   function tests 174
      amiodarone 184b
      hypothyroidism 174, 177–8
   hormones **10**, *169*
      biosynthesis 168–72
      function 173–4
      growth hormone release 77
      receptors 41, *46*, 173–4
      resistance 174
      resistance syndrome 89
      T₄ competitive binding assay
         51
   human chorionic gonadotrophin
      on 149
   hypoplasia 167–8
   radionuclide imaging 61
   see also hypothyroidism
thyroidectomy 180
thyroiditis 175, 176, 189
thyroid peroxidase 170
thyroid-stimulating hormone (TSH)
   88–9, 171, 174
   hypothyroidism 177
   reference ranges **55**
   synthesis *21*
thyrotoxicosis 178, 179b, 188
   thyroid nodules 185
thyrotrophin-releasing hormone
   171
   hyperprolactinaemia 97
thyroxine *see* T₄
tolazide **298**
tolbutamide **298**
total contact casting 327
toxic adenoma of thyroid 184

TPIT mutations 91
transcription of genes 16–17
transcription factors 15, 16–17, 43,
   47
translation of genes 18
transmembrane domains of
      G-protein–coupled receptors
      35, *38*
transplantation, diabetic
      nephropathy 323
transport proteins 24
trans-sphenoidal surgery 80, **81**,
   114
triglycerides 252
tri-iodothyronine *see* T₃
troglitazone 303
trophoblast 149
tryptophan deficiency 222
T-scores, bone mineral density
   205–6, 207
TSH *see* thyroid-stimulating
   hormone
TSHomas 89
tumourigenesis 13
tumour suppressor genes 224b, *225*
Turner syndrome 15, 133, 153, 159
   management 153, **154**
twenty-four-hour urine collections
   calcium 201
   5-hydroxyindoleacetic acid 222
two-hit hypothesis 224, *225*
tyrosine, hormones from 22–3
tyrosine kinase receptors 30, 31–4

ultradian rhythm 13b
ultrasound 57–9
   polycystic ovarian syndrome
      154–6
   pregnancy, diabetes 337
unawareness of hypoglycaemia *276*,
   277
   driving and 339–40
United Kingdom, obesity 344, 346
United States of America, obesity
   346–7
untranslated regions (UTRs) 17
uric acid, insulin resistance and
   290b

urinary catheters, diabetic
  ketoacidosis 281
urinary free cortisol 102
urine collection
  containers 49b
  Cushing syndrome 113
  see also twenty-four-hour urine
    collections
uterus
  fibroids 158
  menstrual cycle 145–7
  oxytocin on 94–6

vagina, menstrual cycle 145–7
vaptans 93
vardenafil 330
variant nuclear receptors 41–2
vascular endothelial growth factor
  (VEGF), diabetes 316
vasoactive intestinal polypeptide
  (VIP) **215**, 220–1
  reference ranges **55**
  tumours secreting 219b, 221
vasopressin 91–4
  corticotrophin-releasing hormone
    and 87
  molecule 8, *11*
  secretion 67

venous sampling, parathyroid
  hormone 202
Verner–Morrison syndrome 219b,
  221
vesicles, secretory 20
VIPomas 219b, 221
viral infections
  thyroid 176
  diabetes 262b
virilization 116, 118, *119*
vision, diabetes 263, 340–1
  see also retinopathy
visual field defects
  pituitary tumours 67–8, *71*, 96
vitamin D 192–6
  deficiency 208–10, 212
  hypercalcaemia 200
  inactivation 193
  reference ranges **55**
  see also 1,25-dihydroxyvitamin D
Von Hippel-Lindau syndrome **123**,
  227

waist measurement 346
  diabetes risk 294b
water
  deprivation test **95**
  homeostasis

aldosterone on 107
  cortisol action 106
  GH on 76
weight gain
  antidiabetes agents 298,
    302–3
  polycystic ovarian syndrome
    157
weight loss, diabetes 263
weight management programmes
  353–8
weight regulation 347–53
Wolffian ducts 130, *131*
World Health Organization
  diabetes
    classification 238–40, 241b
    diagnostic criteria 240–1
  obesity, definitions 344

X chromosomes 15

zinc fingers, steroid hormone
  receptors and 41
Zollinger–Ellison syndrome 220
zona fasciculata 102b
zona glomerulosa 102b, 107
zona reticularis 102b
  tumours 116